Computers in Health Care

Kathryn J. Hannah   Marion J. Ball
Series Editors

Marion J. Ball   Judith V. Douglas
Robert I. O'Desky   James W. Albright
Editors

Healthcare Information Management Systems
A Practical Guide

With 50 Illustrations

Springer-Verlag
New York Berlin Heidelberg London Paris
Tokyo Hong Kong Barcelona Budapest

Marion J. Ball
Information Resources
University of Maryland
Baltimore, MD 21201 U.S.A.

Judith V. Douglas
Information Resources
University of Maryland
Baltimore, MD 21201 U.S.A.

Robert I. O'Desky
RIO Consultant
3408 Balboa Lane
Columbia, MO 65201 U.S.A.

James W. Albright
Bayfront Life Services
701 6th Street South
St. Petersburg, FL 33701 U.S.A.

Library of Congress Cataloging-in-Publication Data
Healthcare information management systems : a practical guide / Marion
J. Ball . . . [et al.], editors.
    p.   cm. — (Computers in health care)
    Includes bibliographical references.
    Includes index.
    ISBN 0-387-97434-2. — ISBN (invalid) 0-540-97434-2
    1. Health services administration — Data processing.
  2. Information storage and retrieval systems — Medical care.
  I. Ball, Marion J. II. Series: Computers in health care (New York,
N.Y.
    [DNLM: 1. Health Facilities — organization & administration.
2. Information Systems. 3. Information Systems — organization &
administration.   WY 26.5 H434]
  RA394.H424 1991
  610'.285 — dc20
  DNLM/DLC
  for Library of Congress   90-10300

Printed on acid-free paper.

© 1991 Springer-Verlag New York Inc.
All rights reserved. This work may not be translated or copied in whole or in part without the written permission of the publisher (Springer-Verlag New York, Inc., 175 Fifth Avenue, New York, NY 10010, USA), except for brief excerpts in connection with reviews or scholarly analysis. Use in connection with any form of information storage and retrieval, electronic adaptation, computer software, or by similar or dissimilar methodology now known or hereafter developed is forbidden.
The use of general descriptive names, trade names, trademarks, etc., in this publication, even if the former are not especially identified, is not to be taken as a sign that such names, as understood by the Trade Marks and Merchandise Act, may accordingly be used freely by anyone.
While the advice and information in this book are believed to be true and accurate at the date of going to press, neither the authors nor the editors nor the publisher can accept any legal responsibility for any errors or omissions that may be made. The publisher makes no warranty, express or implied, with respect to the material contained herein.

Camera-ready copy provided by the editors.
Printed and bound by Edwards Brothers, Inc., Ann Arbor, Michigan.
Printed in the United States of America.

9 8 7 6 5 4 3 2

ISBN 0-387-97434-2 Springer-Verlag New York Berlin Heidelberg
ISBN 3-540-97434-2 Springer-Verlag Berlin Heidelberg New York

Dedication

Marion J. Ball

This work I would like to dedicate to the many individuals who have had a major impact on my professional advancement. I have been extraordinarily lucky in having so many people interested in furthering my career in the field of health informatics. First, I would like to thank my husband, John C. Ball, whose devotion and encouragement have made my entire professional career possible. Second, my mother and father, Erica and Ernst Jokl, both in their own ways have been an inspiration and supporter throughout my life. My two children, Charles Ball and Elizabeth Ball, have done their share to make my career possible. My extended family circle must include Donald A.B. Lindberg, Phil R. Manning, Morris Collen, and Gary Hammon. Without their encouragement and opportunities afforded me by them, I would not be where I am today.

Judith V. Douglas

I dedicate this book to my son Christopher and my sister Beckett, who taught me the value of information in healthcare; to my parents Dale and Frona Vetter, who taught me language and ideas; to my husband Paul and sons Matthew and Justin, who are my life; and to Marilyn Burnett, who turned our manuscript into the pages that follow.

Robert I. O'Desky

Dedications are typically made to people who have assisted us in the past. And in that fashion, I would like to dedicate this book to my mother, Mrs. Ruth O'Desky. However, this book was created to celebrate the potential of the future and with that in mind, I would also like to dedicate this book to my niece and nephew, Aly and Charlie O'Desky. I can only hope that by the time they are able to read and comprehend the book, the technology described will be routinely employed by the healthcare community.

James W. Albright

It is with sincere appreciation that I dedicate my first work to two extraordinary people, Pat Albright and Robert Taylor.

Pat, my wife, is a superb healthcare professional who continues to shape my formal education in healthcare management by demonstrating the compassion and wisdom needed to fully understand the patient care process. Robert, the ultimate teacher, introduced me to the concepts of organization behavior, systems theory and financial management enabling me to comprehend the business of healthcare.

To these two friends and mentors, I say, "Thank you for your patience, guidance and understanding while I learn."

Foreword

William G. Anlyan, M.D.

Chancellor
Duke University

Many forecasters predict that the costs of healthcare will continue to increase with the strong potential for continued erosion of historical patterns of reimbursement. The socioeconomic and political climate of the 1990s will mandate that healthcare practitioners and institutions focus on improved efficiency and effectiveness. The continuing demand to provide reasonably priced, high quality services in a productive manner consistent with escalating expectations of quality assurance can only be met through access to information about what is being done and what works. It is essential that the technology of information systems be applied in equal measure in support of those who render direct patient care services and those who manage the healthcare institutions.

It is increasingly apparent that, in spite of the growth of systems technology in the healthcare setting to date, today's health practitioner and health executive lack sufficient information to structure organizations or practice patterns for enhanced productivity and compliance with quality assurance standards. Practitioners and institutions will need to commit increasing amounts of leadership time and money to the information management resource. A commitment of increased funding to the information management component during times of predictably strained financial resources will mandate a commitment to the principle that information is an essential strategic resource. Traditionally, decisions concerning the cost benefit outcomes of an information system have been based upon its ability to accelerate or to automate an existing process. A systems infrastructure which results in institutional databases must be judged upon its value as a new technology to support information based decision making, and not solely as a means of automating historic decision methodologies.

Existing information management technology is adequate to serve the needs of the healthcare industry. However, much remains to be learned about how to integrate systems so that practitioners and managers can collectively benefit from the advantages of institutional databases. For these changes to occur, institutional cultures and historical patterns of professional practice must evolve to permit information to be viewed as a shared resource. Decisions regarding an institution's approach to information management, and decisions based upon the information being managed, will be major determinants of organizational character and outcome.

A key factor related to the success of managing information systems will be the style of systems leadership and the increased involvement of all systems users in the development and at the application of systems technology. This shared responsibility is integral to the principle that the information needs of the healthcare industry must give rise to new patterns of management, clinical practice, and information systems support. Such responsibility must be shared, not delegated. Success in the 1990s will depend on the extent to which the broad spectrum of health practitioners and managers/executives have a practical understanding of the need for information management and a common commitment to applying the evolving information technology to address the needs of an increasingly demanding healthcare system.

Morris F. Collen, M.D.

Director Emeritus, Division of Research
The Permanente Medical Group

The evolution of healthcare information systems began in the 1970s using large, expensive mainframe computers. In the 1980s, smaller, lower cost minicomputers and microcomputers appeared in many hospital departmental subsystems, and local area networks were developed to integrate the patient data they collected. In the 1990s, advanced computer and communications technology has made available more powerful and lower cost computers, mass direct access storage, high speed and high bandwidth networks, and workstations, which support data selector pointers, barcode readers, text, graphics, windowing, images, and sound. In *Healthcare Information Management Systems: A Practical Guide*, Marion Ball and associates provide healthcare administrators with a very informative overview of the current complex field of healthcare information systems, containing powerful workstations, all linked by communications networks to an integrated database for the patient record data.

The increasingly important role of a chief information officer (CIO) in a healthcare facility can become very evident to a chief executive officer trying to meet the rising pressures for larger, faster, more comprehensive, and more expensive computer based information systems. This book gives a CIO step by step guidelines for planning and managing a hospital information system, and makes an important contribution to the rapidly enlarging field of health informatics. The CIO is responsible for the hardware, software and communications networks of the healthcare information system. This book discusses long range and strategic planning for a hospital information system with a computer based patient record. Generally, the model of choice meets the needs of individual hospital departments with dedicated small computers, all linked by a communications network to a larger central, integrating database computer. The CIO is the best architect of a strategic plan for the integration and connectivity of the many departmental subsystems within a health information system. The CIO also will find helpful the chapters on information system consultants and on vendors of systems.

The diverse and substantive benefits from a properly designed, installed, and operated healthcare information system are described. The system will be essential to meet the ever increasingly complex requirements for utilization review and quality of care assurance. Many suggestions are provided as to how decision support programs can help the executive; and how end user computing can increase productivity. The authors consider information as a resource, just as are people, money, or supplies; and the effective management of all of these resources requires an integrated view of the entire organization. Since hospitals are the quintessential example of an information based organization, in which the information is related primarily to patient care, an efficient information system is indeed essential for patient data to be collected from widely scattered locations where the data originates, and always be accessible in various locations where needed. Thus, a computer based information system is a powerful integrating force in the operation of a modern hospital. The distributed computer models discussed in this book help to preserve the functional autonomy of departments in a hospital, spread out and support decision making, and facilitate the sharing of essential patient information.

A basic focus of this book is to help design healthcare information systems that serve as a decision making resource to produce better, more cost effective patient care; and better, more usable information for hospital administrators and planners. Informative sections of the book discuss the important participatory roles of physicians and nurses and the need to integrate the clinical ancillary services of radiology and clinical laboratory.

This comprehensive book presents the state of the art in the 1990s for healthcare information systems, which presents an opportunity for substantial improvements in providing more cost effective patient care.

Michael J. Mestrovich, Ph.D.

Deputy Assistant Secretary
Department of Defense

Change. The one constant that we can all count on is rampant in the world of information management and technology. Those of us who have labored for a good number of years trying to apply the principles of information resource management to healthcare delivery see the next decade as one of unparalleled excitement and opportunity.

The changes that will occur will not only touch on information management but will extend throughout healthcare delivery institutions and systems. Changes will affect researching, training, personnel productivity, and organization. Perhaps the single most important change, however, will affect the mindset of the healthcare professional team delivering the healthcare technology within the clinical workplace and will force a necessary transformation of that workplace as healthcare professionals utilize the new and powerful tools available to them.

This transformation will not come without pain. The demands on the staffs and institutions will be immense and intense. Some will immediately see the benefits and work vigorously to effect the change. Others will resist and will have to be convinced of the necessity and efficacy of the changes demanded of them. Totally new methods of training and management will evolve out of necessity to cope with the transformation.

Today many dedicated people are diligently working on the strategic plans for information systems, the training programs, the process, and change management concepts that are mentioned above. In the federal sector, both the Department of Defense and the Department of Veterans Affairs have information systems programs ongoing and therefore are beginning to deal with the issues previously mentioned. In the Defense Department that program is called Corporate Information Management (CIM).

The major clinical system within that program is called the Composite Health Care System (CHCS). CHCS has been designed and is operating around the principle of a single patient database for both inpatient and outpatient care. All clinical and ancillary services will have the ability to access that record as required, and as permitted allowing for patient record security. CHCS, therefore, is a totally integrated, clinically based, patient care information system which ties the Defense Department hospitals and outlying patient clinics together through a network allowing access to the integrated patient oriented database.

The medical portion of the CIM program does not stop, however, with just installing a clinically based hospital information system. It has already initiated an examination of the longer term issues of strategic planning, cost containment, resource management, training, and change management as the necessary tools to achicvc the full benefits of automating the healthcare professional workplace. The same issues will have to be examined in other healthcare delivery systems to accommodate the rapidly changing business environment in which health professionals are now working.

This text provides an excellent compilation of thought provoking treatises on a wide range of necessary issues that must be examined as the healthcare profession enters its age of information explosion. I find it comprehensive and direct in assisting both the uninitiated as well as the grizzled veteran in the field. I believe the emphasis on strategic planning, end user involvement in requirements definition and the impact of automation on the clinical setting to be especially helpful.

This book is an enormously practical guide to assist all of us as we seek to provide better access and quality of healthcare at a reasonable cost through the infusion of information technology into the healthcare delivery workplace.

Preface

In this book, Dr. Marion J. Ball, long active in hospital information systems and clinical computing, joins with three colleagues to produce a contributed volume. Her co-editors add their perspectives—Judith Douglas, a Johns Hopkins trained healthcare analyst and planner; Dr. Robert O'Desky, technical healthcare consultant; and James Albright, chief executive officer at Bayfront Medical Center in St. Petersburg, Florida.

Addressed to practitioners of healthcare administration, the book looks beyond traditional information systems. The book suggests how information systems can bring a competitive advantage to hospitals and other healthcare providers. Its viewpoint is not managerial, technical, or clinical. Rather, it is concerned with the role and the use of information in the providing of healthcare.

The book surveys the entire information technology scene that the healthcare professional must address today, from management to practice. No longer is it enough to look only at a single large scale hospital information system and clinical lab, radiology, and other departmental computing areas, each of which is covered in separate books and publications. Nor can the professional note only a few isolated niche applications. The challenge is to oversee an array of computers used in widely different ways. To do this, computing must be seen as a set of tools which health professionals and hospital staff can use in managing and delivering healthcare as an integrated total system.

Healthcare Information Management Systems: A Practical Guide speaks practitioner to practitioner. The emphasis of the book is on practice, on experiential knowledge, not theoretical. More than 40 authors contribute to the book—authors who are confronting information technology issues in practical terms in their own work environments. They come from different professional backgrounds and training, from all regions of the country. They practice in a wide variety of institutional settings, using different systems from different vendors to meet their institutions' information needs. They share the insights gained in their institutions, when they address problems that demand an understanding of both healthcare and technology. They do not have the luxury of unlimited resources; they do not live and solve their problems on the cutting edge. Working in the mainstream, they know the nuts and bolts about what they write. They have worked through solutions, taking what is available and applying it in their environments.

Whether they have made strategic plans or implemented systems, these contributing authors live with their decisions day to day and work within the environment created by those decisions. Some share the experience over a long professional lifetime; others are young and bring new energies and new solutions to the field. Together these authors give us a rich picture of how information technology can be used in healthcare—and how in reality it is being used. It is their contributions which give this book its expertise.

Based on the successes of experienced professionals in bringing information technology to the management and provision of healthcare services, *Healthcare Information Management Systems* gives the reader a competitive advantage in the demanding world of today's hospital, where financial pressures continue to mount. Although associated expenses clearly must be justified, information technology is increasingly being integrated into the delivery of healthcare and is changing the way clinicians, administrators, and other healthcare workers fulfill their mission of providing quality patient care.

To reflect this broad vision and experiential base, the editors asked three leaders in healthcare to offer their viewpoints on what this book has to offer. Anlyan speaks from his experience in the university setting, Collen from the private practice environment, and Mestrovich from the federal sector.

Like *Nursing Informatics,* its predecessor in this series, *Healthcare Information Management Systems* shows the reader "Where Caring and Technology Meet".

Marion J. Ball
Judith V. Douglas
Robert I. O'Desky
James W. Albright

Contents

Section 1—Supporting the Practitioner

Unit 3—Nursing and Information Systems

Section 1—Supporting the Practitioner

Unit 4—Acquiring Information Systems Expertise

Section 2—Managing the Institution

Unit 1—Information: A Resource for Strategic Management

Section 2—Managing the Institution

Unit 2—New Visions of Technological Leadership

Section 2—Managing the Institution

Unit 3—Evolution of Information Management: Organization and Technology

Section 2—Managing the Institution

Unit 4—Buying Expertise

Supporting the Practitioner

This contents array presents the architecture of the book in reader-friendly terms. Use it to get a feel for the thrust of the units and chapters and to quickly select what you want to study in more depth.

Managing the Institution

Unit 1	Unit 2	Unit 3	Unit 4
Information: A Resource for Strategic Mgt.	**New Visions of Technological Leadership**	**Managing the Institution**	**Buying Expertise**
Chapter 1	Chapter 1	Chapter 1	Chapter 1
Administrators as microcomputer users	Surveys of healthcare CIOs	Networking for integration	Insider's guide to consulting
Chapter 2	Chapter 2	Chapter 2	Chapter 2
Planning for information resources	Roles and functions of the CIO	An evolving organizational structure in a teaching hospital	Consultant view of the client role
Chapter 3	Chapter 3	Chapter 3	Chapter 3
Fitting information systems to the hospital culture	Executive search process for a CIO	Information systems in the corporate business plan	Client advice on using consultants
Chapter 4	Chapter 4	Chapter 4	Chapter 4
Connectivity and open architecture	Managing change organizationally and technologically	Management and integration: Challenges for HIS	Establishing good vendor relationships
Chapter 5			
Enhancing financial applications			
Chapter 6			
Methodologies for costing out systems			

Section 1–Supporting the Practitioner

Unit 1—Snapshots of the Future

Unit Introduction

Physicians, nurses, and other practitioners know well that information technology has yet to transform totally the way they care for their patients. Yet the technology is here with the capabilities to support revolutionary applications. This unit describes what the 1990s will bring.

Professor of medicine and computer science, Shortliffe describes his vision of the networked physician, using microcomputer workstations to access information when, where, and how it is needed. Winfree, a healthcare administrator, joins Stead and Elchlepp, both physicians involved in information systems, to share the view of centrally guided distributed systems they have developed in their work at Duke, extending computer power to end users while maintaining vital corporate and information resources. Garling, a physician working in the healthcare software industry, explains the benefits physicians can gain from using information systems in their practice of medicine. Drawing on a long career as a pathologist involved in laboratory computerization, Rappoport looks to future use of barcodes to ensure error free identification of patients, specimens, and medications. An experienced healthcare executive, Schmitz focuses in on decision support systems in the clinical and administrative setting.

What these authors envision will become commonplace in the not too distant future.

1
The Networked Physician: Practitioner of the Future

Edward H. Shortliffe

For the physicians of the 1990s and beyond, computer workstations will be their windows on the world. Much of the necessary technology already exists. Desktop or bedside, in the office or at the hospital, computers can respond to a simple click of a mouse pointing device. Furthermore, physicians are increasingly using computers in their office practices.

In the future, the physician will be able to access the medical record largely by using the mouse and doing very little typing. Moreover, the record will include graphics and images as well as extensive text. Outpatient records will be integrated with inpatient data by using the capabilities of communications networks that link hospitals with the clinics and private offices of their medical staff members. At the same time, the physician—not the hospital—will retain control of the outpatient records for the private practice.

Networking

The challenge is to provide healthcare practitioners access to information when and where they need it and to do so in a manner that minimizes training time while avoiding incremental time commitments. Today, the information the practitioners want to access frequently is available only from sources outside their own institutions. It may be at another medical school across the country or it might be at the National Library of Medicine (NLM). If such resources are available via electronic communications networks, the practitioner can request information in the midst of a computer based interaction with the patient's record—not hours later when the patient is no longer in the office. Similarly, shared national electronic mail networks can tie together clinicians and researchers around the country and link them to Medline from the NLM or from commercial vendors. The technology for such linkages is

3

already available in wide access networks that use dedicated high bandwidth lines or that rely on microwave or satellite transmission.

With national networks for data sharing, the physician wishing to search Medline during a patient encounter and online chart review will be able to request rapid direct connection to the NLM. With adequate system integration, the physician will make such connections with a single click on the screen—no worrying about the phone number for the network or how to log on to the NLM machine. All that should be totally invisible to the user. NLM's Grateful Med has captured this concept; one of the reasons for the success of Grateful Med is that it allows users to insulate themselves from a host of technical and logistical details when they need a bibliographic retrieval. This same concept needs to be generalized to the workstations of physicians and other health workers so that clicking on icons and intuitive manipulation within data management environments will produce the integrated information access envisioned in the scenario for the future that follows.

Increasingly, there are shared national databases in areas of medicine. For example, the ARAMIS database consolidates data on rheumatologic patients that has been pooled from around the United States and Canada for many years. Duke University's Coronary Artery Disease Data Bank allows a physician to indicate certain parameters of a patient, to instruct the system to identify past patients that had these same characteristics, and to request a display of how those patients did under various therapeutic options. The practitioner can then evaluate what the benefits of medical management versus bypass surgery or angioplasty would be in this particular case.

Although such databases may be of interest to a broad cross section of practitioners and patients, they generally will not be maintained at the physician's own institution. With integrated networks, all the practitioner should need to do is click the workstation mouse to request a connection to a remote database.

To create such integrated environments, however, planners must implement a connection between the network installed in the local physician's office or clinic and the hospital network. Similar gateways between the hospital networks and national networks are also required. Such gateways between networks are critical, whether they use physical connections, dedicated telephone lines, or communication via microwave transmissions. Standard protocols for communication and data exchange are also crucial if such gateways are to be capable of handling data that enter from either side of that gateway and of passing those data back and forth in a way that allows machines on one side to read data being sent from the other.

With gateways between networks, physicians who want to access electronic mail, for example, will need only to click on a screen icon and will not need to know that they have just requested access through a gateway to another computer that may be across town. The same functions should be available to them regardless of whether they are accessing the information environment from their office or at the hospital. The computer should be (or should appear to be) essentially the same at both locations. Today, on the other hand, physicians who wish to use electronic mail or similar information resources must generally learn an arcane command language to type at a keyboard in order to make this kind of connectivity occur.

Research, much of it supported by the National Library of Medicine, provides a model for decision support functions that are integrated with the management of patient data. If expert advisory tools exist as integrated components of the data management environment, suggestions, reminders, and critiques can be offered to the physician as a byproduct of routine dealing with patient data. Just as the physician is wondering how to interpret the current status of the patient whose chart is being reviewed or updated, an icon on the screen could be selected, thereby invoking an expert system. Such tools might be running on the physician's own workstation or on shared resources accessed through networks; the physician should not need to be concerned with the precise location of such tools so long as they can be accessed in a facile fashion through a familiar workstation interface.

Handling more than straight alphanumeric data has special implications for technology. Simple graphic displays are well within the power of most computers now in physicians' offices. The technology that meets the requirements for sending and receiving detailed images (such as radiographs or histologic sections) exists today but remains too expensive for most office based practitioners. In fact, it is only beginning to appear in hospitals. Within the next few years, these new capabilities will become affordable and widespread. Physicians will then be able to view photographs or x-ray files and to integrate them into their medical records.

Although much research remains to be done, a unified medical language will make possible medical records which can be shared among practitioners and institutions. Even clinical laboratory information, which may in general seem to be unambiguous, requires greatly improved standardization before it can be accurately shared. Consider, for example, differences in units, normal ranges, and testing methods which may make laboratory data pooling inappropriate or comparisons between institutions meaningless. Even more problematic is the encoding and sharing of the narrative text that is such a critical and extensive part of the medical record. Text material routinely suffers from a lack of standards and of universally agreed upon meaning. Issues about how such text should be entered into medical records await resolution. Until major advances occur in computer based speech understanding—advances which will not occur in the short term—physicians will have to continue to dictate the narrative text for transcription into the record. Standardized terminology, achieved by requiring structured entries of descriptors via the selection of items from menus on the computer screen, has been another approach to this problem. The Unified Medical Language System project, one of the NLM's visionary undertakings, holds great promise, as do other research projects aimed at formalizing the computer based representation of the meaning underlying the terms that are used in healthcare and medical research.

A Scenario for the Future

The following scenario illustrates many of the points outlined in the preceding discussion. It demonstrates the concepts of an integrated physician's workstation, using displays from a prototype workstation interface.* It should be emphasized that the technology illustrated is all currently available, although the fully linked physician's environment will become available only when logistical, sociopolitical, and financial barriers are overcome.

Use of the Office Based System

Dr. James Robinson, working in the office where he sees outpatients, sits down at his workstation and signs on to the computer based office system that he shares with the two other physicians in his group practice in internal medicine (Figure 1). Using the mouse to move the cursor and to select functions, he logs on to his account and identifies himself by a combination of password and badge, designed to give the maximum assurances of data confidentiality. Only he can access his electronic mail, and access to a patient's data is restricted to those health workers who are directly involved in the person's care.

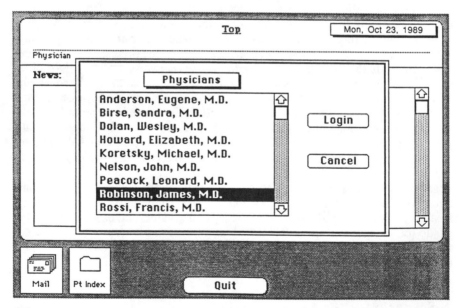

*The prototype system shown here was developed by Joan D. Walton at Stanford University as part of her work on an M.S. degree in Medical Information Sciences.

Figure 1. Physicians' Log In

Once in his particular segment of the networked office system, he gets a broadcast message, entered since he was last on the system, reminding him of the next medical staff meeting at the hospital where he and his partners have privileges.

Dr. Robinson next checks his mail. He is greeted by a screen that displays new messages up at the top (Figure 2). He reads a note from Dr. McGee, a local colleague who is asking him to consult on a patient. They both use the electronic mail facility run by the local hospital and shared by all of the physicians and other staff at that institution. When Dr. Robinson does not find the response he was hoping for from a colleague across the country, dealing with an unusual diagnosis, he decides to pose the same query to a colleagueat the region's foremost academic health center, who is also on the national network the hospital provides for its medical staff.

Scanning his mail, Dr. Robinson remembers to check the October grand rounds schedule that he received in a message in September and keeps online for reference. He then notes that a message of interest has finally arrived from the clinical lab, giving him some recent lipid lab results for his patient, David Jones (Figure 3). Earlier in the week, when he ordered fasting labs for this patient, he requested that the lab forward him the results immediately as well as enter them in the patient's clinical lab database.

With the lab results in hand, he decides to review Mr. Jones' outpatient record. Calling up his patient index on the computer and using the mouse, he pulls out Mr. Jones from his outpatient database. The record includes the notes from Mr. Jones' visits to his office along with data regarding hospitalizations, downloaded from the hospital information system. Such merging of

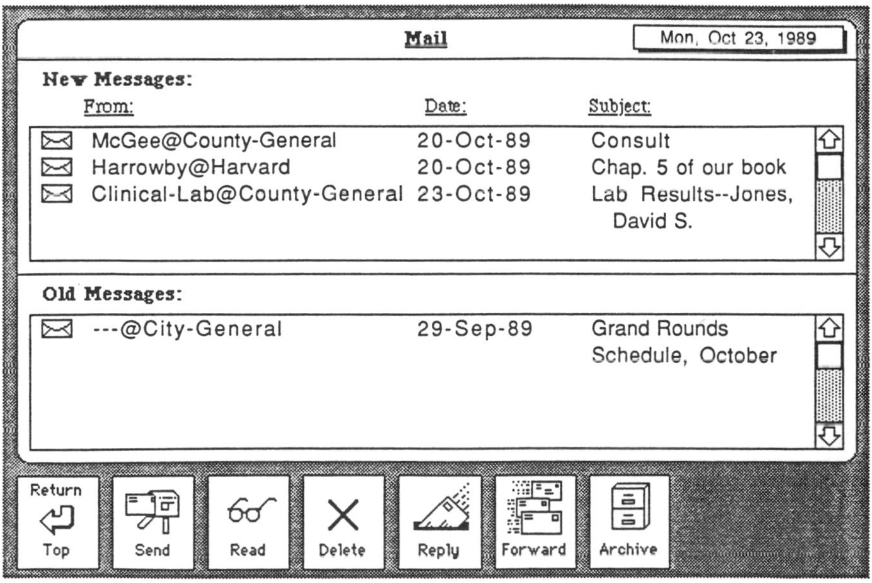

Figure 2. Mail Log

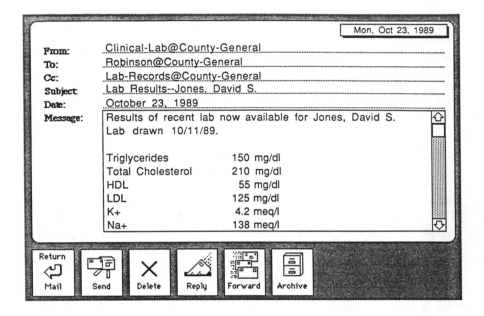

Figure 3. Mail Message

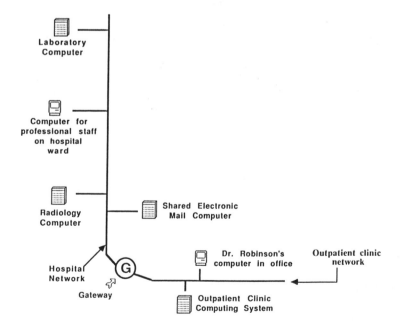

Figure 4. Integrated Network

inpatient and outpatient data is straightforward because of the network connections that exist between Dr. Robinson's office and the hospital at which he practices (Figure 4).

The first screen functions as the cover sheet in a paper medical record. It displays demographic information along with insurance data, current financial details, even a photograph of the patient (Figure 5).

The computer based medical record is essentially a series of endless length "cards." Dr. Robinson moves inside the record by simply selecting the tab on the card of interest. In his system, the cards for initial history and physical can be arranged according to the common practice of organizing by the chief complaint and the history of the present illness, the past medical history and the family history, social habits, review of systems, and the physical exam itself (Figure 6).

For routine progress notes, however, Dr. Robinson prefers the traditional arrangement which organizes the "cards" around the subjective findings at the outpatient visit, the objective findings, the physician's assessment, and plans for the patient's subsequent management (Figure 7).

Dr. Robinson quickly scans the first part of Mr. Jones' record, a problem list of sorts, summarizing his history since he first presented two years ago with chest pain and hypertension. A few months later, the chest pain was diagnosed as angina. The computer based record lists all the encounters with this patient and includes all of Dr. Robinson's notes from the initial history and physical through subsequent progress notes and up to the most recent visit last week, when he ordered the lipid lab work. The record includes a pictorial family medical history. The family tree indicates the patient by an arrow and shows that his father had a myocardial infarction (MI) at age 55 and his sister has an elevated cholesterol (Figure 8). The history, recent lab results, and his most recent x-ray confirm the diagnosis and course of treatment.

He then connects up with the laboratory database and looks at the patient's lipid information. In reviewing the data, he first looks at tables of results. With all the visits this patient has had, he finds it difficult to concentrate on the rows and columns to get a sense of how this patient's cholesterol might be changing over time. So he decides to plot it, placing the total cholesterol and the HDL together on a single graph and displaying their values over time. The graph shows that the cholesterol is starting to fall while the HDL is coming up—this is the treatment goal (Figure 9).

At this point Dr. Robinson may choose to request an interpretation of Mr. Jones' trends (by clicking on the "Interpret" button in Figure 9), thereby accessing an expert system. The advisory tool would not only analyze, over time, the patient's cholesterol and lipid parameters, but also suggest what the NIH guidelines would say for the appropriate adjustment in therapy (Figure 10).+ Such an advice system does not require that the physician follow its recommendations, but provides him with custom tailored access to the kind of information that might be appropriate for this patient's management at this time. Alternatively, Dr. Robinson may decide to use the system to order additional laboratory tests at this point, specifying another routine indirect beta quantification of Mr. Jones' lipids and instructing the system to record the order and to proceed.

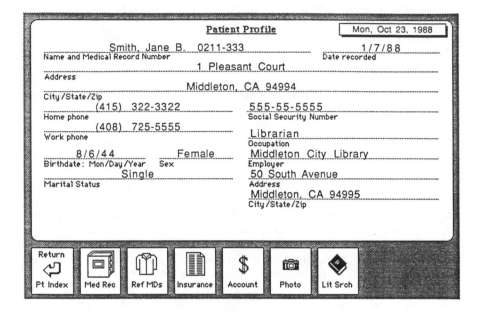

Figure 5. Patient Profile

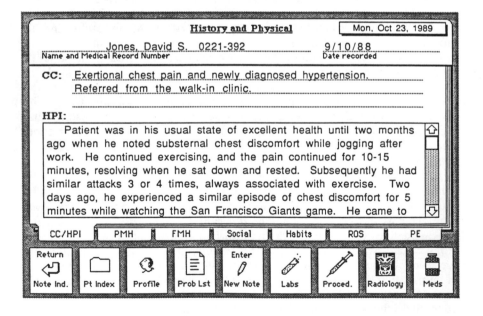

Figure 6. History and Physical

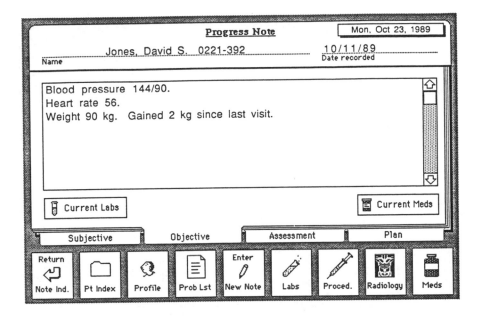

Figure 7. Progress Notes

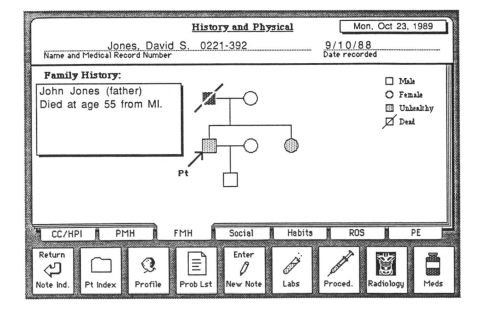

Figure 8. Family History

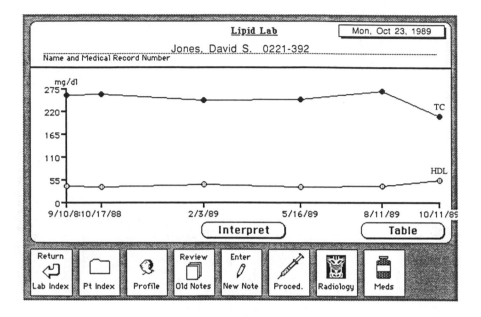

Figure 9. Lipid Lab Report

Going Further Out Onto the Network

The implications of networking shown here extend to physicians in all specialties. Consider the case of Jane Smith, a woman in her 40s followed for many years for hyperthyroidism and peptic ulcer disease. Recently she was referred for a breast biopsy and was found to have carcinoma of the breast. The physician who will be responsible for her treatment must now determine the current recommendation for treatment for a premenopausal woman with this stage of breast cancer. He may choose to seek information from the literature (see the "lit Srch" icon, Figure 11). Using appropriate networks, this facility could provide any of a number of information sources. For example, the physician could do a Medline search or check a full text database to get the full electronic form of the major oncology textbook. Or the physician may take advantage of a new program that critiques his proposed management plan based on an analysis of the relevant literature and the detailed statistics reported in the breast cancer clinical trials (Figure 12).#

From a networking perspective, the literature assessment program works because a gateway from the hospital network ties the physician to the associated medical library. At the library, computer terminals look the same as the

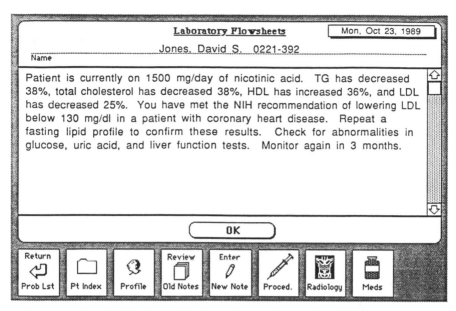

+The output shown in this display is similar to that produced by HyperLipid, an expert system developed by Don Rucker, M.D., as part of his work for an M.S. degree in Medical Information Sciences at Stanford University.

Figure 10. Laboratory Flowsheets

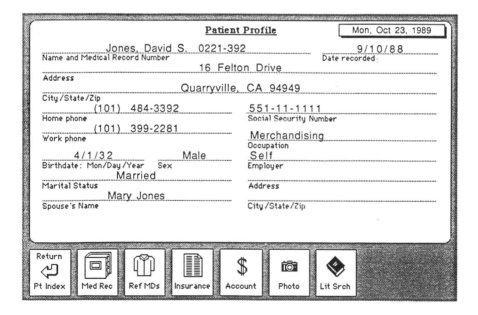

Figure 11. Patient Profile

workstation the physician uses in his office or on the wards. The physician can perform any function from any one of the terminals because they are all networked together and all have access to the same data as long as he identifies himself (Figure 13).

Obstacles

Networking must take into account the fact that individuals want and need control of their own data even when they choose to share them. The distributed computing model, which is increasingly prevalent, allows departments and individuals to run their own computers. The challenge is to make those data available for sharing; this requires the adoption of standards for communication and for data sharing. There has to be an institutional commitment to data sharing and coordination for this kind of interchange to work.

In its report on medical informatics, part of the National Library of Medicine's long range plan, Panel 4 focused on the critical issues included under the rubric of institutional infrastructure and national leadership. Clearly local institutions are not going to create the concepts of integrated networks

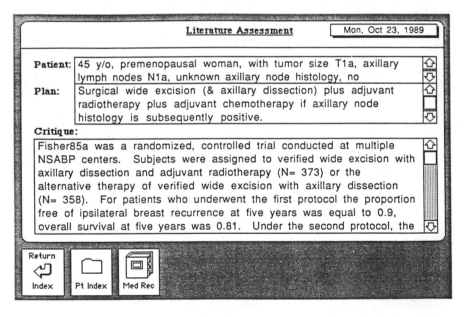

#The output shown in this display is Roundsman, an advisory system developed by Glenn Rennels, M.D., as part of his work for a Ph.D. degree in Medical Information Sciences at Stanford University.

Figure 12. Literature Assessment

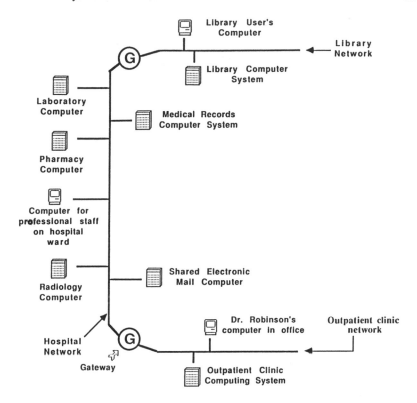

Figure 13. Integrated Network

and data sharing on their own. They can participate, but there must be national leadership to create national biomedical networks for data sharing. It is not up to the researcher to create such environments. No single individual (or even a relatively large academic informatics group) can do so.

The environment can exist only if presidents of hospitals and deans of medical schools, and national leaders at the National Institutes of Health and elsewhere, commit themselves and their resources to its creation. Coordinated programs are essential for creating the necessary infrastructure. The researcher will be a beneficiary of this kind of environment—not its originator. These issues are key to integrated or national biomedical computing environments that use wide access networks. Because most of the necessary technologies already exist, such solutions to logistical problems are the crucial missing ingredients. Their importance to the creation of the future environment envisioned for the physician in this article cannot be overestimated.

Within the academic medical center, complexes of groups will increasingly be dependent upon the capabilities networking can provide. These groups of researchers need to work in a coordinated fashion; they cannot talk at cross purposes. Increasingly, there will be a role for central coordinating individuals who may not be researchers at all but who really understand the milieu of the academic health science center and who can coordinate what goes on in their academic unit with what is provided by the biomedical library (which obviously plays a key role in the integrated environment described here). Academic medical centers also need service computing groups that lay the networks and make sure that standardized protocols allow institutional components to interact with one another effectively.

Researchers and clinicians need service groups that address their computing needs as users and provide consulting when the user says, "I want to buy the right microcomputer, and I have no idea what it is." Right now, too many faculty in medical schools are asking that question, and they have no one to turn to for good, coherent answers, particularly if the implications of the question are, "How do I in fact incorporate this machine into the computing environment here so that I can exchange electronic mail with my colleagues across the country or so that I can share data with somebody else in clinical research in an area related to mine?"

Special attention must be paid to the inpatient/outpatient systems in hospitals within academic medical centers. Probably the biggest schism that exists lies between activities based in medical schools and those in their affiliated hospitals, which often have separate boards and separate administrations. It will be a major sociologic change for hospitals to work actively in a coordinated effort with their associated medical schools. Such cooperative efforts must extend within these institutions as well. Just as the complexes of research groups in the medical school need to be tied by a communications network, hospital departments running individual departmental data systems (notably radiology, pharmacy, and the clinical laboratory) must be linked effectively. Only through such linkages will shared access to data be possible.

With the support of the National Library of Medicine's Integrated Academic Information Management System (IAIMS) program, environments are now being created in which these activities can be tied together (Figure 14). Yet the IAIMS concept cannot go forth without institutional and structural change. With the encouragement of the IAIMS grants program, academic health centers are taking note of the concept of integration. Painstakingly, those institutions are making the changes which will enable the physicians of the 1990s to practice in an integrated environment and to give patients the kind of care that full information access makes possible.

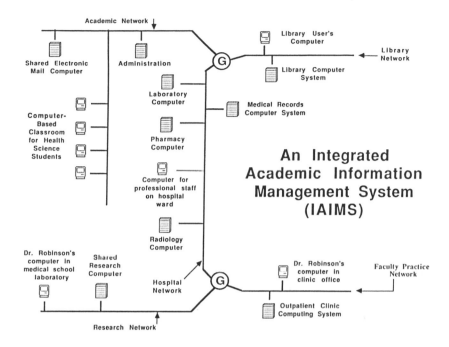

Figure 14. Integrated Academic Information Management System

Acknowledgments

This article is based on a presentation given by the author to the Board of Regents, National Library of Medicine, January 1989. The workstation concept, and the figures in this paper, are taken from Chapter One in the forthcoming textbook by E. H. Shortliffe, L. E. Perreault, G. Wiederhold, and L. M. Fagan, eds., *Medical informatics: Computer application in health care* (Reading, Mass.: Addison-Wesley Publishing Company, 1990).

Questions

1. Many observers have argued that physicians' views and understanding of computing technology need be no more sophisticated than is their understanding of how a telephone works. We use telephones without much knowledge of the underlying technology, and we should be able to use computers too without becoming "computer literate." Bearing in mind the scenario from this chapter, do you believe that the telephone analogy is valid? Explain your answer.

2. As is emphasized in this chapter, simply connecting two computers by a wire does not mean that they can communicate with one another. Consider, and then describe, the layers of conventions (starting with the network itself

and ending with the data to be shared between machines) that need to be agreed upon before the scenario from this chapter will be generally possible.

3. Imagine that a physician wants information on how patients with cancer, similar to one of his own, have responded to each of three different therapies that are currently under testing. He learns that there is a relevant database available at the National Cancer Institute. If he were to manage to connect to this database over a network, describe some of the problems that he might encounter in posing his question or properly interpreting the computer's response. Can you suggest how system designers might help minimize such problems?

4. This chapter argues that the data management needs of practitioners must be smoothly integrated if they are to be truly useful and acceptable. Yet software products have historically been developed as single components, often produced by totally different companies or research groups. How will diverse products be brought together so that they run smoothly in a consistent, intuitive environment, even though they were developed by totally different designers and programmers? What does this tell you about the degrees of standardization and cooperation required? Is there a practical solution given the independence of individual developers?

5. Setting and accepting standards, and coordinating planning for integrated but distributed systems, implies a high level support system for networking and data sharing. If individual system developers cannot create the infrastructure on their own, what might they do to help influence the way in which institutional policy makers and planners view the problem? Consider and discuss ways in which a motivating vision of the future might be effectively imparted to such planners. What are the practical questions one must be prepared to answer in such discussions?

2
Centrally Guided Distributed Information Systems: The Next Step

Robert G. Winfree, Jane G. Elchlepp,
and William W. Stead

Healthcare Computing in the 1990s

The 1990s herald the beginning of the fourth decade of the use of computers in the healthcare setting. Issues concerning the attributes of the next generation of information systems are now evident. The changing landscape of the healthcare system is creating a need for more powerful and comprehensive systems which can offer improved information management. These requirements are driven by the functional needs of institutions and the expectations of increasingly sophisticated system users. Furthermore, they are evolving at a pace which that mandates system solutions be flexible and responsive. New patterns of systems leadership, user involvement, and systems design must be developed and nurtured; and a new generation of systems must be developed that will serve these changing needs.

In the 1990s, the key will be to manage and design information systems in a way that produces the benefits of centralized systems while taking advantage of the power and autonomy of distributed systems. This statement is predicated on the thesis that both standalone mainframe technology and networked unrelated systems will prove inadequate.

The next generation will be one of integrated but distributed information management systems. Developing a management structure to guide the establishment of a systems infrastructure based upon integrated modules will be as challenging as the technical construction of the networks and integration software.

Systems Evolution

The initial use of computers in healthcare occurred in the late 1950s and early 1960s. The dominant—if not exclusive—application was accounting and statistical collection. The 1970s witnessed the introduction of hospital information systems which were designed to address the acquisition and movement of both administrative and clinical data through the increasingly complex hospital environment. Predictably, such systems were controlled by administrative staff, interaction between the hospital information system (HIS) and healthcare providers was characterized by batch reports, and mainframe technology was considered the most viable platform for this extensive network model.

During this period of HIS development, departmental and clinical systems emerged. Departmental support systems (e.g., laboratory information systems) were developed to automate the internal processes of ancillary departments. These systems were controlled by departments, and were not integrated with institutional systems. Clinical information systems were developed in ambulatory clinics or subspecialty areas, and focused on meeting the needs of clinical caregivers. Control was vested in the clinical staff; manipulation of patient records and provision of clinical decision support systems were paramount. Minicomputers and subsequently microcomputers were used as the hardware base for departmental and clinical systems because of their interactive features.

Different types of systems were emphasized at various institutions. In retrospect, it appears that the two factors influencing the relationship of institutional systems and freestanding systems were the extent to which institutional support was present (or absent) and the presence of pioneering information management leadership at the departmental level.

By the mid 1970s, healthcare institutions had begun to realize that the future use of computer technology should focus on producing systems environments which could address the growing overlap between functions required by different sets of users. Developers of HIS discovered they were designing applications that had already been developed by colleagues in different disciplines. Hospital information systems were being redefined to include clinical functions (e.g., drug interactions) and departmental needs (e.g., specimen tracking). Concurrently, clinical information systems were rewritten to incorporate functions such as patient billing.

The experiences of the 1970s and early 1980s have produced a growing awareness that the currently installed base of aging systems must be replaced with a new generation. In the early 1970s, mainframe technology was the only means of providing adequate connectivity, database storage, and processing power to support a hospital wide system. Initial institutional efforts usually focused upon a specific area of activity; systems were typically self contained entities in those areas, such as

- Administrative systems, e.g., SMS or McAuto

- Patient care systems, e.g., IBM's PCS (Mishelevich and Van Slyke 1980) or the Technicon MIS (Childs 1988)

- Departmental support systems, e.g., laboratory and pharmacy

- Decision support systems, e.g., the HELP system (Pryor 1988)

In this classical approach, no one system was able to address needs of all user groups, resulting in attempts to network disparate systems. Proponents of networking standalone departmental systems into an institutional fabric argued that one central database could not provide for local needs and centralized programming groups were not responsive to specific user requirements (Simborg et al. 1983). However, this approach suffered from problems of efficiency and data integrity.

Recent and ongoing developments in software design, network technology, and desktop workstations provide the technological foundation to pursue an alternative approach. Best characterized as a centrally guided, integrated yet distributed information management system, such an approach supports the growing overlap of function among various user populations, and permits transfer of functional capability between systems (Stead 1989).

The Design Concept

The design of the next generation of healthcare information systems must recognize the relationship among the information management needs of a heterogeneous community of users. The multiple participants in the healthcare system can be divided into three user groups for the purpose of analyzing their information management needs. The three categories of administrative staff, ancillary service departments, and direct care providers are not discrete groupings, in that an individual in one group may perform functions associated with another group.

The manner in which the three user groups need to access data can be understood by identifying five categories of data retrieval. The first category is the historical recall of data about a specific patient or study. Accessing data about a current encounter is a second requirement. A third approach involves retrieving data about a subgroup of patients or events based upon one or more common attributes. Access to data for efficient work flow management is a fourth requirement, and the fifth area deals with accessing knowledge databases to supplement clinical decision making processes.

The relative importance of a category to an individual user will vary based upon the primary group identification (administration, ancillary support, and direct patient care). Administrators would predictably place a low priority on accessing knowledge databases, but would emphasize the ability to retrieve historical data on individual patients. Practicing physicians would be less interested in workflow management than colleagues in departments of radiology or laboratory medicine.

Data Requirements

Despite differences in priority, each of the groups needs all five types of information retrieval. This overlap in user requirements validates the thesis that the needs of multiple user groups should be supported by one source of data. New patterns of clinical practice and ever changing methods of reimbursement will influence the architecture of systems.

Two specific examples are the integration of outpatient and inpatient care, and the trend toward development of regional, national, and international medical record databases. Such trends argue that the next generation of systems must be designed to transfer data to and retrieve data from global databases. This prediction is not intended to suggest a monolithic database residing on a massive mainframe. Rather, it suggests that data in multiple forms must be able to flow seamlessly through multiple systems.

The information management needs of the contemporary healthcare institution exceed the capacity of traditional information systems in which one applications package provides all required functions. It is, therefore, important to define the information management needs in manageable components which can be merged to provide a consolidated source of information. There are two ways to achieve that outcome, the first of which is to interface available standalone systems in a manner which permits data exchange. This approach permits all systems to function as related entities, but with the disadvantage that each system must depend upon itself for integrity. Specifically, maintenance of database definition tables, database archives, and database backups must be handled separately on each system.

The second method is to develop a systems mix based upon a set of integrated modules, each of which is designed to work in conjunction with others. Although distributed, a system of integrated modules can be contrasted with a system consisting of standalone systems. A prerequisite for the integrated systems approach is a sophisticated communications protocol between modules. Data transfer between modules with appropriate communications protocols optimizes what each system does best while depending on other modules to perform other functions. Databases can be synchronized by ensuring that a master database and a data editing application are designated for each datum. In other words, although a datum may be stored in more than one database, all updates of that datum must take place in its master database and then flow to all locations where copies of the datum exist. In the integrated model, data definition tables, database archiving, and database backups can be accomplished in an integrated fashion since synchronization is guaranteed.

In a system based upon integrated modules, the database is the software foundation of the system, while the network provides the hardware foundation. Application packages or workstations can be designed to get data from a central source, supplement those data with local data if necessary, and manipulate data to meet the needs of a user group. The central database becomes a black box which serves as a resource for the workstation, thereby providing the benefits of a traditional central system. The workstation can be modified locally to meet local needs for flexibility.

Commercial Systems

Historically and at present, commercially available systems have been developed as standalone systems to meet a particular need. Making such systems function as building blocks in an integrated environment usually mandates significant modification by the vendor. Understandably, vendors are reluctant to make changes which are not transferable to their broader customer base and which fail to contribute to the corporate bottom line. Additionally, the concept of building systems on the foundation of integrated distributed modules is relatively new and untested in the marketplace. The concept changes the criteria for systems selection. It is no longer necessary to find the system that comes closest to meeting all needs. It becomes more important to find a system which does one function well and has been designed with standards in mind so it can be coordinated with other software.

Nonetheless, purchased software can play an important role in developing systems on the framework of integrated distributed modules. In lieu of purchasing turnkey application packages, elements of a tool kit can be acquired which facilitate rapid development of products which can be adapted to the integrated systems environment.

Major systems vendors have begun to acknowledge that providing complete turnkey solutions has produced marginal functional and (from a corporate perspective) financial results. The commercial marketplace is showing signs of accepting the concept of a systems infrastructure composed of integrated distributed modules designed to work together to provide a single source of information. The approach based upon interfacing disparate systems rather than integrating modules, although apparently simple in the short run, does not provide the desired operational benefits.

Management Structure

The key factors related to managing information systems are the style of systems leadership that is practiced and the way in which users are involved in the systems management process. The 1980s witnessed the position of data processing director evolve from departmental status to a corporate level function. At the same time, the movement to distributed systems fostered the perception at the user and (in some instances) management levels that decentralized systems should be controlled by the end user.

In the 1960s and early 1970s, data processing directors were largely viewed as technical staff members and, in most cases, reported to the senior financial official of the institution. During the 1970s, the position of director of data processing evolved from managing computer operations to an institutional role as a department level manager. As institutional information systems became more complex and multifunctional, the role matured, and the concept (and pseudo title) of computer czar emerged. This role was based on the principle that a senior administrator in a central position would be solely responsible for information systems, would understand the problems of data processing, and would control purchases to minimize costs. This approach grew out of the mindset of the early 1970s—a period when technology was expensive and the three major components of a system (processing power, connectivity, and application programs) were virtually inseparable. It was an era when the avoidance of costly errors was assigned a higher priority than the encouragement of experimentation.

The CIO Model

By the middle 1980s, the computing environment had experienced significant change. Desktop processing produced dramatic reductions in cost so that it was neither necessary nor appropriate to centrally control its dissemination. The management emphasis changed from cost containment to information availability, and the computer czar model shifted to the contemporary role of the chief information officer (CIO). At the end of the decade, it was apparent that it was possible to separate the four components of systems (networks, processing power, programs, and databases) and share aspects of those components across functional units of the organization. These events stimulated a rather significant change. The notion of segregating patient care systems (or networks) from administrative or research systems was replaced with a view of institutional systems which could serve multiple uses. Therefore management coordination was required across traditional operating units.

The CIO model requires that, rather than having a data processing background, the institutional systems leader should be well versed in the use and management of information. It is important that the CIO have a systems base (which can be clinical, administrative, academic, or research in nature) that provides staff and systems support. The leadership emphasis is on providing guidance through strategic planning and initiatives rather than control, and reflects a management structure (and style) that is enabling rather than inhibiting.

There are several characteristics of the CIO model that differentiate it from the computer czar role. The CIO must understand how to manage information, achieve a balance between access and control issues, and be able to resolve conflict among user groups on such issues as data creation and ownership. The chief information officer must understand strategic issues, and be a participant in setting institutional priorities. A sound understanding of the institutional mission, strategic planning skills, an appreciation of the need for data integrity, and the ability to make users feel they have a legitimate role in managing a shared resource (data) are key attributes of a successful CIO.

User Involvement

A second outcome of the trend toward the centrally guided, integrated, and distributed model focuses on the user community. As previously noted, this approach fosters a mindset which suggests that control of distributed systems should be vested in the users themselves. Ironically, the expansive, flexible systems environment of the future requires that a level of increased discipline be imposed on the institution. To enjoy freedom of choice, users must abide by institutional standards. This requirement signals the second major systems management issue of the distributed model: involvement of the user in the systems management process.

The user community representation should reflect the character and mission of the organization. Therefore, the approach to involving users in systems management must be tailored to the specific institutional environment.

An academic health center with a threefold mission of patient care, research, and education should involve practicing clinicians, patient care support staff, research scientists, medical educators, and administrative staff. A freestanding hospital would most likely mirror the three user groups of direct care providers, ancillary service departments, and administrators. Academic health centers which are integrally part of a parent university should reach across medical boundaries and involve colleagues from selected disciplines, including library science and computer science.

The functional attributes of user involvement are more important than the structural framework, which could be generically described as a systems advisory committee. Users must be active in identifying and supporting functional needs and areas of opportunity for the institution. They should be charged with identifying how systems should be modified and adapted, an approach which encourages users to support sound system outcomes rather than attempting to bypass necessary development practices. It is important to avoid stifling creativity and innovation. Experimentation is important and constructive even if it is ill defined or entrepreneurial in character, because it can produce good results which can be incorporated into the production system. The need to learn by doing extends to the principle that users should be encouraged to use a system before specifications are formulated. This form of prototyping, though time consuming and potentially costly, can produce significant improvements over time in functional outcomes and learning curve improvements.

Finally, it is predictable and reasonable that users will have difficulty adapting to an institutional focus in the centrally guided, distributed model. Departmental parochialism is natural and must be gradually shaped to an institutional view.

In this context, the concept of a systems advisory committee has proven its value in a variety of institutional settings as an effective management technique. The multidisciplinary committee structure facilitates cutting across traditional departmental reporting structures, thereby bringing together individuals from different backgrounds who share similar problems. This structure permits issues to be evaluated from an institutional perspective, an applications perspective, and a departmental perspective.

The systems advisory committee should serve as a convenor for a number of subcommittees, the composition of which will reflect the role and character of the organization. In the university/academic health center setting, subcommittees should include the functional areas of administrative, patient care management, research, and instructional information systems. As previously mentioned, the two resource areas of information systems technology (e.g., computer science) and library information systems are highly desirable additions to the user driven committee structure. In the traditional hospital setting, subcommittees could be representative of large functional

areas (e.g., nursing, pharmacy, administration, medical staff) or multidisciplinary within the framework of administrative, ancillary service, and direct care
provider categories.

The chairperson (or convenor) of the systems advisory committee in most
situations should be the CIO of the institution, and the committee should be
composed of the chairpersons of the aforementioned operational subcommittees. This model presumes that the CIO represents the enabling rather than
the inhibiting management style, and that committee members embrace the
view that freedom of choice at the operational level is predicated on
acceptance of institutional guidelines and standards. The systems advisory
committee should report to the senior leadership of the institution and, among
other tasks, should be charged with the responsibility for making ongoing
planning and policy recommendations to senior management. Users should
use the advisory committee as a vehicle for ongoing planning activities,
including needs assessment and identification of opportunities. Properly
structured, the systems advisory committee can also serve as a positive
example of the use of information technology by providing data, analyses, and
management reports from existing databases to offices and committees of the
institution.

Conclusion

Healthcare institutions are facing increasing pressures to improve efficiency
and effectiveness. They must also deal with the challenge of meeting
immediate demands for new information management systems at a time when
the existing generation of systems is architecturally 15 years old and the next
generation of systems is at an embryonic stage. Hospitals and other healthcare
organizations must develop a long range vision of the importance of
information systems technology in the institutional priority scheme. Achievement of long term goals will predictably necessitate compromise, and it is
important to avoid middle of the road interim solutions. Properly pursued,
short term objectives can be accomplished without compromising long term
system outcomes. The creation of a progressive management structure to
develop a new generation of centrally guided integrated modules is a challenge
equal to the tasks of developing networks and integration software.

Questions

1. What will be one of the key issues in the design and management of information systems in the 1990s?

2. What are some of the lessons learned between the 1960s and the 1980s?
   Give three examples.

3. What is important in the next generation of design concepts of health
   information systems?

4. Why will we see data in multiple forms flowing seamlessly through multiple systems in the 1990s?

5. How have management structures changed as we move into the 1990s?

6. Who needs to be involved in systems design for the 1990s?

References

Childs, B. W. 1988. El Camino / National Institute of Health—A case study. In *Towards new hospital information systems*, ed. A. R. Bakker, M. J. Ball, J. R. Scherrer, and J. L. Willems, 83-9. Amsterdam: Elsevier Science Publishers.

Mishelevich, D. L. and D. Van Slyke. 1980. Application development system: The software architecture of the IBM health care support/Dl/1- Patient care system. *IBM Systems Journal* 478-504.

Pryor, T. A. 1988. The help medical record system. *MD Computing* 5:22-33.

Simborg, D. W., M. Chadwick, Q. E. Whiting-O'Keefe, S. G. Tolchin, S. A. Kahn, and E. S. Bergan. 1983. Local area networks and the hospital. *Computers and Biomedical Research* 16:247-59.

Stead, W.W. 1989. Building an HIS for the year 2000: An agenda for the 90's. In *Proceedings of AAMSI Congress*, ed. W. E. Hammond, 8-16. New York: IEEE.

3

Physician Utilization of Medical Information Systems: A Prescription for Survival

Andrew C. Garling

Throughout the 1990s, sweeping new regulations in the healthcare industry will require vastly more detailed reporting and monitoring of clinical performance in the hospital environment. Hospitals will be required to meet complex new data requirements or face difficult certification criteria, even loss of accreditation. As the managers of patient information, physicians will ultimately bear most of this data burden.

An extensive year long study of hospitals with a comprehensive computer based medical information system (MIS) found that hospitals with significant physician usage of the MIS are well positioned to succeed in this new era. Factors projecting future success include the following: (1) the data collection tool, the computer, in place; (2) physicians actively using computer based data management; and (3) the hospital demonstrating an essential organizational shift to physician management of the patient information record.

An MIS is defined here as a comprehensive computer based information system that integrates all hospital departments, administrative as well as clinical. The system's physician oriented capabilities include a resulting online realtime patient record with order entry and results retrieval. Physicians who do not use an MIS will be unable to meet the upcoming regulatory requirements, unless there is a rapid shift toward increased utilization of MIS within the hospital environment. Physicians utilizing an MIS are uniquely positioned to manage the upcoming information requirements imposed by the Joint Commission on Accreditation of Healthcare Organizations (JCAHO). The commission's new agenda for change calls for performance monitoring and quality evaluation of inpatient care within the next five years.

Physician utilization of the automated patient information record is emerging not as a choice, but as a mandate for survival in the changing climate of clinical information processing. Physicians must examine this growing trend and assess the suitability of an MIS for their practice environment.

The relationship between physicians and hospital administrators changed abruptly in the early 1980s as the arrival of diagnostic related groupings (DRGs) imposed cost control demands on the healthcare delivery world. Suddenly, administrators and physicians faced similar outside pressures, as DRGs forced them into a dialogue about a timely, quality outcome for the patient.

Prior to the DRGs, the computer had been a helpful tool in both medical department information systems and billing related tasks such as capturing costs and tracking inventory. With the advent of DRGs for inpatient treatment, the information needs of the hospital changed dramatically as it became necessary to defend the charges with clear documentation in order to receive full governmental reimbursement.

Without physician involvement in the selection of an MIS, the eventual success of the system becomes problematic. A continuing study of 221 physicians' use of an MIS by researchers Stephen Jay and James Anderson of the Division of Academic Affairs at the 1150 bed Methodist Hospital of Indiana (Indianapolis) addresses the importance of physician participation. It indicates that if physicians are not involved in the early decision making and implementation of a hospital wide system, they probably will not use it after installation.

"The key to the success of a MIS has to do with implementing it with the full cooperation and involvement of the doctors, not just inviting them to use it after the fact," said Anderson during an address to a physician user group at TDS in November 1988. "Only then will the computers be used, and patient care benefits obtained."

New Era of Knowledge Based Performance Evaluation

In early 1988, the JCAHO reached a new milestone in its agenda for change, by finalizing a draft of the 12 key organizational principles that have been determined to characterize a quality healthcare organization.

Quality of healthcare delivery will become paramount as a future requirement for accreditation. Standards are being developed to enable practical comparisons among similar hospitals. In addition, JCAHO is in the process of developing quality of care indicators which will be used to monitor clinical performance. Preliminary sets of these indicators measuring anesthesia, obstetrics, and hospital wide care are already being piloted in 17 test hospitals, while those for surgical, oncology, cardiovascular units, trauma care, long term care, mental health care, and others are soon to follow.

It seems obvious that this type of data, once gathered by the JCAHO, will be of great interest to other parties, namely consumers, third party payors, major employers, and preferred provider organizations. The Health Care Financing Administration (HCFA), which makes hospital data on Medicare patients widely available, plans to create a data library including individual physician services. HCFA's William Roper has stressed the objective of giving doctors an additional tool to do their jobs.

Using the JCAHO's newly defined common cause quality assurance, it is clear that the microscopic scrutiny of this new evaluation requires more precise and retrievable record keeping on the part of the medical staff. For example, the medical staff will track patterns and trends in care, instead of using the traditional case based approach. This will not be achievable without enhanced computer technologies.

Hospitals are going to have to move quickly to streamline clinical management in order to meet these challenges. For many hospitals, especially those without an MIS, this is not going to be easy. According to JCAHO sources, 59 percent of the hospitals that had full surveys in the 12 month period ending in August 1988 had contingency ratings on the basis of "inadequate monitoring of clinical performance and evaluation of quality assurance."

"Institutions that have a hard time meeting data requirements now, will have an even more difficult time when the JCAHO starts requiring specific data elements," said William Jessee, the JCAHO's vice president for education, in an address to the TDS Executive Forum in February 1988. "A clinically oriented MIS could help relieve this burden."

Facilities unable to demonstrate good medical care with clear, objective data will fail quality evaluation. Hospitals already gathering detailed clinical and outcomes data for quality assurance, peer review, and risk management programs have a head start on this new technology and are positioned to succeed in the upcoming era.

Physicians should be concerned about how hospitals are facing these changes, since it is ultimately the practice of medicine that will be more fully scrutinized. JCAHO Task Force Chairman William Dowling has said that outcomes indicators will help hospitals "look in objective, measurable terms at the manner in which it is organized and managed, and how this affects quality will give professionals new pathways to improving quality" (JCAHO 1988).

Physicians can take a leadership role in managing the changes that are affecting their practices by sharing responsibility with hospital administrators for what lies ahead. To do so, physicians will have to identify the information management tools they need, not only computer hardware but sophisticated software to help them meet the specific changing needs of their profession. The sooner physicians join forces with hospital administrators to develop strategies for the future, the sooner the substantial dollars involved will become an investment for success.

As the principal originators and consumers of clinical information in the hospital, physicians must provide significant input into the selection of an optimal MIS for the clinical setting. Physicians cannot be expected to routinely maintain the information that will be required of them in the near future, if they do not help determine how that information is collected and processed.

This will mean redefining roles within the hospital, as doctors assume more responsibility for managing the needs of the clinical environment. Physicians and administrators must combine their resources in order to achieve the ultimate goals of the integrated computer system, which will give the health-care institution a competitive advantage in the volatile healthcare environment.

Questions

1. What are some of the success factors projecting future success for medical information systems?

2. What are the expectations today regarding quality outcomes for patient care? When did these change? How have these changes affected physicians and hospital administrative staff?

3. What is a danger in MIS development if physician input is not forthcoming?

4. In what way will future MIS systems help meet JCAHO quality measure outcome indicators?

Reference

Joint Commission on Accreditation of Healthcare Organizations. 1988. Task force sights new quality horizons. *Agenda for Change Update* 5.

4
Positive Patient and Specimen Identification

Arthur E. Rappoport

Today healthcare faces critical challenges which information technology can help to meet. Computerized hospital information systems (HIS) have contributed to improved management practices and productivity in financial management and accounting and most recently in administrative decision support. Except for laboratories, clinical units have lagged behind. Only now is patient care beginning to benefit from the capabilities provided by computing and communications technologies.

Machine readable identification systems (MRIS) benefit both administrative and clinical management. By eliminating identification errors and accelerating turnaround time, MRIS promise to improve patient care through maximum quality assurance control.

Capabilities

A global MRIS requires that an HIS be available at nursing stations and other work areas throughout the hospital. The MRIS itself consists of barcode printers, wands, or laser readers connected to the HIS. Increasingly, bedside care systems are being utilized along with the HIS/MRIS.

An Early Model

Developed in the early 1960s, the Western Reserve Care System (Ohio) demonstrated the potential of MRIS. Electronic measurement values from automated and semiautomated analytic devices were linked to the hospital's IBM computer. Analytical subsystem results were integrated into and stored in the patient's medical file. Interim and cumulative reports were printed and delivered to the nursing stations.

A unique feature of that early system was the invention of an MRIS. When tests were ordered, patient identification numbers were also entered into the system. Stubcards bearing a unique printed and punched specimen identification number were attached when and where specimens were collected. The analytical device read each stubcard automatically during the test and merged the test result with the patient and specimen identification numbers.

The MRIS prepared listings for sample collection and instrument turntable loading. It also calculated final results, checking them against quality control standards and producing reliable results in minimal time. Laboratory testing made a giant leap forward to a cybernetic system, increasing productivity.

In that automated work flow, patient labels were still handwritten and subject to being misread or misapplied. To eliminate this potential for error, a patient identification system was created. Upon admission, patients were given hospital bracelets with small pressure labels bearing their hospital number in optical character recognition. The patient identification label was placed on the specimen container, already carrying the specimen identification label generated by computer at the time of requisition. This order entry label displayed the patient's demographic data, the name of the requested test, and the eye-readable hospital number.

Having both labels on the same container ensured that a specimen came from a specifically identified patient and eliminated the possibility of mislabeling. Throughout testing, the original specimen and its similarly labeled aliquot portions remained under MRIS surveillance. Identification was validated through repeated scannings and comparisons of labels. If a variance occurred, a signal alerted staff. By overcoming such human factors as fatigue, inattention, carelessness, or inability to decipher illegible handwriting, MRIS eliminated a major cause of laboratory disaster.

Along with stringent quality controls for reference standards, reagents, instruments, and test techniques, laboratories have used MRIS to improve reliability. MRIS have improved patient care both by accelerating turnaround time and by reducing the likelihood of attributing results to the wrong patient.

Barcodes in MRIS

Early MRIS had to select between many different barcode symbologies available. Today, the universal product code (UPC) is ubiquitous, giving rise to the suggestion, "If it's so useful in supermarkets, it certainly ought to be great in hospitals." The Health Industry Business Communication Council is working to meet that challenge, with the help of the medical community, the American Hospital Association, and major healthcare vendors. The council's goal is to obtain industry wide acceptance of a standard barcode symbology for all functions carried out in medical institutions. Manufacturers of patient bracelets now have the capability to provide barcoded patient hospital numbers as well as the conventional eye-readable data. Acceptance of this technology, hitherto hesitant, seems to be growing as the technology and familiarity with it matures (Longe 1989).

When the American Blood Commission attempted to introduce an MRIS with a barcoded blood bank bag in the 1970s, even the computerized laboratories responsible for operating hospital transfusion services were slow to exploit this technology. Only a few HIS could process this symbology. Limited equipment was available for printing and reading barcode; interfaces and software systems capable of transmitting the specimen and patient identification numbers to the HIS were lacking. Even analytic instruments possessing their own integral specimen identification modules could not communicate effectively with the HIS. Despite these difficulties, the Brodheim report makes clear that MRIS are indeed viable systems and undoubtedly will flourish as time goes on (Brodheim 1979).

Uses in Other Departments

Like clinical laboratories, other hospital professional departments need a system for accurate identification of patients and the materials they generate. For example, radiology departments could benefit from attaching patient identification labels to film cassettes for transfer to the exposed and developed film and finally the film jackets for storage. Imaging devices (CAT scans, ultrasound, MRI) create copious reports and examinations which demand equal accuracy in identification.

EKG and EEG strip charts, cardiac catheter laboratory reports, anesthesiologic data, and other medical records and tracings are also subject to misidentification and would benefit from identification labels applied at the moment of intervention.

With the growing trend toward bedside care systems, the HIS industry has begun to recognize the need for MRIS. Now on the market are barcoded products which attach to hospital bracelets at admission and carry the patient identification number for scanning at any time or place, for transmittal to the HIS and entry directly into the patient medical file. This feature offers opportunities for bedside clinical data input as well as for immediate retrieval.

A Bedside MRIS and Patient Care System

Bedside care systems with MRIS capabilities are now up and running in a number of institutions. Among them are installations at Indian River Memorial Hospital in Vero Beach, Florida, and Providence Hospital in Portland, Oregon, both of which the author of this chapter had the opportunity to observe.

Both are CliniCom systems, with a handheld terminal that hangs on the wall at the head of the patient's bed. This portable, lightweight terminal has an optical barcode reader, a liquid crystal display, and a keyboard. Input/output data are transmitted via shortwave to a radio frequency receiver and in turn by modem to the telephone at the patient's bedside. From there the information is communicated to the system processor, which is linked to the HBO & Company, Inc., hospital information system.

With the handheld terminal, nursing personnel at the bedside can enter medical information using the keyboard for vital signs and other data and the barcode reader for such items as barcoded unit dose drug packets. Time is noted automatically, and transactions can be verified on the terminal. Through password protected access, authorized staff can retrieve and display current and past patient data stored in the HIS, including laboratory, radiologic, pharmacy, and other clinical data relevant to that patient. The system also includes touch screen terminals located throughout the hospital and in the patient's room and backs up the bedside care dialogue with computer generated chart copies. The effect of the system is to expedite diagnostic and treatment efforts by eliminating time consuming paperwork.

The System at Work: A Scenario

The physician initiates the process with a reservation to admit patient Smith to general surgery on next Tuesday, for a cholecystectomy. These data and Smith's demographic information are entered into the admission, discharge, transfer system of the HIS and will await the patient's arrival at the admitting office.

At that time, all of Smith's information is retrieved and verified. Forms are preprinted or computer generated at admission for Smith's signature. The patient receives a hospital bracelet with eye-readable conventional information and the printed and barcoded patient and hospital identification numbers. The same identifiers, in the same formats, appear on all accompanying paperwork (Figure 1).

When the patient is admitted to the floor, nursing station personnel access the HIS to review the physician's orders for the patient, including diet and medications as well as diagnostic and treatment procedures. Any orders not entered when the reservation was made are entered in the HIS.

Each subsequent transaction requires identification numbers for the patient and the care provider. Patient identifiers can be scanned from their hospital bracelets or keyboarded in. Barcoded identifiers for personnel appear on their badges for scanning.

At the bedside, after completing the patient's initial examination, the nurse scans in the identifiers and enters the patient's vital signs and other findings. The nurse administers the prescribed medication, scanning the barcoded identifiers (patient and care provider) and then the barcoded unit dose package for the drug. The system automatically logs the time and transmits the data to the HIS. Accessing the HIS, the pharmacist can confirm that the prescription and its administration were correct.

The HIS automatically compares the entire intervention against the original order entry for correctness and generates a timeline analysis of each step throughout the entire procedure. Again, when medication is given, the system compares the two records for patient identity and drug name, quantity, and time administered. Any discrepancy triggers the display of an error message on the bedside or nursing station terminals. If feasible, the message is accompanied by an audible signal.

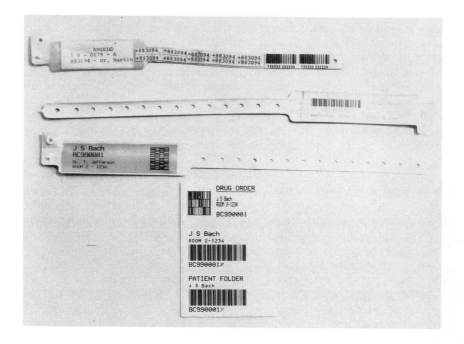

Figure 1. Barcode Identifiers

Coming in response to an HIS generated test request, the phlebotomist checks the eye-readable patient data on the hospital bracelet. A handheld barcode reader and printer like the Pitney-Bowes Pathfinder is used to scan the identifiers on the patient bracelet, provider badge, and requisition. The device also generates a pressure sensitive label with a copy of the scanned patient identification number. The phlebotomist then draws the blood and places the patient and specimen identification labels on the sample container, eliminating the possibility of mislabeling the sample. In a sense, the process links the bracelet at the wrist to a phlebotomy specimen procured from a cubital or wrist vein only a few inches distant. Again, the MRIS notes the time of the procedure and files it in the HIS.

Applications Beyond the Lab

Personnel from other departments, including x-ray, EKG, EEG, and physiotherapy, use the same procedures whenever guaranteed patient identification is required on patient generated samples or paper medical forms. For example, there must be no error in associating surgically removed tissues with a particular patient, but misidentification can occur when several similar operations, such as breast lumpectomies, are performed simultaneously in a large operating suite. All the specimens are transported to the pathologist at about the same time, checked in, accessed, numbered, and processed histologically; stained slides are prepared and labeled. Using both specimen and patient identifiers on sample containers allows MRIS barcode checks along the entire cycle, eliminating the possibility of error. The slides also could bear barcoded labels.

Administrative Functions

MRIS would also benefit medical record departments. Scanning barcodes on forms would eliminate repeated keyboarding of patient demographic data into the HIS. MRIS could facilitate tracking charts throughout the institution by the easy barcode identification of the physicians and departments who had received those charts; record misplacement and loss could be avoided. MRIS could expedite collection and collation of the patient's complete medical record, including various color coded reports (nursing progress notes, consultations, ancillaries, etc.) and outpatient information. With MRIS, storage and retrieval of these records would be expedited, and their privacy would be enhanced, as fewer record handlers would have access to them.

In addition, other administrative areas would benefit from the improved transmission of records as they work to meet requirements for insurance, billing, accounting, and statistics. Clearly, when the electronic patient record becomes a reality—and it assuredly will—MRIS will play a critical role in healthcare delivery.

A Strategic Tool for Healthcare

MRIS will be a strategic tool, as professional associations, the insurance industry, and government agencies work to meet the demand for quality healthcare. As part of its agenda for change, the Joint Commission on Accreditation of Healthcare Organizations (JCAHO) is calling for the identification, selection, and examination of critical indicators in each medical specialty which require professional surveillance, control, and improvement. MRIS could be extremely helpful in searching and evaluating these indicators.

With MRIS, critical analysis of each action (step) made sequentially through the entire hospitalization period would be greatly facilitated. With a bedside care system, data entry would establish the time, nature, and staff person involved in each intervention affecting a patient. In addition to reducing the need for potentially confusing handwritten nursing or progress notes, the system would automatically track turnaround time for procedures. This feature would eliminate the practice of fudging manual data that occasionally occurs when short staffing or other factors prevent staff from completing a procedure at the time specified by the physician.

By providing incontrovertible data through continuous monitoring, MRIS can help avoid criticisms and fingerpointing. Each service provided can be identified along with the barcoded identifier for the individual so that service and times can be documented. The system can alert supervisors if procedures are flawed or are not completed within certain prescribed timeframes.

Through industrial engineering techniques, a faulty procedure can be re-examined and changes initiated. Staff can be educated individually or collectively. When the record shows that the perception is faulty (and not the medical procedure), that perception can be corrected. By thus addressing real or perceived operational shortcomings, errors, delays, losses of critical time, or misplacements of patient samples or records, the MRIS can improve both staff morale and patient care.

This type of automated supervision has psychological consequences for personnel. Although extremely useful in ensuring professional competence, monitoring may create a backlash among personnel. Thus, implementing an MRIS in an HIS requires sufficient time to educate and train the involved staff to overcome potentially hostile attitudes. The system itself can be used to provide such time. Establishing turnaround periods of variable length can accommodate the learning curve for staff and allow the educational process leeway.

Physician attitudes also must be considered. Older doctors in particular may consider automated systems disruptive and be thus reluctant to comply with system requirements, especially given the growing regulatory restrictions imposed by government, insurance companies, and their own professional societies. However, the availability of information at the bedside will convert physicians to the system. They will be able to review the patient's vital signs, fluid intake/output, and medication administration without having to read pages of handwritten nursing notes. Visual retrieval at the bedside of data from ancillary departments, such as laboratory tests and radiology examinations, will expedite medical efforts and the ordering of additional diagnostic or therapeutic procedures. The rapid availability of data stored in the HIS will eliminate the need to call other departments or to hunt through bulky paper records for results.

Instant data retrieval proved its worth in the early 1970s when this author designed an audio response system for his institution. Digitalized touchtone telephones with audio output gave access to HIS stored data and to test order entry, request verification, and result retrieval. The system included a warning system; all stat, abnormal, or "panic" results transmitted to the HIS would automatically trigger telephone notification of the nursing station. The computer voice would spell the patient's name and announce the result it wished to impart. This information was accessible only to employees who entered in their identification number on the touchtone pad to confirm their receipt of the data at that specific time. Nurses and physicians responded enthusiastically to this feature, which eliminated much of the inefficiency that characterizes intrahospital communications. The growth of computer linked voice systems will undoubtedly contribute to the development of like systems, especially when the electronic patient record becomes a reality.

As members of the healthcare team, pharmacists are well aware of and sensitive to the serious problems concerning patient or drug misidentification which can occur when ordering drugs for, or administering them to, specific patients. Positive identification significantly reduces the likelihood of undesirable events since the unit dose bears its own barcoding. Several complete applications have been designed and tested successfully.

The area of materiels management can also benefit from MRIS. Scanning barcodes printed on shipping containers can identify vendors and recognize and record the receipt of supplies and equipment. Similar to the practice in supermarkets and industry, inventory control could be accomplished accurately and rapidly by reading the tapes possessing these data into the HIS. The economics attained by such inventory control practices would benefit the institution not only in its conventional central supply functions but also in pharmacy, dietary, laboratory, radiology, linen/laundry, and other divisions. The number and type of fixed hospital equipment and furniture could be identified and controlled; specified instrument trays could be created for operating room use according to type of operations and individual surgeons.

In conventionally designed hospitals, central nursing stations function as the areas where nursing, medical, and ancillary staffs congregate and where medical records, computer terminals, drugs, and other supplies are located. Innovative new designs almost completely eliminate centralized nursing stations. An individual patient's supplies, medications, and medical records are stored in the patient's room and charting is completed there. No longer located at a distant nursing station and reached by an electric call button, the nurse is readily available to the patient.

Themselves a feature of decentralized computer architecture, bedside care systems are extremely compatible with this decentralized arrangement for patient floors. Together, they can support improved patient care.

The Future

Clearly, MRIS and barcoding technologies can improve both productivity and patient care by providing the data that are needed for monitoring care and ensuring accountability. As healthcare strives to meet the challenges of the 1990s, positive identification can play a key role, ensuring that information is instantly available to the physician and nurse at the bedside—information that is accurate, complete, and protected from inappropriate access. With the advent of the electronic patient record, the benefits of positive patient identification will increase exponentially, transforming healthcare for the new millennium.

Questions

1. What is the main reason to use a machine readable identification system (MRIS)?

2. What could an MRIS consist of?

3. How did MRIS methods improve matters in the lab in the 60s and 70s?

4. How can the medical record department benefit from MRIS concepts? How will it affect the patient computerized record of the future?

5. How would you address the training issue in introducing the MRIS approach to an HIS?

6. Name five areas to which you would introduce MRIS in the hospital setting in order of importance to you.

References

Brodheim, E. 1979. Chairman, *Committee for Commonality in Blood Bank Automation*, Final report, ed. H. Green. Arlington, Va.: American Blood Commission.

Longe, K. 1989. Bar code offers various benefits in health care settings, *HA News* 25(44):4.

Select Bibliography

AHA Case Studies: Hospital Bar Coding.
    Catalogue 101900 1985: *Bar coding in radiology department.*
    Catalogue 101901 1985: *Integrating bar coding into management information system (Materials Management System).*
    Catalogue 101902 1986: *Patient information through bar coding.*
    Catalogue 101903 1986: *A pharmacy utilizes bar code technology.*

Ball, M. J. 1971. *Selecting a computer system for the clinical laboratory.* Springfield, Ill.: Charles C. Thomas.

Boroviczeny, K. G. v. 1989. Die Anwendung maschinenlesbarer Schriften im medizinischen Laboratorium, *Lab Med* 13:101-109.

Harmon, C. K., and R. Adams. 1984. *Reading between the lines: An introduction to bar code technology.* Peterborough, N.H.: North American Technology, Inc.

Keller, H., and R. Richterich. 1972. Identification of samples in the laboratory of clinical chemistry. In *Proceedings of the VIIth World Congress of Anatomic and Clinical Pathology*, 183. Amsterdam: Exerpta Medica.

Knedel, M., P. Schipper, W. Haas, K. Kilian, and H. Krech. 1970. *Ein System zur automatischen Messwertfassung und verarbeitung für klinischchemische Laboratorien unter Verwendung Rechner-lesbar codierter Probenrohrchen.* Munchen: Vortrag Analytika.

Rappoport, A. E. 1964a. Computers could speed processing of hospital patient's lab tests. *JAMA* 190:34.

Rappoport, A. E. 1964b. *Symposium on Computer Assisted Pathology.* Northfield, Ill.: College of American Pathologists.

Rappoport, A. E. 1979. Computers, information retrieval and data storage. In *Laboratory Medicine*, ed. G. Race, 45(4):1-60.

Rappoport, A. E. 1984. A hospital patient and laboratory machine readable identification system (MRIS) revisited. *Journal of Medical Systems* 8:133-155.

Rappoport, A. E. 1986. The use of machine-readable patient and specimen identification to enhance clinical laboratory quality assurance. *Informatics in Pathology* 1:1-15.

Rappoport, A. E. 1987. Computerisierte Laboratoriums (LIS) und Hospital (HIS) Informations Systeme zur Verbesserung einer schnelleren Durchlaufzeit (TAT)." In *Qualitatssicherung im Medizinschen Laboratorium*, ed. K. G. v. Boroviczeny, R. Merten, and U. P. Merten, 147-161. Berlin: Springer-Verlag.

Rappoport, A. E., and W. D. Gennaro. 1969. You get the blood, the computer does the CBC. *Modern Hospital* 113:103-104.

Rappoport, A. E., and W. D. Gennaro. 1982. Advantages of machine readable identification of patients, specimens and documents in computerized laboratory information systems." In *Proceedings of 1st Annual Conference of the American Association for Medical Systems and Information*. Vol. 1, Washington, D.C.

Rappoport, A. E., W. D. Gennaro, and W. J. Constandse. 1967. Cybernetics enters the hospital laboratory," *Modern Hospital* 108:107-11.

Rappoport, A. E., W. D. Gennaro, and W. J. Constandse. 1968. Computer-laboratory link is base of hospital information system. *Modern Hospital* 110:100-3.

Rappoport, A. E., Y. D. Tom, W. D. Gennaro, and R. E. Berquist. 1979. Damming the flood of laboratory data. In *Computing in clinical laboratories*, ed. F. Siemaszko. Tunbridge Wells, England: Pitman Medical Publishing.

5
Decision Support: A Strategic Weapon

Homer H. Schmitz

In today's fast paced environment, healthcare professionals are searching for any competitive advantage that might be available. Ironically, one has been available for many years, but it is frequently unknown, mistrusted, or ignored. This advantage is the appropriate use of the information resource and, more specifically, the transformation of that information into a strategic weapon by use of decision support tools. Use of decision support tools is a vital part of managing the information resource because it provides one of the most powerful techniques for turning the vast amounts of data available in most healthcare organizations into usable information. Therefore, all discussions of the information resource should be understood to include the application of decision support techniques to refine and transform the organization's data into usable information for decision makers.

Decision Support and the Planning Function

Students of organizational behavior tell us that there are certain management functions that must be performed in any successful organization. The number of management functions varies with the author. When they are combined into their basic functions, however, there are three: planning, operating, and controlling. The approach to providing information to support these functions will vary because the information needs of the decision maker vary with the managerial function. For example, the information required to make an operational decision about scheduling a patient is vastly different in form and origin from the information required to make a planning decision about the geographic location of a new business venture. The nature of these data is different, as is the design of the information systems to provide them. This concept has been discussed elsewhere (Schmitz 1987), so it will not be treated in detail here. However, certain basic points should be raised about the nature of the information needed to support the planning function, since that is the area where decision support tools most frequently come into play.

When dealing with information to support the planning function, the timeframe for the focus of the activity is usually future oriented. The nature of the data is that it most often presupposes projections into the future, implying the use of projective techniques such as statistical inference and various modeling approaches including simulation. The decision support model used to provide information in support of the planning function is generally created by the user of the information. That is, each decision in this environment is usually unique and requires a model that considers the individual variables of the specific decision in a meaningful and systematic way. This often dictates that the person making the decision construct the model, or that there be a person within the organization who has access to the information and can formulate the variables into a meaningful decision model. This person has been described as the information resource manager and should reside at the vice presidential level of the organization (Schmitz 1989).

Since the nature of the data is different for each function of management, it implies that there are different systems, or at least different approaches, to serving the information needs for each function. Therefore, in order for this integrated planning approach to be successful, there must be some level of system integration that makes the information from one system available to the other. The organization's total database must be available to the information systems and decision support models that provide information to the decision makers engaged in each function of management. That is, the process is an interactive one that asks the following questions:

- What do we want to do?
- How do we do it?
- Did we do what we said we were going to do?

The first question addresses the planning function; the second, the operating function; and the third, the control function. Obviously the information from one is required by the next in order to perform the task properly.

Figure 1 provides a graphic representation of this process. It is a closed loop, iterative process. The output from one step becomes the input to the next step. This concept demands that the information supporting these tasks be integrated in order to function at an acceptable level.

Approaches to Decision Support

An anonymous author has said, "People would rather live with their problems than have the solution to those problems if they do not understand them." In capsule form, this has been one of the most significant impediments to thewidespread use of decision support tools in the healthcare setting. Healthcare executives have been reluctant to embrace new methodologies for presenting information when they understood neither their meaning nor their application. The potential contributions of these methods were therefore forfeited. Because most healthcare organizations did not have skilled prac-

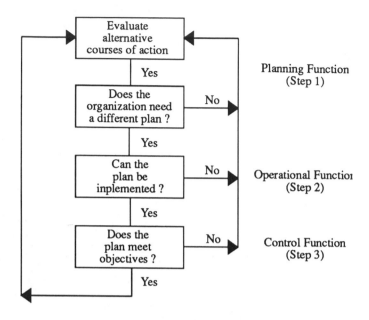

Figure 1. Decision Support Model

titioners in the decision support field, there was no opportunity for executive decision makers to become familiar with the concepts and the results they could produce. This is in contrast to the financial and human resources field where there are generally people on the executive team who can interpret and teach the importance of the insights and techniques for those specialized fields. Alas, the information resources field, including the use of decision support, has traditionally had neither the position in the organization nor the spokesman to acquaint the executive decision making team with the potent strategic weapon that is potentially available to them.

Most other industries have used decision support tools for a decade. It can be generalized that their use has led to more informed decisions and more efficient organizations. Healthcare organizations have generally been reluctant to adopt these methods.

A wide variety of techniques can be used. They range from net present value analysis of an investment's cash flow to the use of the capital asset pricing model to evaluate alternative uses of capital. Other techniques embrace the use of statistical inference methods and management science tools such as simulation techniques, linear programming, and transportation models. All of these methods, and many others, can be applied to the organization's existing store of data to transform it into useful information for a decision maker.

It would be inaccurate to say that there is a single approach to using decision support in the daily activities of an organization. The approach will vary with the structure of the organization, the data available in the organization, the people who develop and use the methods, and the particular tools that are selected for use. Nevertheless, even though there are a multitude of approaches that can be taken to implementing a decision support system, as a concept it is beginning to gain acceptance in some healthcare organizations and should therefore be addressed as an approach to better management of the organization.

Organizational Structure

The traditional organizational structure of information resources in the healthcare setting has been that of a data processing department with a department head reporting either to the chief financial officer (CFO) or the chief operating officer (COO). Their charter has been to solve those technological problems that arise in producing clinical and management reports for the organization. The activity of the department is therefore generally limited to technically oriented hardware and software issues. With this kind of limited focus it is rare for the organization to address data interpretation or system design issues on an organization wide basis. In this traditional organizational setting, the job of the information system manager, and hence of any decision support techniques that might be used, has been reduced to a passive role that centers on technical problem solving. This person has rarely been viewed as part of the organization's executive team.

This narrow view of information management is a terrible and devastating waste of potential for the organization, particularly if there is a qualified information manager in the organization who is capable of providing tactical and strategic insights into the information available to the organization. It severely restricts the potential contribution that can be made and can place the institution at a competitive disadvantage with those organizations that have the insights to manage information resources to their highest potential. By failing to use its information system to its maximum benefit, an institution inexcusably wastes one of its most valuable resources.

The decision support function is important not only for the operational and control functions of management, but especially for the planning function. Managing the decision support function includes the following diverse activities:

- Organizing the data. Most healthcare organizations have more *data* than they can effectively use, but very few of them have more *information* than they can use. The job of decision support is to turn the vast amounts of data into information that is useful to the ultimate decision maker.

- Selecting the models to analyze the data. In order to turn the data into information, the appropriate models must be selected. This can include such traditional approaches as sorting, formatting, extracting, and transforming the data. This also involves using more sophisticated approaches such as statistical inference and management science techniques.

- Interpreting the models' output. It is not sufficient simply to provide the reports to the decision maker. Sometimes there is also the need to interpret and clarify them relative to the assumptions that were used in the model that produced them. This activity would obviously include the active participation and involvement of the information resource manager in the executive decision making process. The reports do not truly become information until they are interpreted correctly.

Available Tools

The focus of this chapter is not to provide a catalog of decision support tools that can be used to transform data into information or to describe how to use these individual tools. Rather, the intent is to acquaint the reader with the potential rewards available if the use of decision support techniques is implemented in an orderly and systematic way and is allowed to become a part of the normal decision making process of the organization. It is furthermore important that the reader recognize some of the pitfalls of improper use and interpretation of these techniques.

There are two types of models used in decision support. One type is the probabilistic model and the other is deterministic. Probabilistic models allow the user to consider a range of solutions. Given the input variables and the probability of their occurrence, the output variables usually take the form of a probability distribution for a range of outcomes. An example of this type of model is Monte Carlo simulation. By contrast, a deterministic model will always produce a single answer for a specified set of input variables. With this type of model, it is possible to change the variables and produce different outcomes for the model, but there is only one answer for a given set of variables. An example of this type of model is a financial profit and loss pro forma.

In dealing with the decision support role, proper interpretation of a model's output cannot be overemphasized. Understanding the interpretation is as important as knowledge about when and how to use the model. It is not uncommon to see executives make decisions based on models they do not understand. For example, decision makers sometimes try to project volumes for the future based on the slope of a linear regression line (trend line), without understanding either the sampling theory behind it or the statistical inferences associated with interpreting the F value that the model produces. They make decisions about averages (means) without understand the sampling theory, the variability of the sample (standard deviation), or the sample's degree of kurtosis (a measure of whether it approximates a normal distribution).

As a final example, decision makers often use personal computer spreadsheets in the mistaken belief that spreadsheets produce a simulation of some scenario they are attempting to project. The personal computer spreadsheet is actually a deterministic model that is capable of providing only a single answer for a given set of variables. It rarely has the capability to give the user a feel for the probability of occurrence for a range of answers. Similarly, the spreadsheet provides little insight into the "correctness" of the answers. By contrast, a true simulation model, such as the monte carlo technique or use of the General Purpose Simulation System (GPSS) computer programming language, provides the ability to specify the probability of occurrence for each of the input variables and then generate a range of outcomes with a probability of occurrence for each.

The reader can no doubt appreciate that interpretation of the decision support model's output is as important as choosing the model itself. If the decision maker does not understand the assumptions of the model or if the user draws inappropriate inferences about its output, the quality of decisions is not likely to be high. It is as easy to make an error in judgment based on inaccurate or inappropriately interpreted information as it is to err because no information is available. Indeed, improper interpretation can be worse than not having the information at all. Having improperly interpreted information at hand can tempt users to believe that their information is meaningful and accurate, creating a false sense of security.

This is not to say that every decision maker must have the expertise to understand these sometimes complex and sophisticated models. It does go without saying that a person is required inside the organization who has the knowledge and ability to function at the institution's executive level and has an understanding of the decision support function that can be imparted to the decision makers. This type of person is not commonly found in healthcare organizations, but when these talents are found and retained, they are well worth the search.

Conclusion

More and more the literature is reflecting the importance of a person able to deliver meaningful use of decision support tools to an organization. This is usually in connection with the management of the organization's information resource. Information is a valuable resource in an organization and is enormously important for the decisions that are made. Inappropriate use and interpretation of decision support models can be dangerous, but appropriate use of these models can be a powerful tool in the hands of an informed decision maker. Chief executive officers and other executives of healthcare organizations can ill afford to ignore such a potent strategic weapon.

Questions

1. Why are data processing tools referred to as strategic weapons?

2. In what areas would timely and accurate information be most effectively used? Give two examples and reasons.

3. Why have decision support tools not been used to their potential up to the present?

4. What is involved in managing the decision support function?

5. Is it worthwhile for a CEO to invest in a person having the skills to manage a decision support system for a hospital?

References

Schmitz, H. H. 1987. *Managing health care information resources*. Rockville, Md.: Aspen Publishers, Inc.
Schmitz, H. H. 1989. Information resource management. *Healthcare Supervisor* 7(2):13-22.

Section 1–Supporting the Practitioner

Unit 2—Medical Care Information Systems

Unit Introduction

Healthcare in the 1980s faced a host of difficult issues, among them the AIDS epidemic and the pressures for cost containment and quality assurance. This unit reports on key areas of medical care information technology applications.

A pediatrician long active in medical computer organizations, Oberst outlines how computerizing the physician's office can benefit the hospital and the patient. A pathologist, Genre shares insights from his experiences in using computerized systems to contend with growing size and complexity in clinical labs. Kessler, also a pathologist, joins with a blood bank supervisor, Flossie, to describe the computerization of hospital blood banks in this age of AIDS. Shannon draws upon his practice of radiology and his interest in medical computing to explain the move toward imaging centers.

Finally computerization has entered the clinical setting to offer actual benefits to healthcare professionals as they care for their patients.

1
Computerized Doctor Office Systems: The Benefit to The Hospital, Physician, and Patient

Byron B. Oberst

The rapidly changing field of healthcare delivery is fraught with problems and decisions. Among these are increasing competition from many sources, increasing costs of providing services, diminishing patient populations in some age divisions, and intrusion of third party entities into the physician/patient relationship. Practitioners must learn management skills not included in their medical school curricula or training programs, and they must deal with the growth of varied and sophisticated patient groups regarding health and health education.

Practice Management

In individual or group practices, there are eight subsets or modules into which practice management can be divided. Each of these modules is both intradependent and interdependent upon each of the other ones.

Four of these modules relate to the business aspects of the practice, and four relate to the healthcare delivery aspects. These applications are (Oberst and Reid 1984; Oberst and Long 1987):

- Business Applications
    Administrative Management
    Accounting Management
    Time Management
    Marketing Management

- • Healthcare Delivery Applications
  - Patient Care Management
  - Physician Management
  - Office/Hospital Management
  - Medical Information Management

Business Applications

The four business applications provide the framework for orderly and effective healthcare delivery. Efficient utilization of resources is dependent upon effective operations provided by good administration. Conservation of monetary resources and provision of an adequate cash stream are based upon appropriate accounting management. The most important but least recognized resource in a practice is the efficient and effective management of time in personnel utilization, physician usage, and patient conservation. Today, survival of a practice is dependent upon the application of basic marketing principles.

Healthcare Applications

The four healthcare delivery applications provide the working structure for patient care. Patient care management includes diagnoses, treatment, and education; physician management deals with patient handling and quality control in the office setting. Office/hospital management involves hospital rounds, movement of patients in and out of the hospital, patient education, hospital DRGs, utilization review, third party regulations, post hospital follow up instructions, and final disposition of the case. Medical information management relates to continuing medical education, national medical database information services, decision assistance programs, filing and retrieving all types of medical information, and a host of similar processes.

System Types

There are three approaches to computer applications for a medical practice:

- • Inhouse computer systems

- • Commercial service bureaus

- • Hospital managed or directed systems (a modified service bureau)

Inhouse Computer Systems. Before making a capital investment in inhouse development, serious study and a complete need analysis are advised. Designed for particular medical practices, inhouse systems can offer greater benefits and flexibility than commercial service bureaus. Generally, the costs of inhouse systems can be recovered through depreciation and better handling of the accounts receivable. Greater recovery of production dollars will result from improved collection procedures and internal monetary controls.

Commercial Service Bureaus. Although the pegboard system may serve the small office, depending upon the number of statements, commercial bureaus are a marked improvement over manual systems for handling accounts receivable in practices with more than two or three physicians. However, commercial service bureaus lack flexibility, and customization entails additional expense. They are costly and unwieldy if charges and credits are not posted in the office with an online terminal. Many service bureaus do not provide close control of the accounts receivable.

Commercial bureaus offer the convenience of easily processing statements, posting debits and credits, having useful statistics available, and several other important features. New features are usually slow to become available and frequently depend upon larger practices desiring the improvements, in which case increased cost factors result.

Hospital Managed Service Bureaus. Hospital bureaus have the same pitfalls as do commercial bureaus. Frequently limited to the physicians on a particular medical staff, they may offer a more supportive atmosphere and dedication due to the affiliation with the medical staff.

System Selection

Selection of a system, whether inhouse or service bureau, should depend upon the following criteria ranked according to consumer interest (Gans 1989): (1) support, (2) flexibility, (3) features, (4) modifications, (5) reputation, (6) installation, (7) references, (8) system costs and other issues, (9) installed systems, and (10) training.

Changes in healthcare today necessitate a lifelong medical record which is more than an archive. The medical record must be interactive to accommodate the growth in patient education and health and wellness programs, both for individuals and in the workplace (Oberst 1988). The physician is the hub of a medical information system. As those hubs, physicians incorporate input and exchange of data between many sources; they have access to an array of clinical computer applications which can assist in the management of the practice. The future will demand more sophisticated approaches to data input, data storage, data displays including graphics, data applications, standardized data exchange, and similar processing needs (Tables 1, 2).

Various computer applications are available, although accounts receivable remain the foundation for the business applications of practice management. The system should offer flexibility and adaptability with user defined features. Simple customization for special needs should not entail increased costs. The system should support upward mobility of the software programs and hardware. Obsolescence should not be the major factor with these changing needs Table 3).

Table 1. Components of the Modern Physician's Information System

1. Insurance Companies
2. Financial Area
        Credit Agencies
        Banks
        Investments
3. Distributors
        Medical Supplies
        Medical Equipment
        Office Supplies
        Others
4. Hospital Care
        Privileges
        Communications
        Patient Care
5. Medical Practice Database
        4 Business Applications
        4 Health Care Delivery Applications
6. Laboratory Services
        Outside Office Tests
        X-Ray
        Diagnostic Procedures
7. Expert Systems
        National Databases
        Drug Interaction Service
8. Personal Needs

Table 2. Present and Future Applications

1. Patient Education
        Computer Assisted/Computer Managed Instruction
2. Clinical Applications
        Patient Assessment
        Clinical Decision Support
        Knowledge Management
        Lifelong Health Record
3. Office Automation
        Word Processing
        Spreadsheets
        Graphics
        Database Management
4. Business Management
5. Telecommunications
6. External Database
        National Library of Medicine
        Bibliographic Reference Service
        Paperchase
        AMANet
        Drug Interactions
        Demographics
        Treatment Protocols

Table 3. Business Application Modules for the Physician's Office

Note: The following applications are NOT listed in order of importance or usefulness.

* 1. Accounts Receivable
* 2. General Ledger
* 3. Insurance Filing and Electronic Claims Processing
† 4. Payroll
† 5. Appointment Scheduling
† 6. Word Processing, Letter Generation, and Mailing Labels
  7. Accounts Payable
† 8. Patient Recall
  9. Statistical Report Generation and Graphic Displays
 10. Database Management and Report Generation
 11. Medical Records beyond the simple archive storage of limited information, problem lists and/or medication lists

[*] Denotes desirability for inclusion
[†] denotes that the program could be very useful and worth the extra cost factors.

Before selecting a system, a study should define the current status of each of the above functions, determine the usefulness of additional applications, and accumulate data relating to ongoing activities, such as the number of patients seen daily, weekly, monthly, and yearly with the attendant processing functions and similar information. This information is central to the development of a realistic request for proposal (RFP).

The use of a computer consultant is debatable for a number of reasons:

- Some consultants have very limited experience with the needs of a medical practice.

- Some consultants have very limited experience with the various software and hardware products which are available.

- Some consultants are value added vendors of hardware with restricted offerings and a limited perspective but can have a very useful product.

- Some consultants do not seek the most useful and cost effective systems to meet the needs of their clients.

- Some consultants are very knowledgeable and worth their value.

Vendors should have a track record of successful operations for at least five to eight years and over 50 installations in various types of medical practices so that their experiences are broad based and their ability to survive in a very competitive situation can be reasonably assured. Vendors should be able to demonstrate that they are financially sound.

Business Applications

Functional Elements

Certain functions are essential to each of the modules described below, which accommodate the accounting aspects of practice management.

Accounts Receivable. Since it is the core of the business applications, essential to all other accounting functions, this module needs to be flexible. User defined features should make it adaptable to the needs of the various branches of medicine. Primarily a billing and mailing statement function, it must meet the necessary accounting specifications and provide audit trails for the posting of debits and credits. Future growth should be provided as well as the ability to handle the numerous write offs and discounts demanded by third party payees, such as copay.

General Ledger. A must for good accounting functions, the general ledger and its functional capabilities are not understood by most physicians, who rely upon their accountants to handle these tasks. The ability to develop cost centers (centers of responsibility) for the allocation of fixed and variable expenses and production dollars is a major need in today's accounting processes. With appropriate coding, the many facets of accounting procedures can be identified, tracked, and accrued. The Medical Group Management Association has standardized the numbering of these various accounts, making it possible for an office practice to do financial analyses based upon ratios comparing certain facts and figures against national averages. These features support cost efficiency studies and allow better monetary control over practice costs.

An important consideration within the general ledger context is the concept of a realistic and functional budget. A general ledger system should provide for the comparison of present period results with last year's budget, and of year to date results with both last year and the budget. These comparisons can serve as a base for planning and projections by providing documented facts and figures.

Payroll. A useful program, payroll should be included in the accounting package. By providing the ability to automate tax withholding and benefit packages, this program saves valuable bookkeeper time, energy, and frustration, especially at year's end. It probably pays for itself.

Accounts Payable. Useful but not essential, this accounting function identifies ongoing bills which must be paid and systematically tracks the discounts businesses offer if accounts are paid within specified periods of time, for example, ten days. Used in conjunction with the general ledger, this program is a cost saving one and usually pays for itself over time.

Electronic Claims Processing. The usefulness and cost effectiveness of this program depend upon the volume of claims submitted. By providing for the quick transfer of insurance claim data, this feature can improve reimbursement turnaround time for services. However, the program is tied to a particular insurance company and requires a separate relationship for each insurance company involved in electronic claims. Each state and each insurance company may need some modification of the software program for the transfer of data. Because reimbursement time for any company should be within 14 days, the software should complete studies to determine that the time period is being met. Refiling of the delayed claim should be an automatic feature of the software package.

Appointment Scheduling. To be effective in a high volume practice like pediatrics, appointment scheduling programs must offer quick response time, a minimum of screens to be accessed, and flexibility to accommodate the different practice styles of the physicians within the practice. Otherwise, patient flow bogs down and chaos usually results. If the appointment program constitutes a bottleneck, the remaining functions of the practice become disrupted and the rhythm of patient care is lost. The program should track and count appointments that are not kept, canceled, or rescheduled. These data represent the amount of time lost; this converts into lost production dollars, which can become significant over time. Before investing in a scheduling program, a practice should see the program demonstrated in a working setting similar to its own.

Job Costing. A little used program which can be useful for accomplishing serious cost efficiency studies, this is not recommended except for special situations.

Inventory Control. This program tracks supplies, expiration dates, shelf life, and similar data. If there is a large investment of capital dollars in supplies, this program is helpful; otherwise, a simple spreadsheet can be adapted to accomplish the same tasks. It is not recommended for universal application.

Use of Business Applications

The essential elements of a good accounting package incorporate the accounts receivable, general ledger, accounts payable, and payroll programs. A practice can manage very well with an excellent accounts receivable program by itself with good accounting supervision and auditing by an external accounting firm with medical practice expertise.

The office personnel should learn to understand their own books and to become self sufficient in most accounting functions. In this manner, the practice learns how to manage its own resources; therefore, the supervision of the office's accounting activities by the accountant moves to a higher plane of involvement and application of expertise for essentially the same monetary costs. This capital expenditure for external accounting supervision and management becomes more cost effective.

Clearly, a good billing system is crucial to the management of the medical practice. Without it, the practice would cease to exist very shortly, as the value of the dollar deteriorates very rapidly after 60 days. Collection procedures, cost efficiency studies, and rapid cash flow are essential for survival. These elements cannot be obtained easily by a manual methodology.

Customer support is crucial to the functioning of a good accounts receivable billing system. This support consists of general training, additional onsite training, modem diagnosis and assistance when problems are encountered, a user exchange meeting for system updates, and other factors. The selection of a system should be based almost as much upon the support which is available as on the contents of the program itself.

The primary disadvantages of a billing system encompass the initial capital investment and changes in behavior required of bookkeeping personnel. There are certain parameters which must be adhered to or problems may result. Personnel are slow to adapt to changes and to leave more comfortable routines. Accuracy is essential and mistakes must be corrected immediately if the data are to be relied upon. Detailed patient information should be obtained at the time of the initial patient encounter for the system to function at its best.

Clinical Decision Support Systems

Clinical decision support programs differ significantly in how they function within the practice environment. Vendor support is much less important than for billing systems. The physician provides all the necessary decision making needed in most healthcare delivery situations. Only a small fraction of the patient population in any given medical practice will require the assistance of additional input, whether by consultation with a colleague or computer assisted programs. However, if a practice is largely consultative, this premise changes; and clinical decision support programs have a practical place. Most medical practices would need to access a support system at infrequent intervals.

The national medical databases with full text retrieval capabilities for books and journals are becoming more useful. From a practical standpoint, drug databases which provide information on drug interactions are the most useful. The National Library of Medicine's Grateful Med access and search software program is the easiest to use and is the least expensive, as no additional gateways for access to the search add to the costs.

Complex medical problems which require extensive study and may benefit the most from clinical decision support programs are usually in the hospital where the medical librarian can be of assistance to the practitioner. In these situations, knowledge management as a decision support mechanism could be of help (Greenes et al. 1989).

The disadvantages of a clinical decision support system are subtle. Cost and ease of access are major hurdles for the smaller practice. Any support system is very hard to utilize during busy patient care hours and tends to disrupt the rhythm and flow of patient care. Access and searches are more easily accomplished during quiet evening hours and weekends, often at home away from the confusions and disruptions of the office. The complexity of access and search techniques continues to discourage most physicians from their use.

However, national databases today provide medical information needed for both patient care and preventive malpractice documentation. Accessing and searching skills are gaining added importance. Reliance upon drug databases is of concern to the Federal Drug Administration (FDA). These programs need to be reviewed for quality control and reliability, through field testing in many situations. A degree of standardization must be achieved before the physician can rely totally upon such programs without hazard.

Clinical decision support systems have yet to be universally accepted. Only then will reliance upon them become the rule rather than the exception. The promoters of these systems still have to convince most physicians of the systems' usefulness in reality as well as on paper.

The Hospital Interface

The interface between the physician's office and the hospital is slowly evolving. With a minimal initial investment, the physician can obtain improved support without capital outlays. Connections to the laboratory, x-ray, nursing station, and intensive care areas can facilitate communications, notably patient progress updates. Physician practices may also benefit from the use of data from the hospital's public relations and marketing departments.

The hospital also benefits. The interface ties the medical staff more closely to the hospital, to the disadvantage of the other hospitals in the community. In the current climate of cutthroat competition among hospitals, such a connection creates a distinct advantage and incentive to utilize a particular hospital and may actually expedite patient care in a more efficient manner. It may help to preserve the hospital patient population base.

Links via networks to the surrounding referral territory and local physician's office would have many advantages for both the physicians and the hospital (Oberst 1975). The system, wherever and whatever, should provide for improved cash control, documentation of various healthcare delivery activities, third party claims processing, and improved patient care with the least cost possible. If local networking is possible, improved communications should be the end result.

Disadvantages associated with hospital based systems tend to reside within the physician's office. With greater dependence upon the hospital computing and administrative staff, the physician may lose some independence. Because the hospital may have greater access capabilities than before, the physician may also relinquish some degree of confidentiality and security regarding the practice's financial status and activities. In addition, because most hospital systems are large and tend to be relatively inflexible, responses to individual practice needs may be dominated by the needs of large practices. Smaller offices may not be given a great deal of consideration. Once an office becomes dependent upon the hospital's computer system, many cost factors and marketing capabilities are removed from the independent management control of the practice and reside within the hospital. This may not be a comfortable situation in today's setting when many hospitals compete directly and aggressively against their own medical staff.

Inhouse systems suffer from space constraints and the resulting need to purge data frequently. It becomes difficult to do retrospective studies with more than two years of data. Storage needs and data input are constant problem areas. Legal problems, confidentiality, and security remain as the most vexing of the headaches connected to any and all systems.

The Future

Future developments should enhance the four healthcare delivery applications of practice management with improved input via optical scanning, barcode applications, voice recognition and/or activated input, natural language usage, and voice messaging. Physician, student, and patient education will be enhanced with the use of hypertext programs in computer assisted and computer managed interactive applications.

Optical disk storage technology should alleviate the problems of volume storage, memory systems, quick access, and misfiling. Read only (nonerasable) compact disk technology should be able to conquer most of the current technical problems and legal objection areas.

These many advances should permit the development of a truly useful longitudinal healthcare record with abstraction capabilities. The smartcard and lifecard technology make two megabytes of memory available to accommodate x-rays, laboratory data, and graphic displays.

There is a major movement within many medical organizations to collaborate to produce a standardized medical record which can be utilized by all parts of the healthcare delivery system in an interactive manner rather than the previous archival, chronological storage of the past. This lifelong record should be capable of being easily transmitted to other facilities and abstracted for essential and critical information. It should indicate potential health problem areas, accumulate individual healthcare costs per problem entity, graph anthropomorphic and laboratory data, and fulfill a host of other needs and desires. With time, this type of record should evolve.

On the business side of practice management, there is a need for worthwhile displays of statistical data and practice activities in graphic form and in an ongoing motif for ease of update. Larger storage capabilities will make the retention of marketing and other worthwhile practice management data easier to accrue and utilize.

With the capabilities now available and those promised within the near future, information management will continue to benefit healthcare practitioners in their business and clinical functions.

Questions

1. How many subset modules are there in a complete practice management system?

2. Should the business aspects of an inhouse computer system include modules for accounts receivable, general ledger, accounts payable, and payroll to be a complete accounting system?

3. Should a serious study be made and a need analysis performed on a medical practice before computerization is considered?

4. Which is the most crucial for the management of a medical practice, a billing system or a clinical decision support function?

5. Do data storage needs constitute a major constraint upon an inhouse computer system?

6. Should a lifelong longitudinal healthcare record be both interactive and capable of being easily transmitted in a standardized format to other parts of the healthcare delivery system?

7. Are commercial service bureaus and hospital service bureaus more useful, cost saving and practical than inhouse systems?

References

Gans, D. N. 1989. Medical group information systems. *Journal Medical Group Management Association* 11:55-56.

Greenes, R. A., D. B. Tarabar, M. Krauss, G. Anderson, W. J. Wolnik, L. Cope, E. Slosser, and H. Hersh. 1989. Knowledge management as a decision support method: A diagnostic workup strategy application. *Computers and Biomedical Research* 22(2):113-35.

Oberst, B. B. 1975. A total health care system as viewed by a private practitioner. *Pediatrician* 4:176-84, 372-82, 383-92.

Oberst, B. B. 1988. Clinical benefits of a life long health care record: Medical documentation update. *Report from the Fourth Annual International Conference on Computerization of Medical Records* 6(3):33-47.

Oberst, B. B. and R. A. Reid. 1984. *Computer applications to private office practice.* New York: Springer-Verlag.

Oberst, B. B. and Long, J. M. (1987). *Computers in Private Practice Management.* New York: Springer-Verlag.

2
Using the Computer to Manage Change in the Clinical Pathology Lab

Charles F. Genre

To realize the medical and administrative benefits that a laboratory information system (LIS) offers, healthcare institutions need to enter carefully into the selection and implementation process. Functional advances that laboratories can realistically expect to see in the near future should influence their choice of systems today.

Selection

The selection of a laboratory information system raises questions which have no absolute answers, but vary according to institution. The first question is simply, "Does the laboratory need a computer at all?" It may be counterproductive to impose a computer system upon laboratories in small to medium sized hospitals which are able to process orders, analyze specimens, and issue and store reports required for patient care without an LIS. Given that labor savings often prove illusory, the expense may not be warranted. No mathematical formula identifies the point at which size and complexity mandate an LIS, but the time comes when every institution should investigate the need for such a system. When the hospital needs to process specimens faster and to provide its departments with cumulative and specialized reports, whether by paper, peripheral printer, or computer screen in realtime, an LIS is warranted.

As laboratories grow, the billing process grows more cumbersome, charges get posted later, and some charges are lost through human error or even human intent. Despite prepaid healthcare, most hospitals continue to do significant fee for service work, especially in the outpatient area. Larger laboratories may acquire a computer to process billing rapidly, completely, and accurately.

Today many hospitals are launching laboratory outreach programs to generate additional revenue and to strengthen the bonds with their medical staff. These outreach programs must provide the same amenities as large commercial laboratories, including in office result printing, clean and legible computer printouts of results, and, most importantly, correct and timely billing. Because this type of outreach program demands computer capability of some complexity, an institution's business plan may mandate acquisition of an LIS.

The plan to acquire an LIS should be approved by the hospital's administrative and financial officers. Always important, cooperation between the laboratory and hospital administration is critical when a major system is selected and implemented, especially if progress does not meet expectations, as often happens.

System Components

Using a consultant if resources allow, the laboratory staff should define the type of system needed, including the number of laboratory sections in the system. Basic systems generally include chemistry, hematology, urinalysis, parasitology, and special function laboratories such as radioimmunoassay, serology, and immunology.

Blood bank and anatomic pathology were not included in many vendors' initial offerings. These laboratories processed comparatively small volumes and physically and/or administratively were separate from the main lab. Moreover, they had a level of complexity that the early systems could not handle easily. As a result, some vendors offer large computer software packages which are less sophisticated in these areas or subcontract with specialized vendors to provide these products in some form of integrated or interfaced package.

Most vendors addressed microbiology in their initial offerings, but were not generally successful. Today, some microbiology vendors offer freestanding microbiology systems with strong instrumentation, data handling, and reporting capabilities. To avoid duplication of effort, these must in some fashion be integrated into the mainframe system, according to each laboratory's needs.

Scope should be defined early in the selection process. Scope of an LIS influences work flow, billing, result reporting, and the completeness of computerized patient data retrieval and analysis. A decision to support outreach programs now or in the future calls for greater computer power as well as more sophisticated billing functions and specimen routing routines.

System Alternatives

Although large hospital chains sometimes select and implement an LIS for all the facilities they control, most hospitals must choose where their LIS should reside. Four alternatives exist, and the system can be

- Freestanding

- Linked to the main admission/discharge/transfer (ADT) and billing systems but issuing its own reports

- Linked to the main hospital system by ADT, billing, order entry, and reporting, but doing all its own processing internally

- Resident on and a function of the main hospital computer

The first three choices are not mutually exclusive and, in fact, may be stages of a single implementation line as the interaction between the laboratory and the main computer function matures. All three give the advantage of the rapid response times provided by standalone systems and the possibility of using the vendor's "bells and whistles" to enhance production. Adopting the third alternative, the linked system which does all its own processing, allows the laboratory to have the best of both worlds.

Placing the laboratory system on the mainframe offers none of the advantages provided by the most integrated standalone options. Mainframe systems are not generally designed to provide the rapid response times that high volume laboratory sections need and expect and are often run by personnel unfamiliar with the operational needs of a laboratory, such as scheduling maintenance and backup to provide uninterrupted service.

Evaluation

Selection of an LIS should be assigned to a small committee, including the director or director's designate, the laboratory administrator, and several other key individuals. The director should head the group and be committed to being involved throughout the selection and implementation phases. Throughout the process, open and honest communication is essential. The hospital's main information systems department must have input to ensure that the LIS can be integrated with the main institutional systems. If central billing is to be done, the finance department must be involved.

Though sometimes controversial, a consultant may be added to the team, for the selection process only or for the implementation and special projects phase as well. The consultant's role is to bring divergent ideas into a coherent whole, know available and suitable vendors, add technical knowledge, and interact with the hospital's information systems division (ISD). In this role, the consultant can help avoid considering a system or configuration with power insufficient to support the current laboratory and its projected expansion. To add credibility to a diffuse and complicated process, the consultant must know laboratories intimately and work closely with the laboratory director and the selection committee.

A member of the committee or the consultant should draft a request for proposal (RFP) describing the laboratory and its present and future needs. Attention should be paid to special projects or needs and unusual circumstances. If the laboratory is attached to a small hospital but has a very large outpatient facility or a special care unit that would skew a vendor's calculations, these should be explained clearly.

The RFP should be sent to all reasonable vendors. A single day should be designated to review the laboratory and its needs with all interested vendors. This review should occur on site, ideally with the vendors as a group. After the predetermined date for return of the responses to the RFP, the committee should identify candidate vendors for site visits.

Site Visits

Visits to all sites should be scheduled to include all members of the selection committee. Critical questions should not be left unanswered because a key visitor is absent. The laboratory should demand that the sites visited equal or exceed its own in size and complexity. More than one site per vendor should be visited, as should all the vendors who appear to meet the laboratory's needs. Given the length of the selection process, the site visit team should record all observations immediately on return from each visit. The site visit team should also involve the hospital's information systems department so that technical questions concerning the LIS and mainframe may be identified and addressed on an ongoing basis. The consultant is also a valuable resource on site visits.

After visits to all sites, the team should identify the finalists. The primary criteria used should center around the way in which the candidate systems satisfy the needs of the laboratory. If the scope and need were adequately identified at the outset, the choice of finalists should be easy. The finalists should be brought in separately to answer questions and to make detailed presentations of their systems to all laboratory sections, including the support areas of venipuncture and specimen receiving. This may take up to three days per vendor and should be performed on site.

A technical investigation of the hardware vendor should be undertaken separately. The hospital's information systems department should be of significant aid in this regard. Meetings with the hardware vendor and its local representatives should be held to discuss the hospital's unique needs for uninterrupted 24 hour service. Of course, the hospital should conduct financial reviews of both the software and the hardware vendors.

A meeting directed by the laboratory and including the information systems department along with administrative and financial officers should be held to jointly review all the finalists. The meeting should be as broad based as possible because broad based support will be necessary for implementation and for future support. Although a winner is usually relatively evident, the laboratory should have the final decision if the finances and system interactions with the hospital's other systems are approximately equal.

The LIS selection committee must understand that vendors are salespersons. The committee should run financial checks on the vendors and investigate all their claims. If the vendor claims the system can be interfaced, the committee should ask to see the interface on a site visit. Under no circumstances should the committee accept the vendor's claims without investigation. The selection committee must use lawyers and hospital administrators to write a contract explicitly stating the terms and expectations.

A clear, precise contract benefits both parties. The lab will know when it has received its product, and the vendor will know in no uncertain terms what to do to be paid. At that time, the installation will be complete and maintenance can begin.

Implementation

Implementing an LIS for the first time is an almost once in a lifetime chance to make long desired systems changes. The challenge is not to computerize an existing manual laboratory, but to use the computer as a new and powerful tool. Throughout the process, one person should clearly be in charge; timetables should be reasonable but definite.

The laboratory needs to analyze everything it does, understand its component steps, and systematically map out its specimen ordering, processing and reporting flow, and billing functions. The laboratory must determine what it wants done. Ordering must be analyzed and tests grouped in a logical sequence. Laboratory tests may be grouped by performing sections, such as hematology or chemistry; request numbers may be given in blocks large enough to accommodate future expansion. Specimen draw requirements must be carefully quantitated so that venipuncture will not be requested to exsanguinate patients for whom numerous tests are ordered.

A computer should not recreate a poorly designed manual system, especially one based on a high exception rate. Sample dispersement throughout the laboratory must be analyzed and appropriate aliquot systems and labels designed. To assist in this process, those laboratory members who will be intimately involved with the decisions should visit several up and functioning laboratories. Only after the choice of an LIS do supervisors really appreciate the problems associated with conversion.

Sample processing predominantly involves internal laboratory functions, but reporting involves the laboratory's customer, the physician. It is essential to pick a representative cross section of physicians to help design the timing and format of the reports. Those working in emergency rooms, intensive care units, and surgical suites should be questioned regarding their needs for result reporting by printer or computer screen. All reasonable requests should be met. Physicians who have had their input honored will be more tolerant of the inevitable disruptions caused by implementing a new system.

The decision to hire a computer supervisor often revolves around whether to get a laboratory person or a computer person. If one candidate has credentials in both areas, is energetic, likes to spend nights at the hospital, and will be there at least two years, the choice is easy. Otherwise, trade offs are necessary. If both the hardware and the software vendors can provide good support and training, most directors tend to prefer a laboratory person. They feel it is easier to teach adequate computer skills in the context of good support than to try to teach a computer person about the requirements for cultures, coagulation, ionized calciums, and so forth. This is particularly true for laboratories installing their first LIS, because for them production and specimen flow are critically important.

For any LIS, a backup system is an absolute necessity. It will be needed, most likely, early in the computerized era. The system should include order back up, accessioning and production, specimen identification numbers, and manual report forms. Most results can be stored automatically on interface buffers with the patient identification assigned. When the system goes live, the results can be automatically uploaded to the accessioned samples. In any case, a protocol should be written and practiced before going live, including requirements for entering results manually if the automatic upload fails.

Replacement Systems

Laboratories implementing replacement systems need to guard against duplicating the old with the new. They should see the process as a golden opportunity to correct past inadequacies. By now, systems have been set and laboratory personnel are familiar with computers. This is the time to reconsider the skills required of the laboratory's computer supervisor. Perhaps computer skills should be considered over laboratory knowledge.

Once all systems have been designed, both the original and the replacement LIS should run in parallel with their existing systems. In this era of cost control, hospital administrators must understand that additional person hours will be needed. The parallel run must include all laboratory personnel on all shifts, including weekend part timers, and all nonlaboratory personnel who will interact with the system, including the physicians. The parallel run should be intense and should last only long enough to get all personnel trained. Prolonged parallel runs simply bore people and use up work hours. These runs should not overlook result inquiry on the screen or printer; not knowing how to work the printer properly will cause havoc, especially at peripheral locations.

The date to go live should be chosen so that the software vendor can provide support and ensure that last minute changes are made quickly. The hardware manufacturer should have on hand a good crew who understands the 24 hour needs of a hospital laboratory. The laboratory director must be present to coordinate the scenario and to make those decisions which inevitably need to be made and made quickly. One person should be present on site for as long as it takes and should have the authority to make decisions when necessary. Few realtime projects succeed if no one or if a committee is in charge.

For both first time and replacement systems, scheduling going live midweek when volume is lower allows corrections to be performed on the weekend and finetuning to be done before the high volume time of the early week. For replacement systems, all samples entering the laboratory are accessioned into the new system at midnight. The two run parallel for several days, allowing the old system to complete all data through a particular date and the new to start on that date. Within the first two days, the majority of results from the old system have been reported. Each laboratory must decide when to cancel the unperformed tests in the old system and reenter them into the new. After one week's duration, these tests are usually in microbiology or are send outs;

reentering them is a relatively small task. Letting the old system complete its tests simplifies seeking results weeks later; tests up to a certain date are known to be in the old system and can be found with minimal confusion.

Benefits

For laboratories of sufficient size and complexity, an LIS is essential if they are to survive and prosper. The system affects literally every subsystem of the laboratory as well as numerous other patient care areas of the hospital. Care must be taken to ensure that these areas are positively affected; a review process should confirm desired outcomes and warn of possible negative effects.

The LIS should organize the inpatient specimen collection process and print patient collection labels in order of rooms to be collected. By specifying the type and number of tubes and the amount of blood to be obtained, the labels assist personnel and speed up collection. Most laboratories find it advantageous to set up a central specimen processing area to receive, verify, and/or accession samples into the laboratory system. Well trained personnel in this area can prevent bottlenecks and detect specimens that are incorrectly labeled or requested. Although they tend to be blamed for misaccessioning specimens, they are often the unsung heroes who guard the system from mistakes generated elsewhere in the hospital system.

Larger laboratories may need more than a single processing area. Because of the diversity and complexity of specimen type and the need to generate numerous plate labels, microbiology often accessions its own sample. Critical care areas such as surgery, intensive care units, and the emergency room may benefit from special accessioning areas and/or dedicated specimen delivery systems, such as a tube system. These are generally less expensive than satellite labs spread throughout a facility.

The computer's impact on specimen analysis will vary by area. Sections which predominantly analyze in a batch mode (therapeutic drug monitoring, etc.) will benefit from automatically assembled batches and printed worklists for specimen arrangement and result entry. The analyzer may be interfaced, but probably should not be unless definite economic gain is realized. In most hospitals, the batches are small enough to be entered manually almost as easily.

In the areas of high volume analysis like automated chemistry and hematology, the impact of the computer can be revolutionary. When interfaced with the LIS, instruments can upload results as soon as they are verified. The traditional worklist simply delays the process of analysis; no longer should technologists be required to wait and load specimens in a particular order.

A bidirectional interface should eliminate repeat accessioning of the test request at the laboratory instrument. Though difficult to achieve with many systems, this type of interface offers real benefits. Also, the design and number of aliquot labels can save considerable time in a busy laboratory. Automatically generated, different colored labels can signify specimen priority ("stat").

At some point during the analytical process, depending upon the analyzer and the number of times it needs to run controls, the result is checked for quality control referable to the specimen. Some of the newer random access analyzers retain calibration for extended periods of time, and results can be verified by a technologist as they are produced after consulting appropriate controls. Though laboratories may accomplish this in different ways, the rule should be to set up a system which will

- Avoid duplicate accessioning of tests as much as possible

- Release properly controlled and verified results to the floors as rapidly as possible

Reporting and Delivery

Report formats and optimal times of delivery should be determined in conjunction with the physicians and the nursing staff. At a minimum, an LIS should provide a cumulative report for all inpatients, updated daily and color coded to eliminate charting difficulties. The need for interim reports varies; high intensity units should have printers and computer screens to provide access to results as soon as they are verified in the laboratory. In most hospitals, the laboratory can generate reports for early morning rounds if compilation time is short. If the LIS is interfaced to the HIS, reports can be generated at the nursing station.

Teaching hospitals offer unique problems. Many physicians are involved and physician ordering patterns are not matured. The first morning paper reports are often pocketed by the earliest resident or intern. Tests are requested throughout the day rather than at normal intervals, effectively nullifying the usefulness of standard paper reports. Acutely ill patients must be moved frequently, making it difficult to route the paper reports to the appropriate location. In such hospitals, paper should not be the sole means of reporting.

An alternate way to transmit the information in its most updated form is electronic reporting on the computer screen. If there is a simple program for patient data inquiry, physicians, nurses, and medical students will all view the computer screen. The ability to print the screen is most helpful. Physicians and house staff often become very proficient at this and can easily and quickly determine what tests have been ordered and what their production status is.

Test Result Archive

If a consistent medical record number is used for both inpatient and outpatient visits, the LIS can easily retain all laboratory data for a patient for up to a year, as determined for each facility. Data retention benefits patients such as the one who appears in the emergency room at 2 a.m. and whose chart cannot be located for any of a legion of reasons. With access to the LIS, the ER physician instantly retrieves the patient's laboratory results for the last year and puts together a pretty good picture from the results and the original laboratory requests. When paper reports are lost from the chart, realtime archive inquiry is often the most rapid way for a clinician to solve a problem. The ideal solution would be an electronic chart or patient database where all results (lab, x-ray, pharmacy) would be stored. In the interim, the test result archive is an excellent use of an LIS.

The benefit to laboratory physicians exclusive of production benefits resides in increased access to information. Anatomic pathologists should have at their fingertips all the previous results from cytology and biopsy for every case on their microscope. Similarly, they should have all the clinical laboratory results for the difficult case which requires anatomic and clinical data correlation for the best diagnosis. Clinical pathologists will constantly make use of past patient data in evaluating current results or in signing out interpretative tests. All laboratory physicians should be able to get result statistics (antibiograms, results of PAP smears, normal values) from the LIS or from data downloaded from the LIS to a microcomputer. A well functioning LIS is an incredibly powerful tool for improving the quality of laboratory physicians' daily work and research.

Laboratory administrative performance is immeasurably aided by an LIS. For example, billing can be tailored to the institution and run either as a standalone function or, more commonly, interfaced to the main hospital billing department. Bills can be generated at the time of request or results, leaving only the question of what to do about tests for which results take a long time to become available.

Audit Trail Data

With an LIS, laboratory administration has an audit trail on each test through the entire process. This provides turnaround time data from request (if interfaced), collection, and verification to result reporting. These data are extremely important in quality assurance and in running the department. If a physician questions the time to acquire a test, the department can investigate the specific incident, including the personnel involved and the actual times involved. In more advanced forms, audit trail data can be used for workload recording and productivity, down to an individual level. The LIS can provide ordering patterns by physician and by medical section; these data can be useful in identifying and changing patterns for purposes of quality assurance or cost containment. Both quality control routines and maintenance schedules can be automated.

Risks

All the benefits of an LIS come with some risk. Hospitals often computerize in fits and starts. Laboratory information systems have been available for a reasonably long time and many hospitals have computerized their laboratories early in the process of automating hospitalwide. Other areas of the hospital may have little or no knowledge of computers and may not really understand the global consequences of an incorrectly written patient medical record number if the name was correct. They may not understand that the result may go to the wrong chart and the bill will go to someone else who may not be in the hospital at all. Computerized billing is a great advance, but constant review of the billing process is necessary because small changes by someone who does not understand the whole process may have amazing ramifications. In production, particularly when using batch methods, worklists may be moved over by one name in a particular direction and the potential for dissemination of many incorrect reports will exist. The laboratory must constantly monitor its processing and reporting and immediately and vigorously investigate all potential misadventures.

The Near Future

What do the next few years hold? System reliability will continue to improve and storage capacity will increase. Laboratory systems will probably use more and more local networks, increasing reliability and versatility. Many of the standalone systems such as those in anatomic pathology and blood banking will be effectively networked into the main LIS. Laboratory systems will concentrate on the laboratory and will make more extensive use of the hospital information system to report and store data, often in conjunction with the other support services.

Reporting will improve significantly. The standard cumulative report will continue because it serves most of the cases. New report formats will be used with increasing frequency. Graphs and trend reports and formats personalized for individual physicians or services will be used. Physician offices and homes will be linked to the computer, either the LIS or the HIS, and data will be more accessible. Hospitals will pursue this as a service for their physician base in an attempt to market themselves and will extend order entry and results reporting to the office or home. Meaningful duplicate order checking systems will be set up to curb unnecessary test requests. Cost data on test requests and on therapeutic choices could be given in real time with potentially significant cost savings for the hospital.

In the near future, test processing will be immeasurably aided by real specimen positive identification, the achilles heel of all clinical laboratories. This, coupled with the next generation of bidirectional interfaces for the highly automated instrumentation, will vastly decrease turnaround time and significantly reduce or retrain personnel. The use of computer generated, machine readable labels will allow the laboratory to automate its specimen saving and retrieval functions. As a result, the test add on function will be more feasible allowing the original hematology and chemistry screens to be reduced in size, another area for possible reagent and personnel savings.

In the near future, the laboratory will automatically accept an order generated by the physician at the patient's bedside and receive a positively identified specimen to put in random fashion on an analyzer which has received the individual test requests downloaded from the LIS. The specimen tube stopper will not have to be popped, eliminating the need for aerosols. After analysis, the tube will be placed in a robot to read the label and construct a save rack. Clerical staff will be able to retrieve the specimen if additional tests are requested. Laboratory sections will be on local area networks with easily replaced hardware greatly reducing downtime from failure. As standardized and improved production areas are created for frequently ordered tests, directors will be able to use their ever dwindling supply of highly trained technologists to concentrate on new and more challenging areas.

Questions

1. What factors favor a laboratory's decision to acquire a laboratory computer system?

2. Who are the key players in the decision making process for a laboratory computer system? Discuss their responsibilities.

3. What are the major benefits of a laboratory computer system for:

   a. the laboratory?
   b. the physicians?

Select Bibliography

Ball, M. J. 1971. *Selecting a computer system for the clinical laboratory.* Springfield, Ill.: Charles C. Thomas.

O'Desky, R. I. 1985. Is there a pathology department computer system apropos to your organization? *Healthcare Computing and Communications* 2:4.

O'Desky, R. I., and M. J. Ball. 1988. Clinical laboratory computerization: A glimpse at the system vendor community and some thoughts on the impact of technology in the next ten years. *Clinical Laboratory Management Review* 2(2):68-76.

Shires, D. B. 1974. *Computer technology in the health sciences.* Springfield, Ill.: Charles C. Thomas.

Siemaszko, F. 1978. *Computing in clinical laboratories.* Kent, England: Pitman Medical Publishing.

Thompkins, W. J., and J. G. Webster, eds. 1981. *Design of microcomputer-based medical instrumentation.* Englewood Cliffs, N. J.: Prentice Hall.

3
Blood Banking in the AIDS Era

G. Frederick Kessler, Jr., and Benjamin Flossie

Even without AIDS, the hospital blood bank would be a highly specialized laboratory, dependent upon accurate and timely records for safe and effective operation. But when the 1980s epidemic heightened concern over AIDS and other blood transmitted diseases such as hepatitis and syphilis, regulatory agencies responded with new requirements for blood banks. All files must now be maintained for a minimum of five years to facilitate look back procedures in the event that either a blood donor or a blood recipient develops one of these potentially blood transmitted diseases. This requires that all blood donors and blood product recipients be linked by a detailed data trail collected and stored in the hospital blood bank.

For years it had been obvious to blood bankers that computerization of the massive amount of paperwork inherent in blood bank management would be beneficial. However, because of special requirements related to the processing and issuing of blood products, blood bank functions differed considerably from those in other clinical laboratories. Successful computerization in the blood bank developed at a much slower pace than in other areas of the hospital. Most computer systems developed prior to the 1980s were either too expensive or too inflexible to meet the requirements of the hospital blood bank.

Blood Banking at the Akron General Medical Center

The Akron General Medical Center Blood Bank processes blood products to meet the needs of a busy 507 bed acute medical surgical hospital. Each month this laboratory issues over 2,000 units of packed red blood cells, platelets, plasma, and specialized coagulation factor products to over 1,500 patients. Good medical practice as well as regulatory agencies such as the Food and Drug Administration and the American Red Cross mandate that careful and accurate records be kept at each and every step of the blood transfusion process.

The blood bank at Akron General Medical Center has four fulltime

73

employees. They are responsible for numerous management and administrative reports including, but not limited to, the total volume of work performed in a given timeframe, billing charges, individual technologist productivity data, and blood use by patient type, location, physician, and diagnostic related grouping (DRG).

Prior to implementation of the blood bank computer, each blood product had to be inventoried, detailed records had to be kept of all crossmatch procedures, and bulky files had to be maintained documenting details of each transaction, which involved thousands of blood products and patient recipients. It is readily apparent that transcription errors in this laborious manual record keeping process could easily result in transfusion of a mismatched blood product with potentially fatal consequences.

Computerizing the System

In 1987, the Akron General Medical Center Blood Bank installed a computerized system utilizing IBM PC-XT personal computers interfaced by a local area network. The network allows common access by each personal computer to a file server, which contains a large memory array of programs and data, much greater than that available to any single personal computer.

This personal computer/file server system offers several major advantages over other types of computer hardware. First, the cost of hardware is much less than for a comparable minicomputer system with a large central processing unit and multiple data terminals. Second, interfacing of multiple personal computers into the local area network allows simultaneous multiuser capability and multiuser access to a common database. Finally, the size of the available memory on the file server is sufficient to allow for all the necessary functions inherent in a fully developed blood bank computer system. This memory is easily expanded as needs increase. The Akron General Medical Center Blood Bank utilizes five IBM PC-XT personal computers interfaced through an Ethernet local area network, with main data storage consisting of 150 megabytes of data on a 3Com file server.

The system software selected was Lifeline II, developed by Western Star Business Systems. Written in Basic, it is a modular menu driven system which allows maximum flexibility in day to day systems operations. The software consists of several program sets, including programs for file maintenance, procedure file maintenance, blood donor, transfusion service, and administrative/management.

File Maintenance Programs

This program set allows the blood bank to define parameters specific for its particular needs such as sources of blood products, lists of technologists performing particular tests, files of physicians utilizing the blood bank, and a catalog of different blood antigens and antibodies important in the blood transfusion process.

Procedure File Maintenance Programs

This module allows the blood bank to maintain files of all tests performed in the laboratory. These programs include parameters which allow the laboratory to define appropriate numbers of workload recording units to be tallied each time a particular test is performed. They also allow the blood bank to define billing charges and other appropriate administrative and management parameters for each laboratory test.

Blood Donor Programs

These programs allow appropriate management of this very important function. Since the majority of our products are collected at the Regional Red Cross Donor Center which services the blood needs of over 80 hospitals in Northeast Ohio, these functions are not utilized at Akron General.

Transfusion Service Programs

Blood Product Reception Programs. Because the majority of Akron General's blood products come from the Regional Red Cross Donor Center, programs are necessary to log in all blood products. The laboratory utilizes a barcode reader for rapid product accession. Products are identified by serial number, product type, source of product, and expiration date.

Product Inventory Program. The computer software maintains complete inventories of each type of blood product including number of days until expiration and unit status to determine availability for crossmatching and subsequent transfusion.

Patient and Component Data File Programs. A patient database is maintained which includes patient demographics (hospital location and clinical service), pertinent administrative data (such as guarantor, home address, age), and critical laboratory information such as the presence of any unusual antigens or antibodies. The computer also maintains files of all crossmatch results on each unit as well as a record of any additional unit testing for hepatitis and AIDS antigens and antibodies, the date and time of transfusions, and a history of any reported transfusion reaction. This data is crossfiled both by blood product component and by individual patient.

Crossmatch Data File Programs. These files store all blood bank product test results including date and time performed and the name of the technologist who completed the test. In the event that a result of a particular test differs from the results of a similar test previously performed on the same patient, the computer notifies the responsible technologist of the problem.

Blood Issuing Programs. The blood issuing process is a complicated and time consuming procedure requiring extensive documentation, both in the blood bank and on the patient's chart. The computer system generates appropriate printed material for the patient's chart, listing the serial number of the unit issued, time of issuance, and space for signatures of all personnel responsible for the blood transfusion. Complete records of the transfusion process are stored in the blood bank and become a part of each patient's medical record.

Blood Disposition Files Program. These files are maintained to document the date and time of the final disposition of each unit of blood, either as the result of transfusion, or through transfer to another institution, or by product expiration.

Workload Functions Program. The computer tabulates all workload recording data as tests are performed.

Administrative/Management Programs

These allow management to generate many practical reports. A sample report might provide a list of all transfusions for a particular month by hospital patient location. Other reports might include a list of transfusions ordered by individual physicians or a list of transfusions for all patients within a particular diagnostic related grouping. These programs allow the generation of many useful and time saving reports, to satisfy both the internal needs of laboratory management and the requirements of hospital regulatory agencies.

Benefits of Computerization

Blood Component Processing and Distribution

In its first two years at Akron General, the computerized blood bank system had a significant impact on multiple phases of laboratory operations, improving the efficiency of routine operations. Barcode readers, direct computer input, and preprogrammed routines have greatly reduced time and clerical errors. In the area of blood component processing and distribution, the tasks of blood product reception, unit confirmation, unit crossmatch, and unit disposition have all demonstrated time savings and error reduction. Overall, the blood bank computer system has reduced paperwork by approximately 75 percent and saved an average of three hours of technical and clerical time per day, or over half of a full time equivalent per week.

The blood bank computer system has also had positive effects on quality of care, most dramatically in emergency situations, when blood products must be rapidly and accurately processed to meet urgent clinical needs. Crossmatches are still performed manually by skilled medical technologists, who enter the results into the computer. The computer then selects and removes the appropriate unit from the inventory, assigns it to the particular patient, retains all crossmatch results, and generates a copy of the transaction for the patient's medical chart. When inventories of rare blood groups run low and patients must be switched to other blood types, the computer will warn the user with a "forbid" message and an audible alarm if a technologist selects a potentially incompatible blood type.

Blood Component and Patient Database

The laboratory computer stores the complete history of each component, including donor identification number, pertinent transfusion history, and all testing data relevant to that unit. The computer system also maintains a file of all patients receiving blood transfusions. This file includes patient demographic data, previous transfusion history, results of all previous blood typing results, and identification of all antibodies present. It notes any special problems that occur during a patient's transfusion. This database has proven invaluable to the blood bank in helping identify patients with potential problems prior to transfusion. The computer checks results performed by the technologist on a patient crossmatch with all of the results obtained previously and immediately notifies the technologist of any discrepancies.

The computerized database has greatly facilitated look back procedures, procedures which have increased in number as the AIDS epidemic has intensified. If a donor or blood product recipient develops AIDS or another blood transmitted disease, it is necessary to match the donor and recipient of each potentially involved blood product. In the event a blood product recipient develops AIDS, the blood bank must perform the look back procedure to identify all components transfused into the patient. The Northeast Ohio Red Cross is notified so that they may check the medical records of all donors of the units in question to determine whether any of these donors were the source of the patient's disease.

Searches which took hours to perform manually can now be performed rapidly, accurately, and efficiently with online database searches. No longer do blood bank personnel conduct time consuming manual searches through 100,000 cards on 30,000 patients, cards stored in multiple locations throughout the hospital. The probability of error, especially in emergency situations, is significantly diminished.

Autologous Donor Service

The concern over AIDS and other blood transmitted diseases is expected to result in an increased demand for autologous blood service, a service notoriously difficult to manage effectively. In 1989, about five percent of the blood products used at Akron General Medical Center were autologous, i.e., drawn from a patient prior to anticipated need, such as elective surgery, and retransfused at the appropriate time. Handled separately from the rest of the blood bank inventory and used only for the donor, autologous blood products are not subjected to the rigorous screening procedures to rule out potentially contaminated sources that the general donor population undergoes.

The greatest problem has been identifying patients for whom autologous blood has been drawn. All too frequently the autologous donor has been entered into the mainstream of blood bank activity and given a unit of bank blood rather than the autologous unit. The donor has thus been denied the benefits of autologous blood products which he or she gave time and effort to donate. Compounding the waste, the blood bank has used a unit of bank blood for the donor, whose autologous blood could not be used elsewhere.

To manage the autologous service effectively, the computerized system labels an autologous unit as such in the blood product files and enters the donor into the patient file as having an autologous unit available. When blood products are ordered on this patient, the computer identifies the patient as an autologous donor and the technologist is informed of the identity of all of that patient's autologous units. The system is also capable of handling the projected increase in autologous donations without adding additional personnel.

Additional Administrative/Management Functions

The laboratory computer system has additional functions that the blood bank has found extremely helpful in managing overall blood bank operations.

Inventory Status Report. This report details the current inventory status of all units in the blood bank. Lists may be generated by ABO Rh type, expiration date, and unit status (e.g., available for transfusion). Inventory management is essential to ensure an adequate supply of blood products to meet anticipated hospital needs while allowing as few units as possible to become outdated.

Billing. Daily billing reports include the patient's name and demographic data, a list of units transfused, and a summary of all test procedures performed. This information is transferred by interface to the hospital fiscal information system for inclusion in the patient's financial database.

Statistical Reports. These are generated periodically and cover all facets of laboratory function. Reports especially helpful to the blood bank include blood product recipient status reports, procedure tallies for workload recording studies, transfusion product use (by patients, ordering physicians, hospital service, hospital location, blood type) and complete reports of all transfusion reactions.

Conclusions and Future Applications

Over two years' experience with a computerized information system at Akron General Medical Center Blood Bank has shown it to be effective in meeting the needs of good medical practice and satisfying regulatory agencies. The system supports routine operations, significantly reducing the probability of clerical errors while reducing time and staff requirements. It maintains extensive files of blood products and patient data, and provides the critical look back feature.

Building upon the system's success, Akron General Medical Center has recently undertaken the integration of the blood bank computer operations with both the main laboratory and the hospital information systems. The major benefits realized so far are threefold. First, this interface allows transmission of patient administrative data to the hospital blood bank. Second, it allows the blood bank to transfer billing information to the hospital financial database; and third, it permits transfer of important patient information such as blood availability to the patient care units.

These and other added benefits will make computerization of blood bank functions an essential part of good blood bank practice and a critical component of responsible patient care as the AIDS epidemic continues.

Questions

1. List a major advantage of the personal computer/file server hardware system as compared to more conventional mainframe or minicomputer systems.

2. Briefly describe how the computerized information system has allowed for more efficient inventory management of blood donor products.

3. List several areas where there has been a significant reduction in clerical errors as a result of computer system implementation.

4. List two areas of blood bank operations where audible alarms have proven very helpful in avoiding errors.

5. Briefly describe the blood bank look back procedure and explain why an increasing number of these procedures have been performed in blood banks in the past several years.

6. Briefly describe a major problem of most manual autologous blood programs and how the computer has eliminated it.

7. List several computer programs that have been helpful in the administration and management of the hospital blood bank.

Select Bibliography

Brodheim, E. 1983. Automated systems in blood banking. *Clinics in Laboratory Medicine* 3:T11-T31.

Brodheim, E., P. D. Cumming, E. L. Wallace, et al. 1984. What are the costs and values of computers in blood banks? *Vox Sanguinis* 47:174-86.

Clark, L. R., J. Parekh, M. Peters, et al. 1984. Hospital blood bank laboratory data processing system. *Journal of Clinical Pathology* 37:1157-66.

Eggert, A. A., M. I. Traver, and T. J. Blankenheim. 1986. A computer based record system for a hospital based transfusion service. *Transfusion* 20:55-65.

McNeelly, M. D. 1987. *Microcomputer applications in the clinical laboratory.* Chicago, Ill.: American Society of Clinical Pathologists Press.

Myhre, B. A., and F. Ritland. 1985. The computer in the blood bank, *CRC Critical Reviews in Clinical Laboratory Sciences* 24(1):21-42.

Reich, L. M., M. J. Mitchell, W. H. Jambois, et al. 1983. A computer system designed for a hospital transfusion service. *Transfusion* 23:316-321.

4
Computer Enhanced Radiology: A Transformation to Imaging

Roger H. Shannon

Introduction

Radiology is an information business. It is one of the core specialties of scientific medicine. In a sense, it is also a part of every direct care specialty, but it has differentiated into a separate field because of the special skills and knowledge that are required to correctly create and interpret images. Many other physicians have also become skilled in aspects of radiology, but few have the fundamental training to appreciate the context in which radiology is practiced or have a command of the subject sufficient to enable them to choose the most efficacious, cost beneficial course of study from a full set of alternatives. Even skilled clinical subspecialists rarely see the number and variety of cases which a radiologist encounters in serving many such referring physicians.

Diagnostic radiology, therefore, is best practiced in an environment of good communication between radiologists and referring physicians, however skilled at image interpretation the latter may be. Good communication in this technical world consists of intercomputer exchange in addition to the many forms of interpersonal exchange to which one has become accustomed. These two aspects of communication will receive further attention in this chapter.

Computers are used in two distinctly different ways by diagnostic radiologists. First, computers are central components of imaging devices such as computed tomographic units (CT), ultrasound (U/S), gamma cameras, and others. Second, computers are the hub of radiology information systems (RIS) for management of administrative and medical information, and for the management, storage, and communication of electronic images (IMAC or PACS).

This chapter focuses on the second use, support systems, commenting on computers integral to acquisition devices only in order to clarify the important and expanding application of computers for radiology support.

The Major Function of Diagnostic Radiology

The core function of diagnostic radiology is quality consultation. Service is thereby rendered to both referring physicians and patients.

The ideal consultation depends on several factors. First, one must choose what study or studies to do. Commonly the choice is straightforward, but often it is not. Choosing may require evaluation of complicated clinical information with preliminary consultation between referring physician and radiologist. Weighing of benefits, risks, and costs is frequently difficult. Order of tests and their timing may be issues. Second, the selected examination(s) must be excellently performed. Good equipment, competent personnel, and individually validated procedures are each critical factors. Third, images resulting from a study should be assembled with all relevant supporting material. Clinical information, previous similar examinations or other concurrent studies, and reference materials are frequently important. These comprise what may be called the information package.

Finally, a timely report should be produced and communicated to the physician(s) who will incorporate the radiological results into the clinical decision stream. The report will ultimately be in writing, but communication of results, opinions, correlations, and suggestions for resolving conflicting conclusions may require immediate personal communication on the part of the radiologist. Formal daily conferences between radiologists and clinicians have become a highly successful convention in many radiology departments.

Consulting is the professional focus of diagnostic radiology. It is highly complex. So too is the setting in which consulting occurs. A two part view of that setting is essential to radiology management or administration. The radiology department itself—a complex, extremely technical, capital intensive portion of the hospital—defines the basic system. Included in the term *radiology department* are the main department and satellite operations in locations such as the emergency room, outpatient clinic, and surgery.

However, radiologic practice as defined here is not limited to the department, but permeates the entire hospital and the clinics of affiliated practitioners. Viewing stations are scattered throughout wards, conference rooms, surgery, and other service areas. Procedures and discussions involving radiologic images and reports are legion. Clinical decisions and procedures are continually influenced by radiology. New information leads to new radiologic studies. It is largely outside of the formal radiology areas that consultations are assimilated by the clinical process and acquire meaning for the patient. The better the communication, the more powerful a tool radiology becomes.

The scope of all these radiologic projections within the hospital and beyond to the outpatient world constitutes the environment, the second portion of the two part view of radiology. The radiology system is embedded in the medical environment. Following the general principle that it is only in the environment that any system acquires meaning, one notes that the clinical process is the essential environment that gives birth to and makes use of radiologic consultation (Grobstein 1973).

Trends and Transition

Rapid Growth

The proliferation of computer support for radiology has been stimulated by two trends. First, radiology has been one of the fastest growing medical specialties for several years. Mushrooming medical knowledge and new, often time consuming procedures have added volume and complexity to radiology's armamentarium. With growth have come subspecialties and larger, more complicated groups of professionals. Most medium size and larger hospitals have spread radiology to several satellites, and the supporting staff has become numerous and varied. Coordination of radiology has become immensely difficult. Manual procedures are no longer sufficient to deal with the volume of detail. Consequently, computer operations have been developed to supplement or replace older methods. The resulting systems are referred to as radiology information systems (RIS).

Changing Technology

The second trend bringing computers into radiology began with the introduction of computed tomography (CT) in 1972 (Hounsfield 1972). CT relies on a computer to capture and analyze thousands of measurements which are arrayed in planes, or slices, that portray cross sections of the body parts examined. These pictures are electronic and are first displayed on devices like television. It is still conventional, however, to transfer these images to film for final interpretation and storage. The methods and technology of CT have been applied to a host of other modalities so that between one quarter and one half of the number of actual images obtained in current practice originate in electronic form (Lodwick 1986).

Newer developments promise the possibility of replacing conventional radiography with electronic images as well, creating the possibility of eventually eliminating film as a recording medium altogether (Saarinen et al. 1989).

Support Systems

To handle these electronic images, additional computers appear to be necessary. Several synonyms designate these systems. Four in popular use are MIMS (medical imaging management systems), PACS (picture archiving and communications systems), DIN (digital imaging networks), and IMACS (image management and communication systems).

RIS were developed earlier than PACS. The former are fairly mature, the latter exist in parts. PACS segments are commercially available, but the filmless department is yet to be implemented. PACS, therefore, are not mature. Current efforts are directed at further development of PACS and at interfacing a variety of existing RIS with the emerging PACS technology. In the early 1980s the American College of Radiology and the National Electrical Manufacturers Association formed a joint committee (ACR-NEMA) to develop standards for interfacing digital acquisition devices to PACS networks. These standards are now being incorporated in industrial design (Lodwick et al. 1989). Numerous other groups are dealing with the problems of data definition and compatibility (Megargle 1989). New findings and controversies frequently appear in the literature. And the state of the art moves forward. Radiology computer support systems are, therefore, in a state of transition that can make choices difficult and the lives of both practitioners and administrators frustrating. However, some difficulty now is justified by the promise of simplified, computer supported management in the future.

RIS and PACS Functions

Radiology Information Systems (RIS)

The typical RIS offers several sets of functions. These include: (1) registration of patients, (2) scheduling, (3) patient tracking, (4) film library management, (5) reporting of results, and (6) department management. Electronic mail, teaching applications, and research functions may be added. Various forms of decision support are also beginning to appear. Although the basic RIS is fairly mature, these systems continue to expand and evolve.

Registration. Registration is the process of initiating the patient RIS record. This is the demographic module. If the RIS is interfaced to the hospital information system (HIS), demographic information is passed to radiology from the hospital master record. If not otherwise available, patient information is entered directly.

Scheduling. Scheduling examinations may vary from a simple computer version of standard paper forms requiring a maximum of clerical effort to sophisticated systems with numerous automated functions which, after checking for conflicts and hazards, automatically schedule at appropriate times. They record examination specific material, notify relevant action centers in the department, produce forms, allocate resources, and create pull notices to retrieve previous studies from film libraries, or implement archive retrieval procedures for PACS storage systems.

Patient Tracking. The patient tracking module follows each patient from arrival to departmental discharge, showing at any moment where the patient is and how close the examination is to being completed. Often technical factors, number and type of views acquired, and other operational and resource use data are coincidentally collected.

Film Libraries. Film libraries are notoriously complicated and difficult to control. These are the centers of coordination for all medically important patient information. Not only are all images, past and present, retrieved, matched, sometimes duplicated, distributed, loaned and recovered, stored, and perhaps displayed; but also associated information which may include demographics, clinical findings, work up consultations, formal interpretations, codes, and follow up with quality assurance (Q/A) information, must be assembled together with the images. Film libraries collect and link the record elements which fully informed radiologists should have at their fingertips in order to perform the highest quality professional work. It is convenient to think of these image and information items as the selective clinical radiology information package (SCRIP) (Shannon 1989). As each item is created, it ideally should be integrated into the SCRIP. Since material is acquired during the sequence of work up, examination, interpretation, decision, and followup, the professional user would never receive less than the current SCRIP with which to work.

Reporting. The notion of clinical information packages naturally leads to consideration of the classic end point of diagnostic radiology—the written report of the radiologist's findings and interpretation. In traditional manual operations, the report is typed on the requisition form, thereby retaining whatever demographic and clinical information has been entered by the requestor. With the advent of electronic systems, many combinations of automated and manual functions were implemented. Independent word processors gained popularity early. Some of these used the submitted paper requisitions, just as did typewriter operations. Others used continuous forms requiring that information on the requisition be reentered. As medical information networks have proliferated, it has become clear that work volume and error rates rise if identical information must be entered more than once.

To take advantage of source entry and to ensure continuity of patient data, interfacing of the various information systems throughout a hospital or medical complex has clear advantages. Possible sources of demographic and clinical information for a radiology reporting terminal include the hospital information systems (HIS) and the radiology information systems into which patient information has already been deposited. Early RIS lacked the power to support word processing without unacceptable slowing of the entire RIS response time.

However, modern systems include good word processing modules and often provide electronic means of distributing reports to wards or other remote request sites. Through a variety of means, progressively more complex and satisfactory integration of functional modules, like word processing, with departmental and hospital wide systems is becoming commonplace. More sophisticated reporting has been followed by such ancillary functions as communication with billing systems, case coding, interesting case cataloguing, and capture of departmental management data.

Management. The final basic RIS module deals with management information. These modules vary widely in their sophistication, but usually provide examination volume and distribution, resource utilization, statistics on timeliness of important functions, and financial information to including revenues.

These six functions—registration of patients, scheduling, patient tracking, film library management, reporting of results, and department management —together with electronic mail, constitute the basic RIS.

Picture Archiving and Communications Systems (PACS)

As RIS have matured in response to the growing need to keep track of materials and events and to manage written records, picture archiving and communication systems (PACS) have emerged from somewhat different origins, but appear to be developing on a course that is converging with that of the RIS. Increased use of digital acquisition devices has demanded that systems be developed to store, manage, and communicate electronic images throughout the radiology department as well as a growing number of other sections of the hospital. Driven by the burgeoning of electronic imaging, PACS have become recognized as an integral and essential component of the inevitable computer based communications environment.

Image Manipulation. In a sense, individual digital imaging devices like CT have always embraced the rudimentary functions of PACS. Computer generated images are displayed on television like cathode ray tubes (CRTs) where they can be manipulated and altered in a variety of ways. For instance, one can adjust exposures or choose only a portion of the full range of exposure and expand it to examine the segment in detail. Edges can be sharpened, or black and white can be reversed to produce a negative image. Future possibilities seem endless. Some will be important new diagnostic tools, others will prove merely curiosities. These display stations are the forerunners of what one calls workstations in PACS parlance.

Communication. Frequently, a second display station which communicates with the main viewing device can be found in a nearby room, allowing monitored image acquisition to continue while previous examinations are reviewed simultaneously at the second site. These multiple viewer configurations constitute rudimentary communication systems, a second element of PACS.

Archiving. Image storage, or archiving (a third element of PACS), has been achieved with magnetic discs in display stations in order to provide rapid retrieval of a limited number of active cases or with magnetic tape for longer term retention of images that did not need to be so accessible. Although these images are fully manageable electronically, convention, an initial need for portability, diminishing but real technological limitations, and a cautious approach to new methods has resulted in recording these same images, for interpretation and storage, on film. The practice is redundant and expensive, and is becoming ever less justifiable in the face of competitive cost for quality electronic images. As the number and types of individual digital acquisition devices have increased, and as more complex and expensive storage technology, such as optical discs, has become available, sharing of support devices and expectation of easier access to images at distributed sites have been natural consequences.

Computed Radiography

With the recent development of reusable, electronically scanned media to replace conventional film radiography, transfer from an environment of physical records to one of total electronic management has much appeal. With this filmless process, images need never be inaccessible or lost. Records can be organized and combined in the best manner to suit a clinical need, and they can be used simultaneously at different sites served by institution wide networks. Retrieval time is minimized, and one can perform a wide variety of image adjustments and manipulations not possible with film. Furthermore, a system duplicating electronic and film images is expensive, making the transfer to a filmless system economically as well as functionally attractive to many PACS proponents.

Transition

In spite of pressures to transfer from film to digital electronics, PACS remain in their infancy for several reasons. First, properly exposed and developed films are very good (Vizy 1989). Second, the ever active tendency for people to avoid change generates resistance which is in part justified by the knowledge that to learn even the best of new ways requires a period of degraded performance until the old skills are sufficiently supplanted by the new. Third, there is not yet a fully developed filmless medical practice environment, but PACS have advanced to a point where the quality of patient care can be protected and pilot programs can be justified because knowledge can only be gained through experience. In the meantime, sections of PACS—certain storage devices, simple work stations, image transmission networks, etc.—are entering the market and seeing clinical use.

Finally, the economics and strategy of transition are not clear. Although costs will likely be greater than hindsight will indicate they might have been, evidence suggests that once the transition to filmless departments has been accomplished, costs of the new image support systems will be competitive with the old (Seshadri et al. 1988). The transition will require the addition of a well developed program for technology assessment (T/A) and a strategy for dealing with human factors, operations, and economics.

Technology Assessment

The problem of assessing whether or not a technology accomplishes what it is purported to do is relatively simple. To detect its unforeseen effects, particularly those that are indirect, is more difficult. Replacement economics also can be microcosted and adequately compared. Here too, the indirect economic effects are more elusive. Perhaps the most difficult, but in the last analysis most important, is the assessment of a technology in terms of its impact on outcome of care to the patient (Lohr 1988). This concept of technology validation in terms of the quality of results has achieved general recognition only recently. Support technology is particularly difficult to assess in this manner because, unlike the direction connection between the patient and individual tests and treatments, the effects of support technology are mediated through many channels, and, therefore, are more general and stochastically more subtle (Shannon and Allman 1988).

PACS in diagnostic radiology, as currently conceived and segmentally implemented, consist of shared digital storage devices, communications networks ranging from local connections to wide area use of satellites, workstations for image manipulation and display, and well managed databases for facile handling of images and associated information. The conception is intriguing, but the future holds more.

The Future

Even as PACS mature, a vision is developing which will serve as the organizing principle for information systems. Many current systems are converging toward a synthesis through which they will become powerfully synergistic in an integrated, computer supported information environment.

Technical Integration

Systems are coming together in two ways. First, now separate systems with similar functional characteristics will be intricately interfaced. Personal computers and their workstation cousins will interact with departmental systems. These in turn will communicate with hospital information systems and the last will participate in still wider area networks which reach out to other offices and institutions with much the same ease as telephone and telefax systems. A somewhat different attempt to conquer discontinuity among existing systems is the popular trend of bringing systems of different modalities together so that symbols, images, and voice can be automatically concerted (Schramm and Goldberg 1989).

Functional Integration

The second type of system convergence involves different classes of functions rather than similar but separate technical systems. Ordinarily the functions alluded to must be accessed independently, often on dedicated terminals at a limited number of sites. Literature and other reference services, decision support systems, statistics packages, and programs to do specialized analysis and graphics are examples of important functions currently inaccessible through most RIS or HIS systems.

Integration of systems in each of the described ways is beginning, but no well developed model is yet available in a clinical setting. Integrating these systems requires research and development in cognition, linguistics, logic, and both software and hardware technology. Some of the work can be accomplished by planning and analysis, but other portions of the necessary knowledge can be gained only from experience. The path to integrated systems is neither short nor easy to travel, but it is destined to be traversed.

Clinical Integration

For diagnostic radiology, assuming that its niche in clinical practice remains substantially intact, integrated systems will provide the opportunity to enter the mainstream of practice in a way that has never been possible. The SCRIP, or information package, can be a practical reality. Participation in work up strategies, performance of examinations and interpretations with full access to relevant information, and the ability to be part of the clinical decision team will bring the full talents of the radiologist to bear on patient problems. The developed potential of radiologic diagnosis and management will contribute to maximizing the clinical efficacy of the medical team.

Summary

Diagnostic radiology is currently so specialized and complex that it has become significantly isolated from the mainstream of medical practice. Both the practice and the management of diagnostic radiology are too complicated to function properly with manual methods. Radiology information systems (RIS) have provided excellent assistance with organization, monitoring, and communication. PACS are emerging as a byproduct of digital imaging modalities and are becoming support systems of importance in their own right. Integration of computer driven information systems is now recognized as a general need of medical practice. Integration of RIS with PACS is receiving much attention. More recently, general recognition that the RIS/PACS combination must be folded into hospital information systems has become established (Shannon 1989). Standalone support systems can then be offered as part of multimodal, general medical information and communication systems. This technology, a proven value in patient outcome, can reestablish the patient's confidence in medical organizations. At the medical organizations' core, imaging will remain a critical contributor to patient welfare.

Questions

1. What are the major components of computer support systems in diagnostic radiology? Include major system interfaces.

2. What are the components of the clinical radiology information package (CRIP), and what is the source of each?

3. How would the CRIP be assembled and maintained in a film based system? In a filmless, digital electronic department?

4. As a radiology manager, what would be your prioritized list and the rationale for choosing which information system segments and interfaces to install? As a medical center manager, how would your list and rationale change? Do the lists conflict significantly?

References

Grobstein, C. 1973. Hierarchical order and neogenesis. In *Hierarchy Theory: The Challenge of Complex Systems*, ed. H. H. Pattee. New York: George Braziller.

Hounsfield, G. N. 1972. A method of and apparatus for examination of a body by radiation such as x or gamma radiation. Patent specification 1283915. London.

Lodwick, G. S. 1986. Radiology systems of the 1990s—Meeting the challenge of change. *The Western Journal of Medicine* 145:848-52.

Lodwick, G. S., et al. 1989. ACR/NEMA Special Session. In *Proceedings of the First International Conference on Image Management and Communication*, ed. S. K. Mun, M. Greberman, W. R. Hendee, and R. H. Shannon. New York: IEEE (In press).

Lohr, K. N. 1988. Quality of care and technology assessment. Edited by R. A. Rettig. Washington, D. C.: Institute of Medicine, National Academy Press.

Megargle, R. 1989. The healthcare information standards coordinating committee. In *Proceedings of the AAMSI Congress*, vol. 7, ed. W. E. Hammond, 400-402. Washington, D. C.: AAMSI.

Saarinen, A. O., D. R. Haynor, and J. W. Loop. 1989. Modeling the economics of PACS: What is important? In *Proceedings of SPIE—Medical Imaging III* (In press).

Schramm, C., and M. Goldberg. 1989. Multimedia radiological reports: Creation and playback. *Journal of Digital Imaging* 2:106-13.

Seshadri, S. B., R. L. Arenson, D. DeSimone, et al. 1988. Cost-savings associated with a digital radiology department: A preliminary study. In *Proceedings of the Ninth Conference on Computer Applications in Radiology*, ed. R. L. Arenson. Philadelphia: RISC.

Shannon, R. H. 1989. IMACS and radiology: Defining the problems. In *Proceedings of the First International Conference on Image Management and Communication*, ed. S. K. Mun, M. Greberman, W. R. Hendee, and R. H. Shannon. New York: IEEE (In press).

Shannon, R. H. and R. A. Allman. 1988. Technology assessment using an informatics framework for medical imaging. In *Proceedings of the Ninth Conference on Computer Applications in Radiology*, ed. R. L. Arenson. Philadelphia: RISC.

Vizy, K. N. 1989. The roles of film in an increasingly computerized world. *Investigative Radiology* 24:503-6.

Select Bibliography

Arenson, R. L., ed. 1986. *Use of computers in radiology: The radiologic clinics of North America*, vol. 24, no. 1. Philadelphia: W. B. Saunders Company.

Mun, S. K., M. Greberman, W. R. Hendee, and R. H. Shannon, eds. 1989. In *Proceedings of the First International Conference on Image Management and Communication*. New York: IEEE (In press).

Section 1–Supporting the Practitioner

Unit 3—Nursing and Information Systems

Unit Introduction

The first book in this series, *Nursing Informatics: Where Caring and Technology Meet*, lays out new roles for nursing in the areas of clinical practice, administration, research, and education. This unit revisits the issues addressed in that book, expanding and updating the information provided there; all contributors are nurses now playing a variety of roles.

Formerly vice president of nursing at a tertiary care hospital and now a university instructor, Tranbarger focuses on how nursing uses computers at the patient's side. Mills, formerly vice president of nursing at a large teaching hospital, collaborates with her successor, O'Keefe, in describing the opportunities that information systems offer to nursing administrators. A leader in nursing informatics, Hannah joins with four of her students and hospital associates, Ross, Gore, Radulski, and Warnock-Matheron; they define the role that nursing must play in developing hospital information systems. Kock clarifies the relationship between nursing and the system vendors, which she observed while involved in the development of an integrated patient information system. Director of a hospital information system at a major academic health center, Marr draws upon her experience in training 9,700 healthcare professionals, over a third of them nurses, to recommend how best to design a computer course for clinical nurses.

The new roles that nursing professionals play are changing the ways that hospitals are staffed and managed.

1

Nurses and Computers: At the Point of Care

Russell Eugene Tranbarger

Hospitals today face many challenges and must address critical issues which grow out of societal expectations of healthcare and biomedical technology in a time of increased financial constraints. For hospitals, however, one constant remains in the volatile and ever changing field of healthcare: Patients are admitted to hospitals to receive nursing care. In fact, this has never been as true as it is today. Virtually every test is now available on an outpatient basis. Surgical procedures are performed in physician offices or surgical centers. Only when the patient's condition requires continuous monitoring on a 24 hour basis is admission to a hospital required.

Nursing Defined

Since Florence Nightingale founded modern nursing in the 19th century, nurses have been at the center of patient care. Almost no one hesitates to define the role of the nurse, not even the toddler who says that nurses give shots or the senior citizen who praises them for giving comfort. Most healthcare administrators and virtually all physicians say simply that the nurse carries out the doctor's orders and assists the physician and the patient. In addition, every state and territory has a law regulating the practice of nursing in that area. The Nursing Practice Act for the State of North Carolina (1978) is typical in its contents:

> Nursing by a Registered Nurse: The practice of nursing by registered nurse means the performance for compensation of any act in the observation, care, and counsel of persons who are ill, injured, or experiencing alterations

in normal health processes; and/or in the supervision and teaching of others who are or will be involved in nursing care; and/or the administration of medications and treatments as prescribed by a licensed physician or dentist. Nursing by registered nurses requires specialized knowledge, judgement, and skill, but does not require nor permit except under supervision of a physician licensed to practice medicine in North Carolina medical diagnosis or medical perscription of therapeutic or corrective measures. The use of skill and judgement is based upon an understanding of principles from the biological, social, and physical sciences. Nursing by registered nurse requires use of skills in modifying methods of nursing care and supervision as the patient's needs change.

Today, nursing involves both simple tasks (administering medications) and highly complex intellectual and physical skills (determining the response of a patient to illness, treatment, and life's events). Each professional nurse defines his/her practice within this framework. The specific nurse's scope of practice varies with education, experience, skill, specialty practice, institutional policies, and so forth. The major common determinants of nursing practice are that it is individualized, continuous, coordinated, intentional, planned, evaluated, and documented.

The Nursing Process

Most educated people know and understand the scientific process of problem solving. Nurses have adopted a modification of this called the nursing process. The elements of assessment, planning, implementing, documenting, evaluating, and reassessing form a self correcting framework for the nurse to use in delivering safe and effective care to patients. Although each nurse may have a somewhat different educational base, all rely heavily on the nursing process.

Nurses tend to view their work as unique, different from the work of other nurses, even from their own work on other days. That is indeed true. Although each nurse does essentially the same thing, context makes it seem very different.

Each work shift in a hospital setting involves literally millions of discrete tasks. Each must be done to the right person, in an acceptable period of time, under prescribed procedures, by approved persons, and in coordination with other people and departments. On a given shift, a nurse may be responsible for up to five employees and as many as 25 patients, each of whom may have a different physician who may or may not be on call. Patients may require any number of medications, intravenous lines, and monitoring instruments. The nurse provides physical care and takes vital signs and other measurements as ordered.

The nurse also provides patient education. With cost containment and diagnostic related groupings shortening the average length of stay, patients face a longer recuperative period after discharge. The nurse is responsible for discharge planning and instructing the patient, family, or home care specialist about care once provided in the hospital.

In addition to paperwork, the nurse prioritizes and responds to any number of telephone messages, taking into account patient events, employee needs, cafeteria hours, patient/family requests and whatever else is occurring on that unit, during that shift, with that nurse.

In short, each nurse deals with a myriad set of signals not unlike a busy air traffic controller at O'Hare or Dulles airport. The nurse must be able to act on the message at the appropriate time and in a semblance of order and often to the satisfaction of many other people.

Computers and Nursing Care

Nursing consumes 40 to 50 percent of the hospital payroll and employs a large percentage of the hospital employees. The critical nature of productivity in this area has accordingly led to the development of computerized systems to assist nursing. Patient acuity systems have been in use for the past 15 to 20 years in many hospitals. These systems help in the allocation of nursing hours of care based on the patients' needs and the hospital's criteria. They develop staffing patterns and generate management reports showing utilization patterns. Often these reports demonstrate opportunities for cost savings through better utilization of hours of care. Some systems also provide quality assurance studies to tie together productivity and effectiveness.

With improved task handling capabilities and increased memory capacities, nurse scheduling systems have become a common computer function. These scheduling systems have improved the utilization of staff, while freeing up nurse manager time previously spent scheduling. The improved schedules have also contributed to staff morale. These systems support nursing in its mission of providing patient care when, where, and at the skill level required, using available resources. These systems form a nursing support net. They do not assist in the provision of nursing care.

Each patient generates voluminous transactions each day. Physician orders generate paper trails to pharmacy, laboratories, radiology, physical therapy, central supply, the operating room, and so on. Each such event also generates charges which must find their way to the patient's bill. Supplies must be ordered from various storerooms to keep the unit stocked, and the costs of these must also be controlled and accounted for.

Hospital information systems provide for these various activities. The computerization of these events usually produces a quicker transfer of the information, leaves an audit trail for problem solving when a failure results, and allows more people to have access to information in an easier way. Pharmacy can receive a list of the patient's allergies without the nurse having to record them and without the pharmacist having to review the patient's record. Many such examples can be found. These systems are indeed helpful to the caregivers. Results reporting, especially of laboratory tests, is very helpful to the caregivers. Overall, these systems generate enormous streams of paper. They do not assist with the delivery of nursing care.

Nursing and the Hospital Information System

Single vendor systems are most popular, with about two thirds of 1,642 automated hospitals reporting use of a single vendor (Gardner 1989). Of the hospitals in the McGraw-Hill 1988 Profile database, 65 percent used one information systems vendor. However, only 33 percent of those hospitals used a single vendor to automate both finance and one or more clinical functions.

Single vendor systems tend to limit choice when more than one automated function is desired. A system may have an excellent patient billing function and good order entry, while offering only mediocre reporting functions.

One way to circumvent the dilemma of variable subsystems of the single system is to network multiple systems. This technology allows the hospital to purchase the best system on the market for each desired function and tie them together into a functional system.

The integrated hospital information system shown in Figure 1 provides for most financial functions and some clinical functions, such as laboratory, radiology, pharmacy, etc. This system allows for departmental ownership of

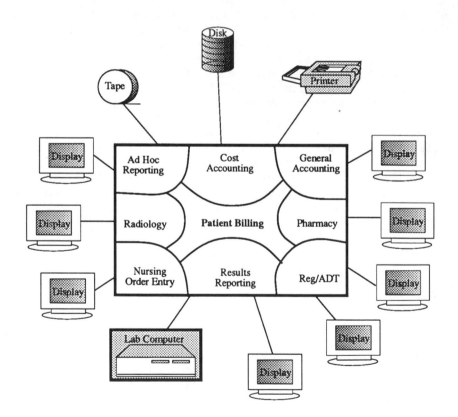

Figure 1. Integrated Hospital Information System

each department's functional purchases and allows for item by item purchase as budget, market availability, time constraints, and strategic need dictate. Each purchase requires that the product be able to tie in to the network and run within that environment.

This integrated approach poses a unique set of problems for nursing. Since nursing is often the connecting link between patient, physician, and department, nursing is usually involved in the transaction. Unless some discipline is applied, departmental functions can operate differently, requiring that the nurse use multiple passwords to access the system. Clearly, the nurse entering the transaction in the computer system must know which system is involved and how that system works. Problems can be limited by keeping things simple, involving nursing in the integration process, and keeping a sense of humor.

Once the decision is made to automate, a plan is essential. Figure 2 represents one hospital's plan for automation. Functions are placed in one of three categories, foundational, operational, or strategic. Together they form an information plan and help all stakeholders understand the goal and where each piece fits in the goal attainment.

Nursing Systems

Nursing's unique role in healthcare mandates its interaction with automated functions. Today's nurse executive can benefit from management decision support systems for patient classification and nurse scheduling as well as payroll and human resource database systems. The nurse providing patient care at the bedside relies increasingly on order entry, results reporting, and automated medication administration records (MAR). Though generally considered nursing systems, these applications do not directly assist in the provision of care. Clinical systems designed for that purpose, which provide decision support and documentation for hands on nursing care, are only now coming onto the market.

Forces in healthcare are accelerating the development and implementation of systems for clinical nursing. Financial constraints and shortages of nurses and allied health and service workers combine to intensify the need for more productive, less manpower intensive systems in hospitals. Competetion, market share, quality of care, liability issues, all cry out for attention and solutions.

Clinical Support Systems at the Point of Care

A clinical support system for nursing must be versatile, able to integrate multiple data sets from multiple sources. Just as nurses collect, analyze, document, and act on multiple pieces of data, any automated system must be able to do the same.

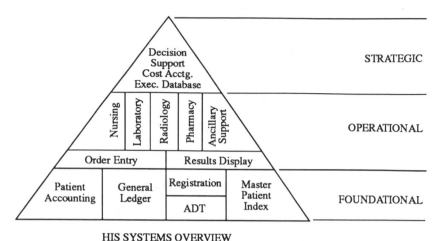

HIS SYSTEMS OVERVIEW

Figure 2. Moses H. Cone Information Plan

Patient Data Collected by Nursing:

- Vital signs: Temperature, pulse, blood pressure, respirations

- Medications: Type of drug given, when, by what route, dosage

- Intravenous fluids: Volume hung, amount infused, rate of flow, substances added, location of access line

- Standard measures: Weight, height, intake and output, response to treatment, laboratory values

- Other values monitored at bedside: Blood glucose, arrhythmia patterns, heart rate, various pressures, times of specific pattern disturbances

Appropriate data elements are included in nursing's admission assessment and updated at regular intervals depending on the condition of the patient. Others are obtained at various points within the treatment process.

A nursing care plan is derived from various databases and is composed of the reason(s) for the patient's admission, problems to be addressed by the caregivers, response of the patient to the care, evaluation of the care, and new directions for care based on the evaluation. These databases are diverse by nature, are located in various places, and require different timeframes.

This diversity of databases places a significant burden on the nurse. After first discovering what needs to be done, the nurse must then visit the proper location for the event, perform the necessary function, and record the results in the proper form in the patient record. One function may cause the nurse to visit five different places, look through several different forms, document the same information in multiple sites, then decide what must be done next. Patient requests, telephone calls, questions, other caregivers—all can be distractions which conspire against the busy nurse during this sequence of events.

Computerization can simplify nursing access to these databases. The challenge is to extend that access beyond the nursing station, where terminals are most frequently located. One solution is to provide the nurse with a handheld terminal to carry throughout the work shift into remote areas of the nursing unit. Another solution is to locate terminals at each patient bed and in central locations on each unit. Although more expensive initially, this solution frees the nurse's hands and eliminates the problem of mislaid terminals. It also provides considerable patient safety. When the correct information is at the patient's side, the possibility of treating the wrong patient or performing the wrong procedure is significantly reduced. The dual location of terminals, one at the patient's bedside and one in the station, allows the nurse to review data with the patient or to do work planning outside of the patient's sight, whichever is most appropriate at the moment.

Regardless of location of terminals or hardware used, computerization offers substantial assistance to the nurse and comfort to the patient. Although expense of systems is a constraint, systems that can enhance the safety of patients and increase the efficiency of nurses can be cost effective in today's healthcare environment.

Estimates of time spent by professional nurse per shift worked on documentation vary from 40 to 75 percent. If each nurse spends just one hour out of each eight hours worked on documentation, the cost of that hour if replaced by a data capturing computerized system will have economic value. Assuming that each nurse averages $15 per hour and that 100 nurses work each day, the resulting figure is $547,500 for the cost of documentation. These assumptions are conservative, given what nurses earn and the size of most hospital nursing staffs. Moreover, nurses frequently do charting after their shift ends. When nurses must stay over to complete their work, not only do costs increase with overtime pay, but also the opportunity for mistakes, especially of omission. Morale also tends to suffer.

Conclusion

The role of the nurse in today's hospital is evolving from assistant to the physician and the hospital, to that of primary caregiver to the patient. Humane care in the era of high technology requires the skilled touch of the nurse. The nursing shortage and the other constraints of finance and human resource availability place further pressures on the hospital to change systems to increase efficiency of the nurse, enhance patient safety, and increase the effectiveness of the caregivers.

Surely, one solution is automation. Hospital information systems can bring real assistance to the nurse and the patient by automating data collection. Providing the nurse with new tools to guide the care process and to manage the diverse databases upon which care decisions are based can be very beneficial. Smart systems using artificial intelligence may help the neophyte nurse to collect and manipulate data, and to reach a decision more effectively and more accurately.

When nurses are able to make better decisions in less time, both patients and the institution are well served. When available technology is applied to the delivery of care to the patient, the nurse experiences a better work life and the patient has a better chance at a healthy life.

Questions

1. What is the role of nursing in today's healthcare environment?

2. What forces in today's competitive environment influence the need for change in the role of the nurse?

3. How can automation technology be used to change the nurse's work habits in the hospital?

4. Can the cost of automated data collection systems be justified?

5. Name other benefits of automated data collection systems exclusive of costs or cost savings.

Reference

Gardner, E. 1989. Finding a strategy that does the trick. *Modern Healthcare* 19(27):28-52.

2
Computerization: A Challenge to Nursing Administration

Mary Etta Mills and Sharon O'Keefe

Nursing administrators need to view information technology as a tool which can facilitate planning, decision making, communication, managerial control, and changes in organizational structure. Information systems can assist nursing administrators in structuring, operating, controlling, and evaluating the performance of the nursing department.

In the past, managers tended to adopt technology and then figure out what to do with the new information and how to cope with its organizational implications. Continuing to react in this manner will hinder the development of systems which ensure that nursing resources are used to accomplish organizational objectives.

Changing Objectives of Nursing Administration

The management and delivery of healthcare services is evolving to new formats. The entire structure of the delivery system is undergoing significant change. Hospitals continue to respond to pressures to reduce costs through corporate reorganization and implementation of labor saving technologies. An increasingly competitive marketplace demands measures which enhance quality of care and provide a service orientation.

These changes have a significant impact on nursing administration, which must increasingly focus on quality, productivity, and flexibility. In the quickly changing healthcare environment, the challenge for nurse administrators has shifted from managing daily operations to mastering change and innovation.

Preparing nursing for the demands of the future requires a massive restructuring of roles and organization. With technology driven control systems, nursing administration can achieve the flexibility and responsiveness of a decentralized system and the integration and control of a centralized organization.

Applications for Key Management Functions

Structuring the Organization

Most nursing departments today follow the bureaucratic model. The advantages of this formal design are that it clearly structures responsibility, accountability, and communication, while helping to reduce complexity and provide stability. Its disadvantage, however, is its tendency to centralize decision making, stifle innovation, and overemphasize tasks and standard procedures.

Information systems that support interactive decision making will allow nursing to move beyond these bureacratic limitations. Integrated databases and analytical models can open up a whole new set of options for structuring and operating the nursing department. Nursing executives will be less insulated from operations because executive information systems will assist them in acquiring the information they need to monitor, coordinate, and control the activities of the nursing department. A flattened organization will result, with fewer middle managers needed to analyze and relay information.

Standard reports and functional reporting systems will be replaced by streamlined qualitative reports on key performance indicators. Available in realtime and not solely at the end of standard reporting periods, these reports will allow for timely feedback to first line supervisors, thus supporting decentralized decision making and encouraging the practicing nurse to invest in the goals of the organization.

Operating the Organization

The primary responsibility of administrators is to ensure that the organization and its resources are managed with efficiency and effectiveness. Three fundamental systems support nursing department operations: workload management systems, workforce management systems, and financial management systems.

Workload Management Systems. Today, nursing administrators are compelled to determine the level of care needed on a given floor at a given time by analyzing patient acuity levels and applying patient classification systems. The delivery of quality nursing care and the justification of costs incurred in providing it require the accurate quantification of workload.

Automated patient classification methodologies facilitate the collection, storage, manipulation, and retrieval of large volumes of workload data. Used in planning for the allocation of human resources, these patient specific data can also be used to

- Identify workload by diagnostic category or product line
- Facilitate analysis of workload trends per hospital stay
- Support costing of nursing services per patient

The information generated by automated patient classification systems assists managers in the allocation of resources, both daily and long term, and in the preparation of budgetary requests.

Workforce Management Systems. Used in matching personnel to workload in the most cost efficient manner, workforce management systems generally include components for nursing personnel management and staff scheduling.

Nursing personnel systems track all human resource planning information necessary to manage the nursing workforce, with a database architecture created specifically for that purpose. Personnel databases can include information regarding every position (availability, specifications) and each individual (employment history, performance tracking, wage and salary history, professional registration, credentialing, educational history). Comprehensive reporting and up to date information on nursing personnel facilitate the effective management of personnel, assist in the recruitment and retention of nurses, and document the career paths of professional staff. They can also assist in providing career counseling, monitoring licensure and continuing education attendance, meeting hospital accreditation requirements, and developing manpower contingency plans in the event of a disaster.

The staff scheduling system uses the database provided by the personnel management system and functions in conjunction with the patient classification system to generate staff schedules based on specific patient care requirements. Because they are driven by the personnel management and patient classification systems, staffing systems can take into account patient need, staff expertise, staff scheduling preferences, and personnel policies. However, the complexity of such systems varies widely, with intelligent systems capable of adjusting staff schedules in an interactive manner on a shift by shift basis.

Scheduling systems assist the nurse manager in maintaining records, monitoring attendance, ensuring compliance with personnel policies, and scheduling time off for personnel. Information is readily available to document work patterns of all nursing personnel.

Financial Management Systems. Operating budgets for nursing departments account for approximately 40 percent of the typical hospital's operating budget. Computers are essential if managers are to effectively control the nursing department budget and accurately plan for new programs. The primary advantage provided by financial management systems lies in their ability to organize, manipulate, store, and retrieve data in preparing departmental budgets and analyzing budgetary variances.

Budget preparation for nursing departments is often a tedious, time consuming, number intensive process. By linking patient classification data and staffing requirements to a budget methodology, the preparation of an annual operating budget can be expedited. Necessary reallocations and adjustments for new programs are facilitated by the use of spreadsheets. "What if" scenarios can be tested to ensure that the budget provides a realistic plan for managers.

Financial management systems provide managers with up to date reports which focus their attention on major variances and potential problems. Nursing financial management systems allow a great deal of flexibility while linking reports to responsibility centers. Reporting can be tailored to organizational level and individual nursing units. These capabilities are critical in today's competitive environment; they make it possible for nursing to respond effectively to the demands for cost control.

By integrating patient classification data, personnel management data, and budgetary data, managers are able to analyze variances and explain budgetary deviations due to price, volume, or acuity variances. Nurse managers are able to target management interventions, designed to produce the desired performance results and to achieve organizational goals.

Information Access and Dissemination

In addition to the systems described above, automation offers nurse administrators the ability to access and disseminate information quickly and easily.

Office Automation Features

Electronic bulletin boards, calendaring, filing, and mail provide a means by which nursing administration can communicate basic announcements, notices, and sets of information to a broad array of nursing managers and staff as well as to support departments. This means of rapid information transfer has provided an ability to manage basic systems communication rapidly, in the short term and without expensive and lengthy paper generation and distribution. Likewise, responses can be expedited and the paper volume reduced. Maintenance of a system of basic nonautomated mail handling, filing, and calendar management can be a time consuming annoyance, although operationally important to administrators. The computer support system reduces the clutter and time associated with this element of management.

Administrative computing further encompasses word processing, graphics, and database management. At this time, most businesses consider word processing basic to their office routine as a means to rapidly produce documents which can be modified without redundant work effort. Graphics capabilities allow the administrator to manipulate and display data. They are especially useful in determining and graphically depicting trends relative to budget management, productivity, and resource flow. For example, critical data elements such as key expenditures, productivity figures from automated management systems, and personnel recruitment and turnover can be routinely input. Using this base, the administrator can visually depict both experiential and predictive trends for use in planning and management.

Local area network technology which links micro/mini/mainframe computers can further enhance both computing and communication technologies by integrating departmental health care computing systems to allow use of distributed data management techniques. This system can help meet informational needs by providing access to clinical research databases, patient management systems, and patient charges.

Telecommunications which provide voice messaging services as well as electronic transmission of data further expedite administrative functions. Automated voice messaging allows callers to record messages and indicate level of urgency so that their call is given priority when the recipient listens to messages received. The system gives 24 hour direct and remote access to the recipient of calls through a code system and provides for the message to be erased, saved, or given a voice response for later distribution to the caller.

Information access is further extended by external linkages to the health science library to provide reference services and bibliographic database management. This may include a microcomputer system to search the Medline database at the National Library of Medicine or a tie in to library resource assistance. The ability to rapidly access information which can help in better understanding issues (such as clinical program plans) or which aid in the formulation and support of databased responses and plans can greatly facilitate the administrator's effectiveness. Realistically, much of what the nurse administrator deals with is intraorganizationally generated data, operations, and issues. Time available to plan and creatively conceptualize is often a luxury making the availability of a rapidly accessible literature base or bibliographic information retrieval and delivery by library resources an asset.

Integrated Systems

The coordinated collection and translation of information to support complex patient care, organizational, and regulatory requirements is of growing importance. Integration provides a cost effective approach to systemwide coverage and an effective way to access and manage information which supports complex decision making.

In an era of resource limitations which include both financial constriction and personnel shortages, efficiency and effectiveness have become increasingly important. Having data automatically distributed into multiple programs for analysis specific to given output generation and perhaps redistribution into still other programs becomes an essential conservator of valuable staff time. Elimination of duplicative information recording, collection, and analysis by nursing staff can reduce the almost 40 percent of nursing time currently spent on paperwork. This in itself will facilitate the use of professional staff in directly delivering or supervising patient care.

In a truly integrated system, all of the functions are designed from the outset to work together. Whether or not this is technically feasible is a subject of debate by vendors. While development continues in this area, interfacing which connects unrelated automated systems has had more success. As a result, some nursing management systems such as patient classification, staffing requirements, scheduling systems, and productivity analysis have been interfaced for automated sequential analysis. The interrelatedness of these programs provides the nurse administrator with information specific to correlated administrative issues. In addition to providing an immediate image of key operational issues, this type of program networking allows planning and forecasting with the use of data based simulations.

Eight system design goals are important to the development or selection of computer systems which support integrated data management:

A Single Patient Database. First, there should be a single patient database. With data residing in a single central repository, integration of financial and clinical data becomes easier.

Integration of Clinical and Financial Data. Second, integration of clinical and financial data should be accomplished so a patient's stay can be reflected in a single, integrated picture.

One Time Entry of Information. Third, there should be one-time entry of information. For example, a patient's demographic data should be entered into the admitting/registration system and these data should update all patient records within the system.

Easy Retrieval of Data from the Database in a Form Defined by the User. Fourth, easy retrieval of data from the database in a form defined by the user should be possible.

Flexibility. Fifth, the system should be flexible. It should be easily modified to meet changing user needs and regulatory requirements and should allow users to easily tailor the input and output components of the system.

Easy Expansion. Sixth, the system should be easily and cost effectively expandable to accommodate increasing terminals, users, applications, and data.

Reliability. Seventh, the system should be reliable and operational 24 hours per day, seven days a week. Contingency backup should be available for all online patient care applications.

Security. Eighth, the system should provide for extremely tight data, program, and terminal security and should be able to restrict access on multiple levels.

Data must be provided which are required to plan, analyze, monitor, and control individual departments, divisions, and the organization as a whole. Computer systems should support and reflect integrated and related functions in the following broad administrative and financial areas:

- Patient billing, review reports, volume statistics
- Budget, purchasing, general ledger
- Personnel, payroll, fulltime equivalents, cost center reports
- Capital planning, expenditure
- Quality assurance, utilization review, case mix, severity, acuity

- New systems to support data analysis as a routine effort
- Budgeting process (planning, development, control)
- Financial statements and all related reports
- Cash report, inventory reports, investment report
- Census report
- Project management reports
- Productivity

Clinical data not addressed here also need to be integrated with financial and administrative data to provide a complete system information base.

Full access of information to the nurse administrator enhances system wide planning considerations. The administrator generates decision support questions for data retrieval and display by information managers or personally accesses the database to obtain information. Given the paucity of planning time available in most daily administrative schedules it may be unrealistic to expect the nurse administrator to directly generate analytic reports. Information systems coordinators are especially useful in this role in addition to systems design, implementation, and operation toward optimally supporting the entire nursing department.

Future Development

Future capability of computer systems in nursing administration will involve designs which provide for enhanced data generation, distribution, analysis, and transformation.

Systems Integration and Networking

The ability to acquire information that optimally represents the status of each of a large number of interacting variables, the outcomes of these interactions, and the probability of future outcomes based on changes in the variables will be the future standard against which administrators judge computer systems. Ultimately the integration of systems internal to the organization will expand to include a need for increased network capability linking internal systems to external environments (i.e., care providers, social and support services, and regulatory bodies). This expanded system will serve to increase resources available for healthcare service and administration.

Marketing functions are one application of programs under current development (Gardner 1989) which link hospital systems to healthcare statistics from many public services. This type of program is designed to offer "specific demographic information to help hospital administrators make decisions about product lines, pricing, staffing and placement of satellite facilities."

Other opportunities exist to link networks to external information bases such as data comparisons for staffing levels, mix, and cost analysis; compensation statistics for distinct local and regional areas; and survey statistics regarding turnover and employment. The availability of these types of data will be critical to the formulation of program plans and strategic directions.

Patient Record

Input of information to the patient record will become a combination of automated patient physiologic monitoring and manual data entry of clinical information. Key physiologic indicators will be monitored against pre-established standards and analyzed for trends and interactions predictive of health status intervention needs. This information would become part of the integrated patient record.

Information specific to patient care orders and process and outcome of care documentation will be entered into the record. This primary database will automatically service programs designed to generate required corollary information. This includes patient classification and acuity analysis, staffing requirements, personnel scheduling, productivity, payroll data, specific patient service charges, practice patterns, quality of management, and risk management monitoring.

Quality Management

As a key program component for clinicians, administrators, and regulators, quality management will be increasingly developed around automated monitoring of predetermined variations (thresholds) indicative of trends in patient care. These trends may be positive or negative and may be specific to individual patients or reflective of patient group experience (e.g., diagnostic categories).

Providing a qualitative base (quality) against which quantitative experience (resource use and expenditure) can be assessed is important. Even more valuable is the early identification of problems and the creation of opportunity to intervene to achieve optimal patient care.

Eventually much qualitative data will be formatted to be compatible with regulatory reporting requirements such as those of the Joint Commission for Accreditation of Healthcare Organizations. This will include programming software to systematically collect, track, analyze, and report clinical and organizational data.

An increasing emphasis on organizational and management effectiveness will expand the current concept of patient care quality to include organizational quality among the specific variables which impact patient care. The development of integrated systems will facilitate automated collection and reporting of these data for internal and external use.

Service Diversification

Major restructuring of the healthcare system will continue to create expanded options for patient care delivery. This has already led to the development of managed care as a means of coordinating services for individuals and groups of patients. Networks which allow systems to interface will be developed to ease patient movement through various types and levels of care providers. This includes such features as appointment systems, progress tracking, outcome measurement, and cost reporting and analysis.

Decision makers will need data based guidance in evaluating and reconciling cost and quality considerations. Current new decision support products suggest that developers are beginning to address the issue of managed care contracts relative to financial analysis. This development effort will need to be more definitively expanded to encompass direct patient service planning and delivery.

Resource Utilization

Every system entails costs and benefits. Many hospital administrators have assumptions that automated systems will pay for themselves in cost reductions mostly from changes in work force requirements (either in numbers or in function). Changes in operating costs concurrent with enhanced patient care and increased provider effectiveness are usually expected. Future development of computer systems, however, will need careful study of the impact of automated systems on workers. The results may provide guidance for job restructuring before the system is implemented. This approach would enable the manager to effectively reduce costs while improving productivity and patient care.

Summary

The role of computer systems in nursing administration is multifaceted. Decision support databases are provided through such means as the reporting of financial accounting and projection analyses, productivity assessment based in patient classification and staffing requirements, and clinical and market based program projections.

Recording and retrieval of professionally oriented data such as credentialing, continuing education, evaluation/peer review, and personal preferences regarding specialty and hours of work are adjunctive to maintaining quality of professional staff and meeting regulatory requirements. Data analyses features which provide the ability to monitor trends in resource (e.g., staff, budget) utilization in relation to patient care requirements enhance the foundation upon which programmatic plans can be made. Information access and dissemination is further supported by office automation, administrative computing, telecommunications, electronic academic reference services, and personal bibliographic data management.

Integrated system elements are critical to optimal administrative functioning. The ability to capitalize on single entry data sets by having them directly support multiple reporting requirements (some analytically based) will conserve valuable staff time. Programs supported by integrated systems include, for example, patient classification, acuity, productivity, quality of care, and financial analyses.

Enhancement of the future capability of computers will involve development of further intraorganizational systems integration and interorganizational networking. Computerized patient records will increasingly be designed to serve as a primary generation point for data required by administrative systems. Quality management at the patient and organizational level will be an area of increased emphasis. Likewise, computer systems will be further developed to coordinate services offered in the diversified care settings created by healthcare restructuring. System wide implications are drawn regarding the need to assess computer implementation costs and benefits and to consider job restructuring as one means of reducing costs while improving patient care.

Questions

1. How can information systems be designed to help nursing to move beyond the limitations of organizational bureaucracy?

2. What are the three fundamental systems which support nursing department operations?

3. How can local area network technology support administrators/managers?

4. What system design goals are important to the development or selection of computer systems which provide information specific to correlated administrative issues?

5. What expectations should nurse administrators have for future information system design?

Reference

Gardner, E. 1989. Finding a strategy that does the trick. *Modern Healthcare* 19(27):28-52.

Select Bibliography

Gardner, E. 1988. HBO software compiles demographic data. *Modern Healthcare* 18(28):42.
Joint Commission on the Accreditation of Healthcare Organizations. 1989. Principles of organizational and management effectiveness undergoing field review. *Agenda for Change Update* 3(1):1-7.
Kennedy, O. G. 1989. True systems integration still far off. *Modern Healthcare* 19(27):54.
Mowry, M., and R. Korpman. 1987. Automated information systems in quality assurance. *Nursing Economics* 5(5):237-44.

Stead, W. 1988. Information management through integration of distributed resources. *Bulletin of the Medical Library Association* 76(3):242-47.

3
Nursing's Role in Defining Systems

Sheri Ross, Marilyn Gore, Wes Radulski,
Ann Warnock-Matheron, and Kathryn J. Hannah

Beginning in the late 1970s, developers of hospital information systems (HIS) began to focus on modular systems. Today, HIS are generally built in a modular fashion (Peterson and Gerdin Jelger 1988). The great benefit of modularity is that a system can be adapted in a number of ways, based on the modules implemented. Consistent with its role and scope, a hospital implementing an HIS may select modules from within an HIS, such as

- Admission/discharge/transfer (A/D/T)
- Order entry/results reporting
- Pharmacy
- Finance
- Inventory control
- Medical records index

Individual modules store within masterfiles the information particular to the functions performed by the department. For example, the finance module stores information on charges for patient stay and services, as well as information regarding staff payroll. The inventory control module may store information regarding cost of items, number of items stocked, suppliers, and ordering of additional supplies. In choosing to implement any or all of these modules, as well as additional ones not listed here, the hospital must make critical decisions regarding system integration. The number and type of modules implemented at an institution will determine the masterfiles to be integrated within the system.

When undertaking HIS implementation, the Calgary General Hospital in Calgary, Canada, identified masterfiles as one of the critical components which provides HIS stability and structure. The hospital focused on developing masterfiles consistent with institutional needs and policy.

As the Calgary General Hospital found, combining a modular structure with a masterfile component results in flexibility. The hospital can develop

114

an HIS consistent with its organization and role. It can adapt the HIS to various departments within the hospital by allowing variations in tests/procedures performed. Moreover, the hospital can improve efficiency, first, through automation itself, and second, through linking related information in the masterfiles. These efficiencies reduce the time nurses must spend on clerical tasks and make that time available to improve the quality of patient care.

To ensure that patient care benefited from the HIS installation, Calgary assigned a special and distinct role to nursing, involving nursing throughout the entire process and creating a new role known as masterfile analyst, a role uniquely suited to and effectively filled by a nurse.

The Masterfile Concept

All HIS contain a component similar to masterfiles, but nomenclature does vary. What are called *masterfiles* in the Unisys PRN 2000 HIS, are *service masters* in the Shared Medical Services HIS and *tables* in the Technicon Data System. Within each system, this component serves basically the same purpose and function, although the information contained may differ.

Although the term *masterfile* is not extensively used in the literature, most often it is defined as an index for large amounts of information on a particular subject for the purposes of storage and accessibility. In a pharmacy system, for example, information may be stored relating to the medications stocked, price, desired route of administration, contraindications for use, drug interactions, and common side effects (Bradish 1982; Strand, Cipolle, and Zaske 1981). Like a filing system, the information is retrieved, utilized, and readily available to be utilized again, either in the immediate or the more distant future. In an HIS, the masterfiles provide data storage, but also are accessed for processing transactions.

Data storage within the HIS masterfiles is provided in hierarchical form, and may be accessed on one or more levels for the processing of transactions (Figure 1):

- Within the hospital masterfiles, information general to the entire hospital is stored. This information includes the valid services, valid financial classes, valid isolation types, and other information of a similar nature.

- Within the department masterfiles, information specific to the department is stored. Examples of this type of information include the department identification, location, telephone extension, and report numbering sequence for the department.

- The procedure masterfiles contain the most specific information representing the greatest number of files within the system. There is a specific masterfile for each procedure, test, or diet that patients may receive. At the Calgary General Hospital, there are 800 diagnostic imaging procedures alone.

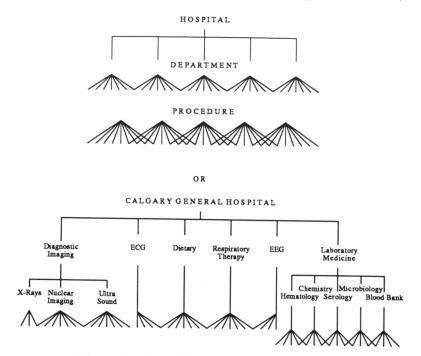

Figure 1. Hierarchical Structure of Masterfiles

The information components are referred to as codes and parameters. The codes represent data accessed within a masterfile (control). The parameters assist in determining the means of processing. To be transmitted, a request must be entered in a manner consistent with the information stored in the codes and parameters of the procedure, department, and hospital files.

Communication Linkages

An HIS provides online communication links between hospital departments. Within an HIS, masterfiles provide flexibility in the processing and communication of orders throughout the hospital. Completion of order entry for a single procedure at the nursing unit level produces notifications or requisitions in all indicated automated departments. Figure 2 compares manual and automated order processing.

Prior to automation, the coordination of such a test or procedure was accomplished only by placing numerous telephone calls. Misinterpreted or misplaced messages, often the result of poor telephone communications, could ultimately result in delaying completion of the procedure.

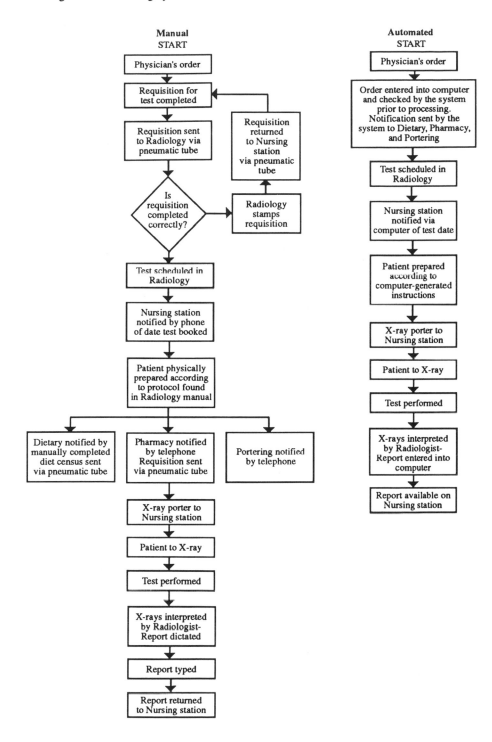

Figure 2. Comparison of Manual and Automated Order Processing

Accuracy of Input

Masterfiles indicate all required entries related to a specific test or procedure. This is accomplished by the codes and parameters stored within the masterfile. The codes may be as rudimentary as "Are height, weight, and blood pressure required for this test?" If YES is entered as the parameter related to the codes of height, weight, and blood pressure, these information pieces have to appear on the request entered into the system. If the entry is incomplete, processing stops and the person entering the orders immediately receives an error message highlighted and flashing on the screen. Ideally, the error message indicates the specific code and parameter where information should be added, deleted, or altered (Figure 3).

Incorrectly entered and processed information can potentially have adverse effects on patient care in the hospital setting. To prevent errors from occurring, flags can be set in the masterfiles. The ability of the system to inform the user of incorrect entries ensures validity and consistency among all users. In addition, the control and processing functions serve as concurrent audits of each request for quality assurance purposes.

The masterfile structure has the additional advantage of allowing information to be altered with relative ease, without difficult and time consuming programming changes.

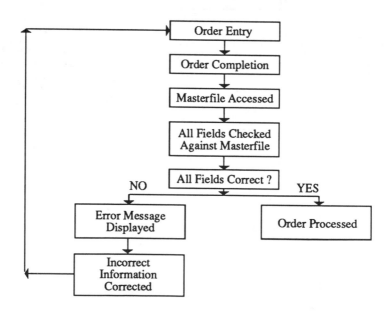

Figure 3. Order Entry Feedback Loop

Developing the Masterfiles

Technical Process

At the Calgary General Hospital, the decision was made to begin by communicating information for patient care; thus, the modules first installed were for admission/discharge/transfer (A/D/T) and order entry/results reporting. The procedure masterfiles developed for these modules can easily reach up to 2,000 procedures, depending on the size and scope of the acute care hospital. The benefits of automation are apparent when time and effort involved in manually coordinating that number of procedures are considered.

The procedure file for a computerized tomography (CT) of the abdomen demonstrates the coordination of events that occurs when a single procedure masterfile is accessed. Automated departments receiving orders entered from the nursing unit include dietetics, diagnostic imaging, pharmacy, and central stores. They then initiate appropriate action related to the CT. On completion, a report of the CT is sent to the nursing unit. The interaction provides evidence of the efficiency factor of automation.

The experience at Calgary General suggests that the most efficient implementation of an HIS establishes the A/D/T module prior to automation of order entry/results reporting. This enables registration of the patient within the system to allow lateral communication to occur across modules. The link between the two modules is the patient's registration number within the HIS.

All departments involved must enter into a collaborative effort when masterfiles are developed. Generally, this is during the pre-conversion phase of the implementation process, when learning is occurring across all disciplines regarding

- The system itself, its potential, and limitations for use

- The group process involved in assuming a project of such magnitude

Relearning also takes place, as departments closely examine how requests are handled manually and how departments interact. This phase before conversion is the time to determine the feasibility of automating those interactions.

Group Process

This collaborative group cannot succeed without strong leadership, capable of building trust and confidence among individuals with varied perspectives. Such leadership is critical in ensuring that the conclusions of the group will benefit the institution as a whole and that support is at hand once implementation is under way.

Individuals from different departments will view the functions performed within the hospital in varying ways. The administrator and upper level managers will have more global or macroscopic perspectives than individuals functioning solely within a department. Even within departments, staff may have a very clear understanding of how their area performs various functions but may be unfamiliar with how those functions support other departments or overall hospital functioning.

An understanding of the automated system's capabilities and a review of interdepartmental interactions provides a basis for developing the masterfiles. The hospital masterfiles contain information that may be accessed by all modules and departments; departmental masterfiles also contain information frequently accessed by most of the HIS modules. Since all departments will access these masterfiles, they should all have input into the development process. The process adhered to in establishing hospital and department masterfiles will assist departments in subsequent development of procedure files, if necessary.

Protocols should be established to control the method by which masterfiles are entered into an automated system. The use of a procedure coding form can facilitate this process. The form can be a representation of the online screen where codes, parameters, and flags are entered for procedure masterfiles. Ideally, an individual who possesses a clear understanding of how the system functions and how masterfiles were established would possess the skills to complete the procedure coding forms.

When entering masterfile information into the system, the codes, parameters, and flags can be set or entered exactly in the manner in which they appear on the forms. The actual task of masterfile entry may be completed by a data entry clerk. However, the chance of entry error is greater if this task is delegated to an individual who was not involved in the development phase of the masterfiles or who lacks comprehension of system functionality. A stringent review process should be followed to ensure integrity of the masterfiles.

Testing

Following data entry and verification of the masterfiles, the testing of the files is a crucial requirement prior to their release for use by HIS users. Evaluation of the functionality of the masterfiles should also determine whether or not the software performs as expected or as documented by the vendor. Testing of the masterfiles should be done according to a well developed and detailed plan that determines whether

- Established parameters yield predictable results. For example, a procedure masterfile with "once" set in the frequency field should generate only one requisition, given that other appropriate flags have been set.

- Established masterfiles are functional. For example, the masterfiles should operate in synchronicity with pre-implementation system analysis, recommendations and/or newly established operations, and current hospital policies and procedures.

Patient case scenarios can be used to test the functionality of the masterfiles. For example, actual ordered tests from the nursing unit areas to the department can be used to test diagnostic imaging masterfile procedures. A detailed matrix can be developed to evaluate expected outcomes relative to the codes and parameters set in the masterfiles. Expected outcomes and actual outcomes are listed horizontally across the top of the matrix; each department that assisted in developing the masterfiles should review the test plan and expected outcomes to ensure their validity.

Following their review of the test plan, the involved departments should also actively participate in the testing of the masterfiles. Entering the orders to test the procedure masterfiles and documenting the outcomes in the matrix will assist in ensuring that hospital procedures and policies are adhered to. To ensure that patient safety is not compromised, the masterfile test must also validate each code/flag and parameter set.

Without question, the testing process will take time and may prolong the implementation phase. However, there is nothing more devastating to the implementation of a product than the threat to the safety of patient care and the loss of confidence if it fails to meet user expectations or to maintain institutional policies.

Maintenance

Although masterfiles generally need few alterations once established, maintenance may be required for varying reasons. If the testing phase succeeded in ensuring that the masterfiles released to HIS users are functional, the changes after implementation will be minor. The dynamic nature of the hospital environment often necessitates alterations in the masterfiles to accommodate changes evolving in patient care. However, even minimal changes taking little time may have significant impact upon the system. Policies and procedures for maintenance must be established so that the integrity of the masterfiles is preserved at all times.

A formal procedure for requesting required changes should be established, with a standard form to ensure that notifications for changes requested are documented and received in a consistent manner from all departments. The form should require the signature of an individual designated by the department to authorize requests. The departmental designate can also act as the contact person should questions or concerns arise from the requests. Ideally, one individual should receive, review, and process requests.

Coordination is required when departments request implementation of changes or enhancements, as in all other phases of the process regarding the masterfiles. Earlier, in the development phase, coordination is required to link within the system the various roles departments assume in performing tests or procedures. Coordination is also significant in the consideration of policy and procedural changes. As the number of operational automated systems increases, questions arise regarding their implication in legal matters. Thus, policies related to the automated system assume paramount importance. All policies must establish communication channels as well as link those with responsibility for initiating changes.

The development of automated information management systems necessitates alterations to previously established (i.e., manual) ways of performing functions at the nursing unit level. These alterations must be reflected in written form, governing, for example, the processing of physician orders or the recording policies.

Clearly, wherever automated systems are installed, security is of concern. Because the masterfiles contain information that is vital to the operation of the hospital, restricted access to the files is essential. Individuals who do not understand the ramifications associated with altering the files could jeopardize both the care of the individual patient and the well being of the institution.

The Masterfile Analyst Role

For all the considerations mentioned above, the development, integration, and maintenance of masterfiles within HIS necessitates nursing involvement at all stages of the process, beginning at the earliest phase. This need can best be met by creating a masterfile analyst function and officially designating a position to fulfill this function. Ideally, the individual selected for such a position should have demonstrated experience in the system development phase as well as a macroscopic hospital perspective. Of course, involving nursing in the development phase would assist in satisfying the first characteristic. The second characteristic—the global perspective—is inherent in nursing. In the designated role of masterfile analyst, a nurse can perform the duties and responsibilities involved in every phase of the process.

In the development phase, the masterfile analyst is responsible for maintaining patient care as the focal point when the processing of transactions is addressed. Through education and experience, the nurse has a unique understanding of the roles various departments play in completing tests or procedures. Historically, it has been the responsibility of nursing to coordinate manually the patient's activities during hospitalization. Individuals from outside nursing are often aware of the responsibilities other departments have in the process. Nursing, however, is aware of each involvement and provides invaluable input in implementing HIS modules and masterfiles.

In the maintenance phase as well, a nurse offers special characteristics appropriate to the masterfile analyst position. The ability fostered in nursing education to analyze information and to develop problem solving strategies based on that information has been cited among the attributes enabling nurses to work within systems (Jaekle 1988). Other traits nurse educators endeavor to develop within their students are interpersonal skills and a dedication to the role of patient advocate. These interpersonal skills, refined through experience gained at the patient's bedside or in nursing management, are relevant to the masterfile analyst, who must work to negotiate issues by incorporating the input of several disciplines simultaneously. Nurses are also characterized by the ability to practice diplomacy and to make decisions based on limited information or in unprecedented situations, abilities helpful to masterfile analysts. All of these abilities assume added significance because hospitals translating to automated systems tend to lack personnel skilled in systems development.

The role of nursing in HIS implementation and masterfile development is critically important if those activities are to achieve their goals for patient care. As care givers and patient advocates, nurses are keenly aware of the impact that decisions related to hospital operations can have on patient care. During development and after implementation, a nurse functioning as masterfile analyst can determine whether practices should remain consistent or be altered when the change is made from manual to automated systems. Throughout, the nurse/masterfile analyst can serve as change agent and suggest alternatives that uphold the interests of the patient.

An appropriate reporting structure for the nurse/masterfile analyst position is critical to its success. Reporting outside of nursing allows no capacity to speak for and represent the nursing perspective and no capacity to influence and bring about change within the nursing division. Individuals reporting within the nursing administrative structure as specialists in the area of systems are warmly received by the nurses functioning at the unit level. In a role clearly rooted in the evolving field of nursing informatics, the nurse/masterfile analyst can communicate the concerns of the nurse at the unit level to the computer staff, using technical language they can understand. The mutual respect between nurses in these two very different roles produces a rare relationship conducive to solving problems and providing high quality patient care.

Summary

Clearly, many benefits can be derived from the masterfile component of an HIS. Information needs can be met regardless of the hospital's particular organizational structure, and the system can be adapted to various departments within the hospital. Building on the linkages provided by the HIS, the masterfiles can link common features while allowing for variations within specific units in the types of tests or procedures performed. High level automation benefits nursing, the other departments involved, and thus the hospital. Even more important than efficiency gains, however, is the enhancement of patient care.

By acknowledging the role of nursing in integrating patient care and assigning the masterfile analyst function to a nurse who reports to nursing, the hospital makes a vital step toward ensuring that the system implementation is smooth and that patient care is always held in the fore.

The flexibility that HIS and the masterfile approach allow is especially important in the healthcare sector, which must keep pace with technological advancements, alterations in practice based on new research findings, and changes in the patient populations served in hospital settings. Moreover, within a single hospital or among several, different departments handle similar transactions in a variety of ways. The complexity of healthcare services offered demands the functional capabilities of masterfiles and the global perspective of nursing.

Questions

1. What are masterfiles?

2. What should nursing's role be regarding masterfiles?

3. What are the benefits of masterfiles?

4. How are masterfiles arranged within the HIS?

5. How can system security related to masterfiles be ensured?

References

Bradish, R. A. 1982. Changing an automated drug inventory control system to a database design. *American Journal of Hospital Pharmacy* 39:1502-5.

Jaekle, B. 1988. The role of nurse as system's analyst. In *Nursing Informatics*, ed. M. J. Ball, K. J. Hannah, U. Gerdin Jelger, and H. Peterson, 103-5. New York: Springer-Verlag.

Peterson, H. and U. Gerdin Jelger. 1988. Hospital information systems. In *Nursing Informatics*, ed. M. J. Ball, K. J. Hannah, U. Gerdin Jelger, and H. Peterson, 182-9. New York: Springer-Verlag.

Strand, L. M., R. J. Cipolle, and D. E. Zaske. 1981. Cost of developing a computerized drug file. *American Journal of Hospital Pharmacy* 38:1334-6.

4
Nursing's Relationship with Information Systems Vendors

Linda Kock

The relationship that a healthcare institution has with a software vendor can significantly affect the implementation of applications and programs. The probability of success is increased if those people involved assume the responsibility for creating positive business relationships rather than wait for them to happen.

Historically, business relationships usually have been formed between the vendor and the purchasing department or the information systems department. However, when organizations pursue total integrated systems in the area of information systems, as healthcare institutions are doing today, the actual user department needs to be heavily involved in establishing positive working relationships with the vendors of information systems.

Frequently, when a healthcare institution is purchasing computer applications, the emphasis is placed on the tangible aspects of system selection, system design, and product comparison. Little attention is given to the interpersonal dynamics and interactions that affect the success of any acquisition.

This chapter deals with one nursing department's role in relating to the software vendor by being involved in the selection and implementation of a totally integrated hospital information system.

The Parkview Memorial Hospital Experience

Located in Fort Wayne, Indiana, the Parkview Memorial Hospital has 600 beds and reported 159,284 patient days in 1988. Parkview Memorial is a general, not for profit hospital. A tertiary care facility with inhouse emergency room staff and critical care units, it offers a full range of medical and surgical services.

125

Background

Until 1985, the nursing department at Parkview Memorial had not been involved in the world of CRTs, personal computers, screen design, and downtime. Many of the nurses were quite content to leave it that way. However, some of them were more adventurous and curious and wanted to enjoy the benefits of fast turnaround of information and less paperwork. When they saw these benefits accruing in some of the larger ancillary departments like laboratory and radiology, they decided to develop a position for a patient care systems coordinator. This nurse was responsible for bridging the gap or breaking the language barrier between the data processing department and the nursing department.

Nursing requires organization, interpretation, and processing of copious data routinely. Through formal education and clinical experience, nurses are expert investigators and problem solvers. These attributes, coupled with an understanding of the hospital environment, make nurses invaluable assets in promoting automation in healthcare (Donne 1987).

At the time Parkview began to select an integrated system, their laboratory system was the only standalone system interfaced to the mainframe. The accounting system was several years old and, with increased federal reimbursement regulations on the horizon, had outgrown its functionality. Radiology had a system developed inhouse about six years earlier. The dietary department's system had been developed inhouse about a year prior, with the involvement of the individual who later became the patient care systems coordinator representing nursing. Diet orders and floor stock items could be ordered online by the clerk at the nursing unit.

Nursing was in the process of working with pharmacy to develop a pharmacy system which included multiple nursing functions. After about two years' work, the system had been implemented in the pharmacy department, but the nursing functions in the system had not yet been implemented. The other ancillary departments of cardiopulmonary, respiratory, rehabilitative services, social services, and central services had no automated systems.

The nursing department began to push the data processing department to develop something useful to nursing as the hub of all patient order and result communication. A committee of nursing representatives identified functions that were needed or wanted. Priorities were then set according to which functions would result in the most significant time savings. After reviewing these needs with the laboratory and radiology departments, nursing submitted their requests to the data processing department.

Since the laboratory and radiology departments had online departmental systems, the decision was made that the best and quickest way to get benefits for nursing personnel was to make results on those systems available online for nursing. This proved to be positive in many ways:

- Minimal technical time made results available on the nursing units
- Nursing personnel learned to interact with the CRT without fear of losing information

- Nurses and unit clerks were stimulated to want more functions made available
- Phone calls between the laboratory and the nursing units were noticeably reduced

Developing the Vendor Relationship

System Selection

In the fall of 1986, the administrative direction of the hospital was to pursue selection and purchase of an integrated hospital information system rather than to continue inhouse development which had been minimal to that point in time.

The selection team consisted of the patient care system coordinator, the director of the information system department, the vice president of finance, and a representative of nursing administration. The process of system selection began with the development of a detailed application specification list. Specifications were prioritized with the input of various nursing representatives, information system personnel, and ancillary department personnel. Criteria were set by the administrative information system steering committee.

Because of the type of hardware being used, the field was narrowed to two of the major vendors. These two finalists were then critically reviewed. One method used to evaluate the two systems being considered was to conduct a series of reference checks.

A set of questions was developed for a phone survey of current users of each system. The users to be contacted were selected by nursing from a total list of users provided by each company. Two nurses completed the majority of phone calls. Some of the questions asked were:

- How long have you had the system installed?
- What departments are implemented?
- Describe your satisfaction with the system in regard to functionality, support, education.
- Did you complete a cost benefits analysis?
- What is your experience with downtime?
- What departmental systems did you have to interface with?
- Who completed the interface, your institution or the vendor?
- If you had it to do over, what would you do differently?

The part of the total product that the nursing department was particularly interested in—nursing orders, care plans, and charting—had not been implemented fully in any hospital. Therefore, nursing had to rely heavily on the information received from the hospital that was the alpha test site for the product.

Neither vendor being considered objected to the reference checks, a fact that added to their credibility. Though time consuming, it proved to be a valuable selection process. Certainly, "for a decision of such magnitude, it should be worth the trouble, and yes, even the expense" (Randall 1988).

Contributing to the decision about which system was more appropriate for Parkview Memorial were site visits to several of the users with whom the committee had made phone contacts. Each company's vendor representatives, who accompanied the committee members on the site visits, made the arrangements and assumed responsibility for the costs of the visits. In addition to fostering a relationship among the committee members and the vendor representatives, the site visits were particularly helpful in supplying information on how the systems being viewed worked. To take the best advantage of the site visits, a list of questions was prepared in advance and used as a guide when talking with users on site. The author was favorably impressed by the vendor representatives' willingness to absent themselves from discussions with personnel at the site; this practice was seen as evidence that the vendor was exerting no influence on answers the visitors received.

During the product demonstrations and the many meetings clarifying what the product would do, the business relationship continued to develop. The author and perhaps other members of the selection committee had a skeptical attitude toward vendors, and suspected high pressure salespeople of being interested only in the sale and not in satisfying the customer. This perception was dispelled through the many meetings that were held to select the system that would most appropriately meet Parkview's needs.

"Vendor support throughout the term of the agreement seems to be the thrust of most vendors' marketing efforts. Development of a long term relationship (a marriage as some would describe it) is based upon each party participating in such a relationship" (Andrew 1989).

Negotiations

Following the selection of HBO's Clinipac system, the hospital and the vendor entered into a series of meetings to negotiate various terms of the contract. Throughout this process, the nursing representatives remained integrally involved in the discussions. Items specified in the contract dealt with such key areas as

- Implementation support
- Education/training needs
- Participation in future enhancements

Since the decision had been made to develop screens for the current design for applications already installed, Parkview Memorial opted for a two year implementation plan. Convinced that they would need less support later in the implementation stage or that they would need to implement the smaller ancillary departments, the hospital focused on the upswing of the learning curve. The resulting contract called for intensive support during the early phase of implementation.

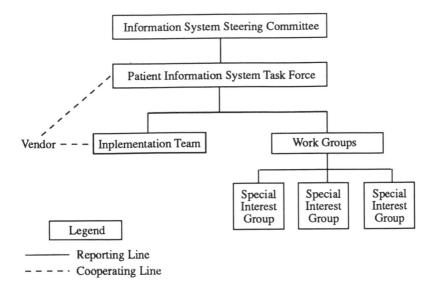

Figure 1. Project Organization

Maintaining the Relationship

Implementation

After a yearlong selection process, Parkview Memorial purchased a total information system. Now ready to develop a detailed implementation plan, the hospital identified an organizational structure to be used for communication flow and decision making. The intent of the structure was to involve all the departments in defining and resolving issues (Figure 1).

The information system steering committee comprised the vice presidents of finance, patient care, medical staff, and ancillary departments, and the director of information systems. This group provided the overall direction for the project. Policies were made by this group based on recommendations from the patient information system task force, which met monthly.

The task force membership included department directors from laboratory and radiology, the vice presidents of patient care and medical staff, the patient care systems coordinator, the project manager from information systems, a management engineer, and the patient care system project director.

The implementation team was the technical group that met weekly. Membership in this group included two programmers, a programmer analyst, a management engineer, the patient care systems coordinator, and the information systems project director.

The departmental work groups were composed for the most part of users from nursing and whatever department was being worked on at the time. The representatives from nursing, including both registered nurses and unit clerks, would gather input from their respective peers either in their own unit meetings or through special interest groups representing the various specialties in nursing, such as obstetrics, emergency care, intensive care, and psychiatry. By establishing work groups, the organization plan fostered the development of a network linking large numbers of soon to be users.

In the first six months of implementation, the same vendor support representative was on site an average of three days a week and functioned as a team member. On occasion, meetings of the task force and the implementation team benefited from the representative's technical expertise and indepth familiarity with the product in solving program issues.

When Parkview Memorial was ready to go live with the first departments, two vendor support persons assisted with the multiple, round the clock training sessions required for approximately 800 patient care personnel. At this point in the process, the relationship between vendor and hospital was particularly intense. Vendor support representatives were almost perceived as hospital employees, and the business account manager from the vendor company visited periodically to maintain contact and provide any additional direction or support needed from his level.

Benefits

As the vendor representatives became better acquainted with Parkview Memorial Hospital and its staff, several positive outcomes occurred:

- The vendor was so favorably impressed by the pharmacy system the hospital had developed inhouse that they purchased it to make their line of products more complete.

- The hospital worked with the vendor to develop some new enhancements of their current product.

- The hospital was viewed as a premier institution in the hospital marketplace and was asked by the vendor to accommodate several site visits for potential customers. Site visits can take some time, but it is time well spent because it gave Parkview the opportunity to network with counterparts in hospitals all over the country.

The experience at Parkview Memorial is proof that integrated systems are possible in healthcare, and that nursing must play a role in their selection and implementation. Process and structure are indeed important; but mutually beneficial results require efforts on the part of both the vendor and the buyer to foster a positive business relationship and constructive human interaction. Involving nursing, the end user and the hub of patient information, as an equal partner is a critical step.

Questions

1. Why is it important for nursing to be involved in system selection as well as system implementation?

2. What are some questions that might be asked in a software product reference check in addition to those listed in the chapter?

3. How are people made to feel part of a team?

References

Andrew, W. F. 1989. Current trends in HMIS: Part II. *U.S. Healthcare* (March):35-8.
Donne, M. 1987. Nursing opportunities in information management. *Computers in Healthcare* (April):49-52.
Randall, A. 1988. Reference checks—How good are they? *U.S. Healthcare* (December):35-6.

5

Technology Assisted Training for the Clinical Nurse

Patsy B. Marr

To become part of a technologically advanced medical environment, nurses must master the new skills required to manage the computerized hospital information system. In most cases, nurses either have not used such systems before, or have had minimal exposure to them. Yet nursing effectiveness is directly related to the speed and accuracy nurses bring to this core communications vehicle. The assimilation of nurses into the culture of the computer is essential not only to patient care but also to the well being of the care givers themselves.

Understandably, many people approach new technology with apprehension. Any training program designed to help nurses learn to use a hospital information system must therefore be positive, based on sound adult learning theory and appropriate goal setting. The learning environment must encourage openness and self pacing.

Nurses need to emerge from training with a grasp of the basics and an enthusiasm for learning more once they are back in the clinical setting. Further, nurses need to be sensitized to the issues of patient confidentiality, password security, and quality control. When fully experienced with such systems, nurses can become part of the change process itself, helping to enhance the use of such technology. In short, the training of system users needs to be as advanced as the system itself.

Training Theory

A sound training program is based on adult learning theories. Foremost among these concepts is that adults want to participate in their own learning process and want to help shape their own goals. Other considerations in designing the program are that adults want to learn in order to meet work needs and that they tend to relate new information to relevant experiences (O'Conner 1986).

132

Accordingly, in the design of a hospital information system, computerizing the manually documented nursing process will help the nurse relate the familiar to the new and different communication technology. For example, a computerized chart can be made to resemble a sample patient chart from the manual era before the system. Similarly, other items can be made to resemble their earlier counterparts, such as supply or laboratory requisitions, medication administration forms, and nursing work documents like the patient kardex or nursing unit activity report. This enables the nurse to make the connection between the computer as a communication tool and day to day unit activities.

Certainly the most successful training programs are computer driven, with numerous pathways from which to select the level of detail a learner needs. This ability to interactively manage diverse data on the computer itself is a recent technological development popular with the adult learner.

Training Program Goals

At the conclusion of training, nurses should have a basic understanding of the relationship of the hospital information system to the functions of their specific jobs. It is not realistic to expect them to be fully skilled upon completing the training course. That comes only with practice in the clinical area. But the training goal has been achieved if the participating nurses understand the principal functions managed by the system and the essentials of how to use those functions.

System orientation and hands on training should occur not more than two weeks before the nurses will put this learning to use on the job. While the centralized course offers overall concepts that are reinforced through practice examples during training, it is through the daily use of the system in the clinical setting that computer skills and the finer points of system capabilities are learned. Some learning occurs through trial and error, but experienced nurses on the unit serve as the most valuable resource.

Training Environment

The ideal setting in which to learn basic computer skills is a room designed specifically for this purpose, a quiet environment with indirect lighting to prevent glare on terminal screens. A typing chair, with both back and height adjustments, is essential. The terminal is best positioned on a surface at a height that is comfortable for data entry as well as screen reading. Data entry and retrieval may be by touch screen, light pen, keyboard, or a computer mouse, the small touch device with multidirectional arrows used for selecting specific functions or data.

It is helpful to have the training center close enough to the clinical units to be both convenient and separate enough to limit distractions. The right location will allow the trainer and trainee to focus on the concepts and content of the training program. A clinically trained instructor should be either in the room or readily available to answer any questions. Many hospitals have found that more questions are related to clinical content in the system than to the mechanics of using a computer.

Most training is accomplished by use of programmed instruction manuals. Recently, however, training has moved to the computer through the use of interactive learning modules. These modules present general concepts, specific examples, and immediate feedback, enabling the student to experience an environment that approaches real life. This method allows the adult learner to actively participate in the learning process at an individualized pace and provides opportunity to measure progress toward goals (O'Conner 1986). Not only is this the method preferred by students, but it has added benefits. Institutions that have moved from programmed instruction manuals to computer based training have reduced their training and instructor time and have improved training quality (Perez and Willis 1989).

Finally, it is important to create a learning atmosphere of trust, respect, and helpfulness. Nurses learn by connecting new information to past knowledge; a comfortable atmosphere allows the students freedom to express concerns, questions, or apprehensions they may have about the system (O'Conner 1986). Training can encompass much more than the simple use of the system when nurses are taught by an experienced nurse instructor who has sophisticated clinical and organizational knowledge in addition to system expertise.

Quality Control in Training

The major areas of concern in maintaining quality control include accuracy in using a system, the timeliness of data entry, and completeness of system documentation. Depending upon the specific system, there can be predetermined program edits that prevent inaccurate or illogical data from being entered. In hospital information systems, however, the use of these edits is minimal because of information complexity. Most systems enable the user to view information as it is being collected and to correct the error at that time. Other systems offer only a final review of data immediately before entry, enabling verification and/or deletion and correction.

The importance of timely data entry is more difficult to convey to nurses than the importance of accuracy. Historically, except for medications, nurses have always charted at the end of their shifts rather than sequentially throughout the shift. With the installation of a hospital information system, it is often expected that this will change. It seldom does. What usually happens is that whatever charting patterns existed prior to computerization are replicated when the system is installed. It is also difficult to monitor compliance with timeliness. Some systems accommodate data entry time guidelines which, when exceeded, produce management reports that can be used to help monitor timeliness. With the current trend of placing terminals at each patient bedside or in every patient room, there is preliminary evidence that documentation is occurring at or nearer the time of the event (Halford et al. 1989).

The third area of quality control addressed in the training program is completeness of documentation. Even though the examples in the training modules emphasize documentation standards, it is daily follow up by nursing leadership that addresses the completeness issue. This quality control item is so closely related to the standard of care delivery that only expert clinicians can do the monitoring.

Two more factors must be considered when addressing quality concerns in a training course. First, printed documentation carries a sense of finality and not to be questioned accuracy. New practitioners must be specifically instructed to question a printed medical order entered by a physician just as they would a handwritten order. They should not assume that a computer generated order is unquestionably accurate. The computer does not alter the nurse's professional obligation to question and to verify any order.

Second, new users of the hospital information system must be advised to go slowly in the system until their skills are well developed. When nurses finish the training program and begin to work with a seasoned user in the clinical setting, they often feel compelled to match the experienced user's speed. But speed will come. Training must emphasize accuracy rather than speed.

Maintaining Confidentiality

Converting the patient record from a handwritten document to a computer generated document changes the procedures to be followed in maintaining patient confidentiality. Policy, however, does not change. The institution continues to be responsible for maintaining the confidentiality of the patient's health record.

With manually generated documents, there is only one copy of the data, located in the patient chart on the nursing unit. To access these clinical data, care givers go to the unit and identify themselves as having approval to review and/or responsibility for caring for an individual patient. With computerized data, access is different. The information may be accessed from any terminal in the medical center. Patient records may be reviewed by any healthcare team member who has permission to access that category of data. Depending on the parameters of code assigned, a team member can privately review data for any patient in the system at any given time, regardless of who is responsible for the care of that specific patient.

This makes it mandatory that users of the system never share their sign on code with anyone. Training must make it clear that each sign on code uniquely identifies an individual to the system by name and title, gives approval to carry out certain system functions, and provides access to patient data appropriate to the user's title and job function. It is the same as a handwritten signature, and attaches the person's name and title to all patient clinical data entered into the system. Because various groups of the healthcare team have access to this large clinical database, the professional obligation to maintain patient confidentiality must be reinforced with every individual.

Introducing Changes to Seasoned Users

Hospital information systems are never static. Drugs are added and deleted from the formulary, new radiologic procedures are developed while others become obsolete, and items obtained from central supply change with the current vendor. Since system programs have the capability to require specific information entry before the user proceeds through a given function, regulatory mandates can be met through system design. These mandates include the source of patient referral when a patient is admitted, clinical indication for doing invasive radiology procedures, and management reports for patients waiting for nursing home beds to become available.

If, in the initial design of the system, a standard protocol is followed for certain symbols and sequences of logic, then new capabilities added to the system can be readily communicated to users. Two major methods are used to inform staff of changes. The most common one is a system newsletter addressed to the affected user groups, including a description of the new function, an example of the change, and the date and time the change will become effective. The other method, which may be used in conjunction with the newsletter or as a standalone, is to insert a message or help screen in the appropriate system module to tell users of the change they are about to encounter. This screen is left in the system only until all users have had an opportunity to become proficient in the new function, a process that usually takes two to four weeks. Only rarely is a change so complex that system instructors need to meet with users to demonstrate the added capability. An integral part of training should include information on how system changes are communicated.

Seasoned Users as Change Agents

Mature systems have seasoned users as change agents. They are a rich source of new ideas and creativity for system functions that uniquely benefit the user. Their involvement promotes system ownership, pride in contributions, and motivation for bigger and better system functionality. When this environment emerges, it must be nurtured and encouraged in order to take advantage of the added value (Marr 1988).

Often, user committees are formed to create ideas. In most cases, the nursing committee proves to be the most dynamic in generating ideas. Nurses who are comfortable in hospital culture, knowledgeable in the practice of nursing, and skilled in the use of the system become proactive system users, not reactive users. In a real sense, such nurses become part of the institution's training and development process.

Hospital information systems are dynamic, changing communication tools. Nurses must, therefore, be students of the system, keeping abreast of its changes and even participating in them. Properly trained and actively encouraged, nurses can come to regard the system as a tool integral to their professional practice.

Questions

1. Name one or two adult learning theories that are useful in teaching nurses to master hospital information systems.

2. How soon before nurses use the computer on the job should they receive training?

3. Why is it important to have a nurse instructor available even when system training can be self instructional?

4. What are two or three quality issues to be addressed in a hospital information system training program?

5. What is different about maintaining patient confidentiality in a computerized environment?

References

Halford, G., M. Burkes, and T. A. Pryor. 1989. Measuring the impact of bedside terminals. *Nursing Management* 20:41-5.

Marr, P. B. 1988. Successful implementation of a hospital information system. In *Nursing and Computers; Third International Symposium on Nursing Use of Computers and Information Science*, ed. T. Lochhaas, 781-6. St. Louis, Missouri: C. V. Mosby Company.

O'Conner, A. B. 1986. *Nursing staff development and continuing education.* Boston: Little, Brown and Company.

Perez, L. D., and P. H. Willis. 1989. CBT product improves training quality at reduced cost. *Computers in Healthcare* (July):28-30.

Section 1–Supporting the Practitioner

Unit 4—Acquiring Information Systems Expertise

Unit Introduction

To realize a return on investment in information technology, healthcare institutions must ensure that their staff become competent users. Training is an essential part of the equation, yet often is overlooked in the demanding implementation phase. This unit focuses on encouraging physician and other end user involvement.

Victoroff, a family practice physician in private practice, and Timm, manager of a medical informatics center in a suburban hospital, relate how they set up a computer "store" to expose physicians to microcomputer applications. An information scientist involved in teaching nursing informatics students, Sutherland proposes an organizational structure supportive of healthcare professionals as end users of computing. An internist, Peterson stresses the importance of physician use of computers and highlights the role of information systems in quality assurance functions mandated by the Joint Commission on Accreditation of Healthcare Organizations.

The power of computing to improve patient care can not be realized until it is diffused and integrated into the practice setting. Educating healthcare professionals is key.

1
An Approach to Physician Computer Exposure

Michael S. Victoroff and Terese M. Timm

Contemporary medicine depends on computers the way 19th century farming depended on horses. In hospitals, virtually every department relies on computing in one form or another. Health workers, from nurses to cooks, find data terminals indispensable to their jobs. Ironically, doctors have been among the last to employ computers in their care of patients. Or more precisely, most doctors have not made direct use of the information handling functions of computers.

Certainly in clinical research, radiology, intensive care units, anesthesia, and other high tech areas, physicians use embedded microprocessors as casually as they use the electronics in microwave ovens and automobile ignitions. Although information is central to the practice of medicine, physicians have been slow to modernize their information management tools, compared to other knowledge workers.

This situation should not be tolerated. Medical care at every level suffers grievously, and needlessly, from poor information handling. The sooner a consistent, integrated, comprehensive health information technology can be adopted, the better the care of patients will become. Computer terminals should be as familiar in examination rooms as stethoscopes. Physicians should become as comfortable with automated clinical information and decision support as they are with human consultants and printed literature. The illegible, static, irretrievable, elusive handwritten chart deserves to go the way of the buggy whip. But before clinical medicine can catch up with 25 years of progress in information systems, profound changes will have to occur in the attitudes of physicians about computers.

Doctors and Computers

Most doctors still associate medical computing with the billing systems often found in their colleagues' offices. They are unaware of the dozens of medical software programs available in areas that reach far beyond accounting, into the heart of clinical medicine. Nor are they familiar with the scores of general purpose programs that could be usefully employed in patient care settings.

While doctors have been cautiously waiting on the sidelines, software has become more relevant to medical care. And computers have been getting smaller, more powerful, cheaper, and easier to use. Medical computing is on a trajectory where availability, acceptability, accountability, and liability will carry it the short step from practical to necessary. When the signal comes to start the new rules in medicine, will physicians be in shape to play the game?

It is not a big leap from laboratory reports that merely flag abnormal values to reports that list causes of abnormal values. Computers have already shown themselves to be comparable to expert clinicians in their ability to diagnose abdominal pain, depression, and rheumatic diseases, prescribe antibiotics, interpret pulmonary function tests, and manage electrolyte disorders. And they are superior to humans at tasks like identifying drug interactions, calculating drug doses, and analyzing diets.

The field of medical informatics promises to give us scores of such expert systems within the next few years. But there is no need to wait for these advanced applications. We can see the value of clinical computing now. Today's computers show their greatest strength in information storage and retrieval—the most basic aspect of modern medicine.

Medical record storage, drug information and interactions, automated histories, diet calculators, and patient recall systems abound. Not all are reliable or accurate, but they will be so soon enough to establish standards. Clinical reference material is easy to access, both on the desktop and in remote databases like the National Library of Medicine's. These references provide information much more up to date than texts and more accessible than journals. Patient and professional education programs are numerous. These are only a few of the applications currently available. It has already been proposed by one consumer lawyer that the failure of a doctor to employ a drug interaction program in certain settings constitutes malpractice.

If this represents the handwriting on the wall (or the CRT), it is imperative that physicians learn to evaluate, critique, operate, and develop the automated systems they will be using in clinical medicine. It behooves every practitioner, hospital, medical school, professional society, and healthcare institution to advance the cause of medical computing out of simple self interest. But what strategy will take medical informatics, like transistors 40 years ago, from laboratory curiosities to full scale service?

How will physicians develop the expertise to use automated clinical systems as they become the standard of care? How much technical sophistication will they require, to operate them? Will doctors use such programs blindly, as they use the controls in elevators? Or will they be responsible for second guessing the work of programmers? What liabilities attach to the use of these new tools? How will patients accept them? How will they affect the costs of healthcare? These questions will not be answered by an abstract, armchair expert approach.

Experience with technological evolution suggests that only direct, so-called dirty hands experimentation can advance the discovery process. The authors predict that the time when major hospital and university departments of medical informatics will be commonplace and necessary is just around the corner. Here, as in departments of radiology, postgraduate physician specialists will provide clinical consulting services to their colleagues, carry out research and development, and pass judgment on evolving standards and products.

However, if the future is clear, the path toward it is not. The following describes one hospital's approach to the problem of recruiting its medical staff to the cause of medical computing.

The Usual and Customary Quagmire

St. Joseph Hospital in Denver, Colorado, realized that getting physicians involved in medical informatics was the key to advancing from administrative information systems to clinical information systems.

A 551 bed, tertiary care, nonprofit hospital operated by the Sisters of Charity of Leavenworth, Kansas, St. Joseph Hospital is part of an eight hospital system located west of the Mississippi River. St. Joseph has an active staff of 500 physicians, mostly subspecialists. It operates a residency program of 100 residents in areas of family practice, internal medicine, surgery, obstetrics and gynecology, and dentistry.

The hospital already had in place a fairly extensive computer information system. A Burroughs/Unisys mainframe served approximately 600 data terminals, providing accounting, order entry, result reporting, and other typical clerical and financial functions.

A scenario ensued that is so classic among hospitals it has become virtually a standard of practice:

- The department of computer information services carried out an extensive analysis of its future needs, drafting a model and a strategy for implementation.

- A search for an off the shelf solution was carried out, with the predictable conclusion: "No one else's system will work for us as well as one we design ourselves."

- On the advice of consultants and the vendor of the existing system, the hospital recommitted itself to a heavy investment in what was called state of the art mainframe technology, along with the requisite staff of programmers, who announced unrealistic target dates for implementing such a large and enhanced new system.

- Potential users had little comprehension of the functions of the system to be built, or the basic process of software design. Nor did the programming staff have any appreciation of the operations in most of the departments affected. Neither group had much of a notion of how to collaborate with the other. The target dates were transformed into cost and time overruns. The system had major problems, and it was everybody else's fault.

• Except in an ex officio capacity, physicians had been excluded from the planning process. It was decided that the system would have its foundations in the existing clerical and financial applications, with clinical functions becoming appended eventually. By the time the medical staff became involved, most fundamental design considerations had already been set in concrete, disabling much of the potential of the system for clinical uses.

When the designers looked to the medical staff for advice, they made disheartening discoveries:

• Physicians were mostly oblivious to the operations of the existing hospital information system. They tended to be suspicious of computers on principle, ignorant of their current value, and unaware of the degree to which they already depended on them.

• Furthermore, the medical staff as a whole was uninterested in clinical applications software, uninformed about its potential value and liabilities, and incompetent to judge proposed applications when presented with them.

• A minority of doctors were actively interested or involved with clinical computing. But they tended to be isolated, and their interests ran to microcomputers rather than mainframes. Moreover, the most knowledgeable tended to be skeptical of the hospital's intentions and capabilities, and were reluctant to be drafted for design assignments.

The hospital concluded that the typical physician was ill equipped to participate in the design of a clinical information system. Worse, physician resistance would probably be the main obstacle to the installation and use of the system, once it was available. And yet, physicians were essential elements in the informatics strategy—they could not be bypassed or neglected.

St. Joseph determined that its future in clinical computing was being impeded by a critical shortage of computer literate physicians. Importing a new medical staff was impractical; the only option was to find and develop computer sophistication among the doctors available.

The Project in Medical Informatics

Through the inspiration of one or two farsighted members of the administration, St. Joseph made physician computer education a priority. The hospital

CEO inaugurated the project in medical informatics, and supported it with direct personal oversight, an expedited budget approval and purchasing process, and vociferous public enthusiasm which reverberated throughout the hospital management structure. Without this level of support, it is unlikely that the project would have succeeded.

An advisory committee defined a set of initial goals:

- To expose as many of the medical staff as possible to medical applications of computer technology, raising the level of knowledge and skill within the medical staff with respect to computers in medicine

- To lure the computer knowledgeable physicians on the medical staff into the open, and encourage them to take the lead among their colleagues

- To demonstrate and test innovative applications which might enhance the hospital's quality of care, effectiveness, and reputation

- To encourage physicians to experiment with computer applications in their own practices, hoping first to link and eventually to capture computer dependent doctors within the web of the hospital's computer network

The long term intent was to recruit or create a cadre of computer knowledgeable physicians, who would contribute to the planning and development of future informatics activities within the hospital, and to secure a symbiotic relationship with a medical staff reliant on hospital computing services.

To accomplish this, it would be necessary to survey the medical staff concerning its current interests, use, and expectations of computers in medicine. The plan was to identify factors inhibiting computer interest and use among physicians, and to devise antidotes to them.

The committee's first step was to recruit one of this paper's authors, a family practice physician on the staff with extensive experience in microcomputer applications in medicine. He was hired by the hospital as a consultant in medical informatics, with the assignment of proposing a plan to accomplish the goals above. The intent was to make this a temporary position, a decision which in retrospect may have sacrificed some benefits.

The core of the proposal was the creation of an office of medical informatics. This paper's other author became its manager, the medical informatics assistant. She was a hospital radiology quality assurance coordinator who had previously done work for a developer of medical software.

The project began with these assumptions:

Microcomputers would be the keys to physicians' hearts.

- PCs offered an immediately comprehensible, minimally threatening, attractive introduction to computing.

- PCs were ubiquitous, affordable, and already in the hands of a significant number of physicians. Clearly they represented the basis of future medical workstations.

- PC software was affordable, easy to teach and learn, and useful in physicians' offices. A wide variety was available for MSDOS and Macintosh hardware, including examples of every type of application imaginable, for both medical and general purposes.

The best way to improve the attitudes, skills, and practices of the medical staff would be to provide opportunities for concentrated, multiphasic, individual exposure to microcomputers in a supportive, low pressure setting.

- Every physician curious about medical computing would have an opportunity to put his or her hands on a keyboard. The aim was for maximum availability with minimal waiting time and no bureaucracy.

- The concern was not whether the visitors mastered Pascal programming or spent their time playing Space Wars. If doctors started using computers for any purposes at all in their own homes and offices, they could start using terminals in the hospital.

The plan was to approach the medical staff by honest seduction, not covert coercion. The intents and aspirations of the project were straightforward.

- Opportunities would be presented on a silver platter. Learning computers would be made attractive and convenient.

- Physicians would be enticed by a wide variety of interesting applications at every level of aptitude.

- No one would be forced or put on the spot.

- The staff would have as much free and painless access to knowledge-able consultation as could be provided. Medical informaticians would be computer evangelists, inspiring enthusiasm and promoting interest. The center would use outside experts to supplement knowledge when this was necessary.

The obvious setting in which to execute this plan would be a storefront office, as prominent as possible within the hospital, supported by lots of public relations and outreach.

The Center for Medical Informatics

So a computer playground was built for doctors. The center appropriated a conference room on the main corridor of the hospital's ground floor, immediately across from the doctors' dining room. It was furnished opulently, with matching oak carrels, chairs, and bookshelves. A bulletin board displayed announcements of educational opportunities in medical informatics. Literature racks held popular personal computing periodicals and pamphlets. A blackboard on one wall was usually covered with diagrams and discussion notes. Software was protected in a locked metal file cabinet, but manuals were kept on open shelves over each of five comfortable workstations. There were two plush chairs and a small coffee table, which invited casual chats.

The desire was to make the shop look as nice as Computerland, and for the same reasons. Tentative computer shoppers, whatever their expertise, are reassured by competence, elegance, and efficiency. After all, the aim was to associate these very qualities with computers.

The bookshelves contained a broad selection of manuals, journals, catalogs, books, software guides, buyer's guides, reviews, videotapes, and articles pertaining to general and medical computing. The collection addressed all levels of interest, from advanced programmers to neophytes.

Extensive files on medical billing systems, clinical systems for patient care, continuing medical education, and manufacturers' brochures on every software product obtainable were accumulated over time. The authors became familiar with a wide variety of programs and demonstrated them frequently to visitors. Before long, volunteers contributed by testing and reviewing hardware and software packages, and reporting on them.

The center's hardware consisted of initial hardware purchases totaling $22,380 that included:

- 1 PC XT (clone) with a 20 MB drive
- 3 PC AT (clones) with 20 or 40 MB drives
- 1 Macintosh SE with a 20 MB drive
- 1 Compaq Portable 286 with an 80 MB drive
- 1 Intelligent PC/workstation connected to the hospital mainframe (Convergent Technologies B-25)
- 1 IBM AT in a moveable workstation located in the doctors' dining room

All the PCs had EGA monitors. In addition, a variety of printers, modems, mice, and other accessories were purchased. In direct contravention of standard institutional practice, the authors deliberately used a variety of vendors representing both brandname and generic computers. This allowed potential buyers to learn something of the differences between sources. Systems in the center were loaded with selected software for demonstrations and self study. The portable computer was loaned to physicians who wanted to evaluate software for a limited time in their offices or at home.

Naturally, the software library was the major attraction of the center. The medical software library would allow physicians to explore the widest possible variety of PC functions. In contrast with their experience purchasing hardware, the authors were pleasantly surprised at how far the initial software budget of less than $8,000 could be stretched. A firm antipiracy policy was observed, but visitors were urged to spend as much time as they liked, working with programs in the center.

Categories on hand initially included 56 general purpose software products (from word processors to DOS utilities) and 48 specialized medical programs, including several demo packages designed to show features of full scale billing systems. These included:

- Spreadsheets, both brand name and shareware

- Database management programs, from simple to top of the line; from general purpose to specialized

- Word processors, popular and obscure

- Medical education and CME packages

- Communication packages

- Graphics

- Larry Weed's Problem Knowledge Coupler

- Medical decision support systems

- Drug information and drug interaction systems

- Patient recall systems

- Medical records systems

- Patient education systems

- Every demo disk the authors could lay their hands on

- Plus an ample selection of games and amusements

Access to remote databases such as AMA/Net, CompuServe, PaperChase, DXplain, etc., was made available. Reference services were coordinated with the hospital librarian, who was extremely supportive of the center's activities.

The center was staffed officially from 7 a.m. to 3 p.m., but often activities kept the authors there after 5 p.m. and on weekends. A key was available after hours for physicians who wanted to work independently. Scheduled appointments accounted for a small percentage of the visitors; most were walk ins. Like a neighborhood saloon, the center soon developed a following of regulars.

Besides the center itself, medical informatics claimed a section of the main hospital bulletin board for announcements relevant to computers in medicine. Announcements and news about the project were published from time to time in the medical staff newsletter.

One aspect of the plan involved "putting a computer where the doctors would have to trip over it." A moveable workstation was furnished containing a PC loaded with a variety of software that was available from a simple menu. This station was installed in a prominent corner of the doctors' dining room/lounge, with a poster inviting doctors to experiment.

In addition to activities within the center itself, the authors ran a busy outreach program. Discussion groups and demonstrations by experts in the medical information field were organized. Presentations were given at medical staff and departmental meetings, research projects by house staff were encouraged, and the authors proselytized at administration meetings, attended CIS planning and training sessions, and visited physicians' offices.

The Budget (1987)

Hardware	$ 28,757.03
Software	$ 5,019.38
Publications	$ 647.69
Office Supplies	$ 1,713.55
Personnel:	
Informatics Consultant @ 2,167/month	$ 8,668.00
Informatics Assistant @ 1,500/month	$ 6,000.00
TOTALS	$ 50,805.65

Early Statistics

Within the first four months of operation:

- 497 visits by physicians and hospital employees were logged at the center

- 69 software packages, books, and manuals were borrowed

- 17 physicians were known to have purchased software packages after demonstrations and discussions in the center

- six programs were formally reviewed by physicians at the center's request; dozens more unsolicited reviews were collected

- four physicians purchased computers and made major changes in their office practices as a direct result of information discussed and gathered in the center

- five more physicians requested consultations with the intent of installing medical office systems

- at least 50 knowledgeable physician computer users among the medical staff were discovered

A users' group formed around the leadership of those knowledgeable physicians. This group eventually supplied experienced individuals to all committees and departments of the hospital requiring assistance in medical computing.

In addition, it was observed that about half of the center visitors were novice users. The rest ranged from experienced users to experts. At least one physician per week visited the center for the first time. There was an average of six to ten visitors per day. An average visit lasted 20 to 30 minutes. Over 300 hours were spent in individual and small group teaching and in consultation with physicians, in a period of four months.

Attending physicians used the center extensively. Residents, teaching faculty, clinical and administrative staff, outside consultants, vendors and developers, and staff affiliated with other Denver hospitals soon came to know of the Medical Informatics Center's existence and purposes.

The center functioned as matchmaker between potential customers and outside vendors, system integrators and consultants, even networking physicians to physicians. It became a gathering point for people interested in computers, at every level of expertise. Surveys were conducted of computer usage and attitudes on the part of the medical staff. These findings were extremely helpful in refining the emphasis, activities, and budget.

Medical Informatics worked in close cooperation with CIS and other hospital departments to coordinate microcomputer and mainframe training, research, and development. Affiliated organizations (large medical group practices) consulted the center on informatics projects of their own. A tremendous grassroots interest was discovered within the staff. St. Joseph Hospital became identified as a leading proponent of medical computing in the Denver area.

Within less than a year, the project had not only met all of its initial expectations, but had exceeded them in almost every category. In addition, benefits were realized in a number of areas that were originally unforeseen.

Accomplishments and Observations

This dedicated center assisted physicians and hospital staff in acquiring basic knowledge of microcomputers and familiarity with potential applications of computers in medical practice.

The components of microcomputer systems appropriate for office use were identified, and products found to be acceptable for several categories of medical applications were recommended. Many physicians perceived this as a very valuable service.

Formal presentations were made to the departments of family practice, medicine, and surgery, describing the center and its purposes. The authors were called upon to advise the admitting office, anesthesia, CIS, diagnostic imaging, emergency room, family practice, laboratory, medical education, medical library, medical staff office, ob/gyn, pathology, pharmacy, physical therapy, and surgery on specific issues in microcomputer hardware and software. Every session produced a small wave of new visitors to the center.

The local Kaiser Permanente group involved the Medical Informatics Center in a project on screening and follow up of women for breast cancer. Kaiser's anesthesia department used the center's equipment and facilities to encourage computer use among its staff. Another large group practice used the services extensively in its development of medical management software.

Several physicians who normally did most of their work at other hospitals were so impressed by the facility that they began to shift some of their patients to St. Joseph. One internist sent his office manager to the center to evaluate word processors they were considering purchasing.

One surprise was that there were fewer requests than anticipated for the loaner computer system. Instead, most of the physicians who were on the brink of deciding proceeded with the purchase of their own hardware, after experimenting with systems in the center.

Many visitors to the center were knowledgeable users, interested in upgrading. They highly valued the availability of a wide variety of software that they could evaluate without being pressured by salespeople.

Lessons

The purpose of the project was not to test whether physicians might be interested in using computers—it was already decided that they should. The question was how best to introduce computers to physicians; how to fascinate them with medical computing the same way they have been fascinated by other medical technology, for example, diagnostic imaging.

The authors believe that the chief obstacle to progress in medical informatics is lack of physician demand for new information tools. Partly this is because many tools are not yet perfected, and partly because doctors are not aware of how soon this time is coming. To break this inertia, hospitals can advance the cause by intensively exposing physicians to computers, encouraging their adoption, rewarding computer skills, and providing opportunities for use and research.

The authors also believe that hospitals whose physicians have a strong commitment to medical computing will eventually benefit from increased prestige, attract leading edge professionals, lower operating costs, deliver better care, enjoy higher morale, suffer fewer errors, and expect a host of other advantages.

But it is not easy to introduce physicians to computers. Physicians must be drawn into the informatics strategy of the hospital at the earliest possible stage. These physicians must have the kind of experience that can only come from time in front of a monitor. Getting them there requires appropriate bait.

In this context, the authors conclude that the boutique approach to computer education is an extremely constructive way to introduce medical informatics to physicians. By extension, there is no reason why this approach would not work with nurses, administrators, or lawyers, for that matter.

It takes a considerable investment to bring computers to a passive audience. Halfhearted efforts will fail; there is an ignition point that must be reached for the investment to produce any yield. But computers are alluring when presented in the right context. Although the center encountered mild degrees of compuphobia, there were not many physicians who were intimidated by the technology, its shortcomings, or the rigors of keyboarding. Doctors have a deep enthusiasm for automation, balanced by sensible skepticism and appropriate reserve.

Most susceptible doctors seem to be waiting for something exactly like what this program and facility offered: a low pressure, high visibility, officially sanctioned, lavishly equipped facility where learning took place in whatever style the doctor chose.

The first six months of the center's operation were its most productive. Then the contract with the physician consultant expired, leaving the entire responsibility for operations in the hands of the assistant. Then the workload heavily pressured the remaining staff assistant, forcing the curtailing of many promising activities.

The presence of a professional peer seemed to be vital to the popularity of the facility among physicians and to its growth. When the consultant contract terminated, new business slowed down significantly, although regular visitors kept coming.

A computerwise, practicing physician with good teaching skills should be the anchor of this kind of enterprise. Especially when it comes to proselytizing before medical staff meetings, a fellow clinician has a much better chance of selling new ideas than some not a peer would.

While having a physician consultant frequently available in the center was essential, the informatics assistant was the indispensable factor that made the whole project work. One on one tutoring proved to be a far more effective way of introducing physicians to computers than independent study or group sessions. Continuity equals credibility for any new undertaking.

The authors feel that another factor in the center's success was the adequate initial hardware investment. Many visitors mentioned that the generous availability of workstations made it easy to drop by and experiment without standing in line, making an appointment, or feeling that others were impatiently waiting or watching. New visitors, novices and experts alike, always approached the PC tentatively. Computers were left—lots of them—quietly waiting like coconuts filled with rice used to trap monkeys. Curiosity finally prevails, the hand is inserted through the little hole, and then the fistful of goodies makes it impossible to let go: the victim is captured.

If It Could Be Done Over....

Although those involved with the Medical Informatics Center are extremely gratified with the overall success of the project (which continues), there are some things that could have been done differently, in retrospect. The authors would

- Staff the center 12 hours per day if possible. The most popular times are early in the morning, when physicians would stop by on rounds, and at the end of the workday. Noon was also busy.

- Advertise the center's presence even more extensively.

- Urge the hospital to make the physician consultant position permanent.

- Seek third party funding (grants, etc.) for special projects, such as a speakers' program, hardware and software shows, workshops, and other events that were often requested.

- Devote more attention to medical billing and accounting systems. The authors deliberately chose to make these a low priority, being interested in clinical applications first. But many of the visitors wanted discussions and assistance in office management and accounting systems.

- And it would have been desirable to have even more time to research available programs and technologies, to take field trips, collaborate with other Denver hospitals, link up with activities at the University of Colorado and the medical school, pursue issues in computer law, and continue meditating upon the potential of these new tools, relishing the exhilaration of being on the working edge of medical informatics.

Questions

1. Can national medical databases be used to help educate physicians on the viability of employing computers in their practice?

2. Do you feel that the failure to employ computer facilities could be ground for malpractice in the future?

3. What situation could require the implementation of a computer familiarization/operation facility?

4. Can this storefront approach be extended to computers besides PCs? What other things besides computer terminals and PCs should be included within the facility?

5. Should billing systems, spreadsheets, etc., be made available to the potential users of the facility?

6. Are there any alternatives to the type of facility described in this paper that can be used to educate physicians to the potential offered by computers?

Appendix A. Job Description, Medical Informatics Assistant

Qualifications

1. Familiarity with current EDP principles and practices, and hospital information systems.

2. Experience in the healthcare environment; preferably clinical training in a health profession; hospital experience.

3. Fluency in the MSDOS operating system. Fluency or at least familiarity with Apple Macintosh. Experience and/or training in microcomputer operations, hardware, and software; general familiarity with medical computing applications.

4. Teaching skills; demonstrated ability to teach at all professional levels; microcomputer teaching experience.

Mission

1. Serve as the principal assistant to the Director of Medical Informatics.

2. Manage the Informatics Resource Center.

3. Provide staff support to administrative activities of the Office of Medical Informatics.

Daily Responsibilities

1. Staff the Informatics Resource Center:

   a.   Initially the sole staff person; eventually the supervisor of other staff members.

   b.   Make sure facilities, software, and equipment are kept orderly, secure, and available.

   c.   Keep the essential records of the center.

2. Take a major role in the training programs of the center.

3. Assist the director in carrying out the responsibilities of the center.

   a.   Basic duties will include keeping catalogs—on computer—of hardware, software, and supplies used in the project; organizing literature, brochures, and references to products of interest to physicians (tracking the lending library); keeping track of the budget; arranging meetings; taking messages and serving as librarian to physicians with inquiries; handling correspondence; and other secretarial tasks.

   b.   Provide basic technical support to users by knowing how to set up a demonstration for a physician, solving common problems with hardware and software over the phone or in person, and taking instruction from expert technical personnel in the solution of more complex problems.

Appendix B. Position Description, Director of Medical Informatics

Qualifications

1. A physician with current clinical experience.

2. Familiarity with current EDP principles and practices, preferably hospital information systems.

3. Fluency in the MSDOS operating system (and preferably also with Macintosh); experience and/or training in microcomputer operations, hardware, and software; thorough working knowledge of medical computing—especially clinical applications.

4. Skill and experience in medical education; teaching experience in medical informatics.

Mission

1. Assume primary responsibility for the development and administration of the Office of Medical Informatics, its facilities and operations.

2. Take a major role in the long range planning for medical informatics activities.

3. Act as liaison with other departments (library, MIS, etc.).

4. Keep abreast of progress in the field.

Daily Responsibilities

1. Establish and supervise the management of the Informatics Resource Center.

2. Establish/manage/coordinate the training programs, software development, and consultative services of the center.

3. Provide timely reports on the status of all projects, utilization, finances, progress toward goals, and recommendations for the future.

4. Develop and administer the Office of Medical Informatics, its facilities and operations.

5. Take a major role in the planning of hospital informatics activities.
   Act as liaison with other departments (library, MIS, etc.).

Appendix C. Software in the Center for Medical Informatics

Too numerous to name each product.

The Medical Informatics Center has purchased and has available for use over $6,000 in software for the IBM compatible and Macintosh computers collectively. To demonstrate a variety of software and demo products, there is always more than one type of product in each category. Categories of the software include:

General

Spreadsheets
Database management systems
Word processors
Outlining programs
Communication packages
Graphics
Time managers
Personal information systems
Menu programs
Utilities
File and system backup programs
Diagnostic programs
Editing programs
Bibliographic reference programs
DOS tutorials

Medical

Medical education case studies
Medical education tests
Larry Weed's Problem Knowledge Coupler
Drug interaction programs
Patient record systems
Patient recall systems
Medical record systems
Patient education programs
Drug information programs
Medical decision support systems
Patient questionnaires
Online database resources

2

New Roles and New Skills to Support Informatics in the Hospital

David E. Sutherland II

Recently healthcare information specialists taking a graduate course were asked, "What do you see as your role in hospitals in the future?" Experienced in the analysis, design, and implementation of information systems in the healthcare field, these specialists gave diverse responses, suggesting an unclear picture of the role of healthcare informaticians in modern hospitals. However, they did share a view of healthcare informaticians as pioneers exploring a new and challenging terrain.

Healthcare Informatics

This terrain is composed of a jungle of forces compelling dependence upon complex technologies. Never before have the interdependencies of the healthcare industry been so closely intertwined. Technology is being asked to address a number of concerns. As personnel costs rise, technologies, with their decreasing costs, are viewed as a means of gaining control over costs. More sophisticated technologies are expected to provide the capability to convey accurate and timely information to patients, third party payors, and health professionals.

Yet today healthcare informaticians are armed with only a rudimentary knowledge of this terrain. Until they have a bigger picture and a clearer understanding of the roles and skills they need, their role in healthcare will be limited.

Hospital administrators must be made aware of the role information and its supporting technologies play in modern healthcare. Some administrators may become healthcare informaticians; some will remain users of the technologies; others will become users. Clearly, administrators must be educated in the uses of information technology, with special attention to the information functions of the organization. Their understanding must be kept current, once established.

"Papers have been written and programs developed, but little agreement exists as to the roles informaticians are to play or what skills they require" (Ball et al. 1989). To ensure the optimal use of information technology in healthcare, support must be forthcoming for informaticians, a new breed of professional in today's healthcare setting. This support must be based upon an understanding of the informatician's roles, as determined by key aspects of given healthcare settings. Once roles are defined, specific skills can be identified and appropriate support mechanisms established, including the building of a technically competent healthcare staff.

Roles and Skills

Why are information specialists needed? As Zuboff explains in *In the Age of the Smart Machine* (1988), the information phenomenon involves "informating" people, or the process of providing information that empowers decision makers at all levels of an organization. As the demand for timely decision making increases in the healthcare industry, the need to informate people also increases. To enhance information use, knowledge of information systems must transcend the organization. Leaders must be developed who have the skills to fulfill the roles critical to information use. Roles and skills are distinctly different. Roles address methods of operation, or how individuals get their jobs done. Skills are the knowledge individuals bring to specific settings.

Information specialists need to redefine their roles and skills. In the past, their role has been that of technician, solving technical problems and living in a technical world. In the future, hospital information specialists will function to fulfill three critical roles, namely the roles of

- Catalyst
- Change agent
- Technician

In the past, skill sets were related to the specific technology being worked with. In general, technicians knew specific programming languages, operating systems, and, to a lesser extent, data communications. They lived in a closed technical world and knew very little about the work functions of the organization for which they were developing systems. In the future, healthcare informaticians will need skill sets which include technical skills, skills in communication and human relations, and a deep understanding of the work functions being supported.

An appreciation of the dynamics of information systems will be essential for all employees in the hospital setting, including information specialists, administrators, clinicians, physicians, and technicians. By informating the organization, hospitals will be able to actualize benefits, benefits that will go far to achieve maximal cost efficiencies and resource utilization. But in order to informate the organization, a new understanding of the roles of all employees and the interdependencies of these individuals will be necessary.

Peter Keen has forwarded the notion of the hybrid in information technology management (Keen 1987). Under this concept, an informatician should possess

- Content knowledge about work functions
- Technical knowledge

The amount of knowledge individuals should have in either of these areas is dependent on what they do within the organization. For instance, a person working with users of a computer system should have a deep understanding of what these users do (the content of their work) and may not need a strong technical background. On the other hand, an individual involved in planning local area network configurations should have a very strong technical background and may not need to know so much about the content. Both categories of skills should be addressed when planning roles for hospital administrators dealing with information technologies.

Informatics Support for Administrators

Understanding the needs of professionals in healthcare informatics requires a knowledge not only of the healthcare industry in general, but of the needs of a specific institution in particular. As a hybrid in the organization, the informatician serves as a bridge between the technology and the users of that technology. The informatician should be the one to address the needs of healthcare administrators through designing educational programs and support structures consistent with

- The organizational infrastructure

- The specific informatics needs of the organization

- The realities of work situations and ability to attend classes

Organizational Issues

The organizational infrastructure includes the reporting lines (course of interaction) in the organization, the hierarchy of the organization (ranks, titles, etc.), and the work flows, including data and information flows. If the hierarchy has evolved over the years to serve organizational purposes, reporting lines will generally be very clear. These lines should not be overlooked in the process of educational design. Although these reporting lines and workflows may be a topic of study at some point in time, they should definitely be taken into account and most likely honored as a support structure is established. Only then, when all three elements are taken into consideration, can an organization truly benefit from the use of information and associated technologies.

Planning for the role of informatician raises two several critical questions. The first, "Where should that individual reside in the organizational structure?" leads to a second, "Who should have what information systems skills in the organization?" The answer to the second question relates to the breadth of knowledge in information systems and the necessary skills. Organizations may have a small number of individuals who act as internal consultants for information systems questions. Alternatively, information systems knowledge and skills may be spread throughout a given organization. This latter structure can be difficult to manage. Identifying who in the organization has the knowledge may be a prerequisite to getting the answer to any question. In general, however, the informatics function resides at various levels in the organization and at various points at each level.

Program Model

A model hospital informatics program is useful in defining questions of role and structure. Under this model, the hospital has a vice president for information systems (VPIS) who reports directly to the president of the hospital. Reporting to the VPIS are six information systems specialists (ISS), each of whom is assigned to a clinic head. Within each function of each clinic, an individual has been identified as an informatician. These individuals carry on their specific functions in the clinic settings as well as help their clinic to function by understanding its information needs.

Informaticians across the organization continually monitor information needs in an informal manner. They observe working situations and assess problems and opportunities. Within each clinical area, the informatician meets periodically with functional staff to formally request ideas and seek clarification on specific points. Subsequently, the informatician submits these points to the information systems specialist for the clinical area.

The six information systems specialists are responsible for the analysis, design, and implementation of systems to support each clinic. Each information system specialist does so in conjunction with the other specialists and with the vice president for information systems to design systems which meet the clinic and hospital needs. They maintain a knowledge of all systems within the organization, including the overall system architecture and the interdependencies of these systems. Once a system need has been identified, the specialists produce a proposal for the system. The proposal is taken to a systems review board made up of the vice president for information systems, the chief operating officer, and the heads of the various clinics. The review board either approves or rejects the proposal.

As the model makes clear, the vice president of information systems, the information systems specialist, and the informatician share similarities as information systems professionals. However, there are differences as well. For example, informaticians do not require the depth of technical knowledge the information systems specialists possess, but they are characterized by a functional expertise not needed by the specialists. A skills matrix highlights these distinctions.

Matrix of Roles and Skills

The roles and skills of vice presidents for information systems, information systems specialists, and informaticians can be grouped and placed in a matrix along the two dimensions identified by Keen. These two dimensions can be further broken down into subcategories for hospital administrators.

The technical dimension includes breadth of experience, measured by the numbers and types of technical projects the individual has worked on. This may equate with seniority, but not necessarily. Many senior systems people have not had broad experience in systems areas. This dimension also covers currency of technical skills, as evidenced by the types of technologies the individual is comfortable with and how recent these technologies are. For instance, individuals who have written COBOL for their entire career and know very little about newer programming languages do not have current technical skills.

The dimension describing content refers to the level of understanding an individual has about general hospital operations and areas of specialization which support patient care. Many systems people know relatively little about the functions of the organizations they support. In addition, content also includes organizational skills, a skill set which includes planning, administration, and control.

Appearing in the matrices is an assessment of the level of skills and the roles (Figures 1 and 2) for each of these three professional categories. As the matrix illustrates, each category is characterized by a different need for skills and roles. Completing such a matrix (Figure 3) can be a valuable experience for institutions addressing informatics. Findings can be refined, and distinct technical and content skills can be specified. By customizing this assessment to reflect their own institutions, healthcare organizations can grow their hybrids to meet their specific needs.

Informatics and the Future of Healthcare

Only when skills and roles such as these are developed with specific healthcare organizations will more efficient and effective service be possible. Until then, healthcare cannot benefit fully from information technology. New skills and new roles hold the key to using powerful new technologies.

Vice President of Information Systems (VPIS). Responsible for the systems decision making process, the VPIS is aware of the strategic plans of the hospital and ensures that the strategic plan is supported by a well planned technology architecture. A technical visionary with a thorough knowledge of the operations of the hospital, the VPIS must be able to work within the constraints of the organization and adjust plans accordingly. The skills essential to this position include planning, budgeting, management control, and systems architecture.

SKILLS MATRIX

TITLE

Vice President, Systems	Information Systems Specialist	Informatician
Planning	Planning	Software Packages
Budgeting	Budgeting	Systems Analysis
Technical	Technical	Needs Analysis
Hardware	*Hardware*	
Software	*Software*	
Communications	Systems Analysis	
Administration	Systems Design	
Human Relations	Project Management	
Personnel		

Figure 1. Skills Matrix

ROLES AND SKILLS MATRIX

SKILLS	TITLE		
	Vice President, Systems	Information Systems Specialist	Informatician
TECHNICAL 1. Breadth of Experience 2. Currency of Technical Skills			
CONTENT 1. Hospital and Functional (clinical, lab, etc.) Skills 2. Organizational Skills			
ROLES 1. Catalyst 2. Change Agent 3. Technician			

Figure 2. Roles and Skills Matrix

COMPLETE ROLES AND SKILLS MATRIX

SKILLS   TITLE

	Vice President, Systems	Information Systems Specialist	Informatician
TECHNICAL			
1. Breadth of Experience	5	3	1
2. Currency of Technical Skills	4	4	1
CONTENT			
1. Hospital and Functional (clinical, lab, etc.) Skills	3	4	5
2. Organizational Skills	4	4	3
ROLES			
1. Catalyst	3	5	3
2. Change Agent	2	4	5
3. Technician	3	4	1

0 = no need for this
1 = minor importance; small degree helpful but not necessary
2 = minor importance
3 = basic competence needed
4 = high level of capability required
5 = absolutely essential; critical requirement

Figure 3. Complete Roles and Skills Matrix

Information Systems Specialist (ISS). A decision maker, the ISS must weigh the requests for project development and put these requests into a case for review by senior managers. The ISS is responsible for

- Systems specifications
- Systems justification
- Project management
- Systems maintenance
- Systems implementation

Each area requires a set of skills; most frequently, an organization will have a number of ISS who are assigned specialized responsibilities.

An ISS serves as the information system designer, managing the analysis of systems opportunities and the construction of the system. Together the ISS manage development teams in the more technical area of the information systems department. The most technically proficient ISS are designated system developers who are responsible for the information system process and for meeting the specifications identified by the ISS team.

Three other functions are characteristic of ISS. As change agents, they work with their area of functional responsibility to plan changes to be effected by the implementation of new information technology. As catalysts, ISS always look for ideas to be implemented and ways to garner support for high priority projects. As technicians, ISS understand the constraints of different technologies as well as the constraints of the existing architecture.

Informatician. Functioning within the clinic unit, the informatician is a nurse, physician, or other practitioner whose main role is as a healthcare specialist. These individuals undertake the role of informatician as a secondary responsibility, in support of their primary clinical functions. They have what might be considered a marginal level of technical ability. Generally, they understand microbased and some mainframe applications and assist professionals in their functional units in setting up and maintaining personal or small group applications. As far as more complex systems needs are concerned, they are aware of and utilize the proper channels for systems requests.

Informaticians need complete knowledge of the functional units in which they reside. They play the role of change agents and, to a lesser extent, technicians. As catalysts, informaticians work with others in their clinical units to forward systems needs and to assist with systems implementation processes.

These new roles are critical if healthcare is to realize the benefits that information technology holds.

Questions

1. How can the availability of information assist administrators in the performance of their duties?

2. What are the three critical roles that the information specialist should assume in the future?

3. Is there an alternative to the CIO structure of hospital organization available to future administrators?

4. Define an information position and use the matrix included in this chapter to evaluate a potential applicant.

References

Ball, M. J., J. V. Douglas, and J. L. Zimmerman. 1989. Informatics education and the professions. *Journal of the American Society for Information Science* 40(5):368-77.

Keen, P. J. 1987. Roles and skills for IS organization of tomorrow. *ICIT Briefing Paper*. Washington, D.C.: ICIT Press.

Zuboff, S. 1988. *In the age of the smart machine.* New York: Basic Books.

3
Computerized Hospital Information Systems as a Tool in Quality Medicine

Peter Peterson

Many physicians face the question of whether or not to use the computer as a practice tool. This is especially true in hospitals that have computerized hospital information systems with physician oriented patient care applications. Although concerns persist in some quarters that computer use may be tedious or inappropriate, or even place the physician at risk, computerized hospital information systems offer the physician significant advantages over manual information processing methods, and ultimately benefit patient care.

Four specific advantages may be expected: (1) direct access to patient information, without relying on ancillary staff; (2) direct order entry capability, thereby reducing manual steps and potential for error; (3) authorship potential, for entering preestablished quality assurance standards or personal order sets, and for storing current specialty diagnostic and treatment information; (4) protection for the physician through automatic, thorough documentation of patient care activities.

Physicians rely heavily on tools to perform their daily tasks. To them, the stethoscope is as essential as a wrench is to a mechanic or a brush to a painter. In recent years, most major professions have adopted the computer as a new tool. Architects and engineers now draft their designs on computer screens; bankers work in a virtually paperless industry. Medicine, in particular, has become a dazzling paradigm of microchip technology, from handheld glucometers to magnetic resonance imaging (MRI).

Still, the use of the computer in its most fundamental configuration—as an information collection and processing tool—is curiously lagging in medicine. Vast amounts of mundane information are generated and consumed daily in the clinical environment using, in most cases, antiquated pencil and paper methods that were developed decades ago.

With diagnostic related groupings (DRGs), denied admissions, threats of Medicare sanctions, and discounted care for HMOs and PPOs, it sometimes seems as though using computers is just another complication for doctors. It means changing styles of practice that have been with them since medical school. It means taking the time to learn how to use an automated system, which can be very frustrating and time consuming.

As computers increasingly become a part of the clinical landscape and more and more physicians are being asked to use them, what are their choices? Physicians can still, of course, refuse. Or they can take the lemons and learn to make lemonade.

Using a Hospital Information System

In 1982, a total computerized hospital information system (HIS) was installed at Porter Hospital in Denver. A TDS HealthCare 4000 System, it offers extensive patient care, as well as financial and administrative applications. As physicians and other medical staff interact with the system, patient information is automatically organized and distributed throughout the hospital to manage orders, schedule patient care activities, and report results.

There is a minimum of typing on the HIS, because interactions take place using a lightpen to make screen selections on predesigned menus. Printers are located throughout the hospital so that hard copy can be produced for reference or for the patient's paper chart.

Doctors were invited to use the system because the hospital realizes significant cost savings when physicians enter their own orders, freeing up nurses' time. Savings are also realized by eliminating problems such as lost lab slips, duplication of effort and poor handwriting, which can lead to inefficiency and errors.

But the questions asked by physicians were, What the computer would do for them? What would it do for patient care? Would it make them better doctors? Over time it has become clear that the HIS offers a number of applications that directly benefit physician practices.

One useful feature of the system is the screen with patient lists. This allows an easy check on where patients are located in the hospital, which is especially helpful if they have been transferred since last seen.

Retrieving lab data through the HIS is also useful because it saves time. For example, the lab results on a patient can be obtained from any terminal in the hospital. This avoids the familiar "could you please hold?" syndrome of calling the lab or the nursing unit. By directly accessing the data, it is possible to get in and out of the HIS with the results in far less time than it takes to call for them.

The real highlight of the system, though, is its order entry capability, which is as beneficial to doctors as to the hospital. This takes a little more time to learn than the retrieval of information, but the effort pays off in accuracy and expedience. A physician's order entered directly into the HIS bypasses as many as ten manual steps as it is instantaneously transmitted to its endpoint. Consider what this means: no calls back, confusion, delays, or errors.

Order entry in the HIS becomes especially attractive when physicians have terminals in their offices. Doctors can access an inpatient record, review lab data, and enter orders directly into the system during a quiet moment between appointments or at the end of the day. This offers real convenience and flexibility to the busy physician.

Patient Care Benefits

The benefits of a HIS are maximized when its capabilities are directly applied to patient care. For a physician, this can be achieved by standardized order entry through the use of personal order sets (POS), and by using the HIS as a reminder system, or a filing cabinet for useful medical information.

A proponent of computer use in medicine and a major figure in medical informatics is Dr. Lawrence L. Weed, who introduced the problem oriented system of medical records and SOAP charting in 1965. Dr. Weed has advanced the idea that it is impossible to keep all facts in one human mind. The memory system is the method most physicians have relied on from the first day of medical school, yet the current volume of medical knowledge overwhelms the memory. Because of this, reminder lists can be helpful aids to the memory system for both differential diagnosis and treatment of a medical problem.

The computer can be used to store information from texts, journals, and clinical meetings. Then, if the memory system fails, or if a physician wants to look up something, or be sure that all possible diagnoses or treatments have been considered, the relevant screens can be accessed from a terminal in the office or hospital. The information is much more available on a computer screen than as clippings filed in a desk drawer.

In a recent example, a patient with diarrhea and a fever of 105 degrees was admitted. Because information from a department meeting handout had been previously entered in the computer, appropriate treatment was started while waiting for the infectious disease consultant to arrive. The consultant subsequently agreed with initial therapy and the patient benefited from prompt treatment, since an approved standard was already in the computer.

Another example is acidosis. It can sometimes be difficult to remember all the causes, especially for physicians who are tired or stressed. By having a differential diagnosis list in the computer, there is a back up system available to ensure that all possible causes have been considered. More causes can be added to this list as they come up, or as additional readings bring more to mind. Diagnostic criteria such as the pH required for a diagnosis of renal tubular acidosis can also be included.

Dr. Weed has made a related point, that if standards of patient care are preestablished, then every patient should get that same quality of care under all circumstances, regardless of the time of day, or the stress or fatigue level of the medical staff. No one would argue this objective, yet it is far from a reality in the present healthcare system. If physicians are tired or stressed or in a hurry, it can impede their ability to give good care.

One way to help guarantee consistent standards of care is by using POS that have been entered in the HIS. Accessing a menu of orders for a given problem eliminates concerns that something could be forgotten. Individual orders or "all of the above" can be selected with the lightpen, and they will print out within moments in the lab or pharmacy. In this way, patients can count on receiving consistent, high quality care because orders cannot be forgotten, lost, or even delayed.

POS can also be used to schedule procedures for the following day on the HIS. For example, if a chest tube is to be put in tomorrow, an appointment is made with the nurse, the POS is accessed, and orders, which are lightpenned onto the screen, are automatically distributed to all relevant departments. The next day everything is waiting when the doctor arrives. There is no wasted time while the nurse looks for the proper dressing or calls central supply to obtain supplies.

Nurses like the HIS too, because it frees up their time. The HIS creates more professional staff relations in this type of situation, which contributes to an enhanced, positive working relationship.

Since the Joint Commission on Accreditation of Healthcare Organizations (JCAHO) and the government have established specific standards of care for various problems, it has become essential for doctors to follow certain treatment guidelines or their charts will fall out in the audits. These standards and additional hospital quality assurance protocols can be entered in the HIS as POS. Besides being thorough, using POS ensures that treatments have been precisely documented and can be easily accessed in the event of an audit or malpractice suit.

This style of practice has been described as cookbook medicine, but the implied pejorative should not keep physicians from using a good system that works well for both them and their patients. Clearly POS are not suitable in every treatment situation, but most doctors have standard orders that would work well as POS. The proof is in the results, and with POS patients can count on well thought out, detailed strategies for both diagnosis and treatment of their illnesses.

A study performed in the Methodist Hospital of Indiana in Indianapolis, a 1160 bed community hospital, has cited a number of advantages to using POS and departmental order sets (DOS) compared to general order entry in the HIS. These include a 20 percent reduction in the time hospital personnel are involved in order entry; a 30 percent reduction in terminal usage; and a 40 percent reduction in undetected errors. The findings show that on the average, using a POS saves physicians more than ten steps in completing the orders on a patient (Anderson et al. 1988).

Discussion

The computer can be an invaluable information management tool that helps physicians deliver well documented, consistent, quality medicine. By using POS, preestablished quality standards can be met, which is not true of a system that depends on memory. Of course, mistakes can still occur using an HIS, but these are typically due to human error in information entry, not because of bugs in the machine or software.

It is important for those still skeptical about computerized medical information processing to realize that the computer does not wrest control of patient information away from the doctor. If anything, the HIS helps physicians take control of their practices, because virtually all patient care information is literally at the fingertips. With the HIS, up to the minute information can be obtained on any inpatient 24 hours a day, without relying on staff to report this information. Order entry and results retrieval ar< instantaneous processes. Delays and inefficiencies associated with phor calling and manual information processing are no longer factors in the patie care equation when using an HIS.

What does the HIS not do? It will not correct errors in doctors' judgment. It is not the same as artificial intelligence which supposedly thinks for its users. Most doctors do not need artificial intelligence; they need reminders for differential diagnosis and treatment. As a tool that manages this information, an HIS is more efficient than manual methods, and produces tangibly more positive outcomes for both the doctor and the patient.

With even more government and JCAHO regulations on the horizon, the importance of an HIS to the hospital and the physician can only increase. Physicians will face even greater pressures. Stricter standards will require more thorough, clearer documentation of patient care. It is not reasonable to expect the traditional manual system to succeed in properly managing the information requirements of the next decade. Today, computers are successfully managing vast quantities of information in all the other major professions. Physicians need to use computers in medicine to supplement the outdated memory system, to protect themselves, and to provide the best of care to patients.

Questions

1. What potential advantages does the computer offer to the practicing physician?

2. Why have physicians been reluctant to use computers?

3. How can a medical record system that has been computerized assist the physician?

4. Will computer systems eventually lead to cookbook medicine?

5. Do physicians need the artificial intelligence systems that have evolved over the past decade? Explain.

References

Anderson, J. G., S. J. Jay, S. F. Clevenger, et al. 1988. Physician utilization of a hospital information system: A computer simulation model. *Proceedings of the 12th Annual Symposium on Computer Applications in Medical Care*, 858-61. Washington, D.C.:IEEE.

Section 2–Managing the Institution

Unit 1—Information: A Resource for Strategic Management

Unit Introduction

Healthcare institutions must involve both their governing bodies and management in creating more and better information. High level decision makers working to provide high quality healthcare must regard information as a strategic resource. This unit scans the range of issues which decision makers must address as they acquire, implement, and manage information systems.

Harlen and Magraw, both vice presidents for patient care management at a 518 bed medical center, explain the advantages microcomputing can give to practicing administrators. Drawing on experiences in higher education and an academic health center, Penrod presents a strategic planning model for information resources. Melvin, an information technology consultant, joins with McLoone, a hospital CEO, in delineating the effect of technology on organizational structures; both operating in countries with national healthcare systems, they provide insights into managed care. Trained in computer science and now chief information officer for an 800 bed, four hospital system, Gabler discusses the use of open networking architecture to support and integrate decentralized departmental systems. A certified public accountant, formerly a hospital administrator at a major teaching hospital and now a consultant, Ryckman sets forth trends in financial systems and proposes strategies for the successful introduction of new applications. A healthcare economist, Malec reviews methodologies for assessing benefits and effectiveness in cost justifying information systems.

To meet the demands of the 1990s, healthcare institutions need skilled professionals who in turn need the best tools available, both for managing those institutions and for providing patient care.

1
Computer Literacy: An Advantage to the Administrator

Kevin J. Harlen and Thomas W. Magraw

Since prospective payment replaced cost based reimbursement, hospitals have had to operate in an increasingly competitive environment. The dramatic change in reimbursement methodology has encouraged, if not forced, hospitals to take on more of the characteristics of traditional businesses. To survive and to thrive in this environment, hospitals and their managers must be able to gather accurate, timely information to put to use for both operational decision making and planning purposes. Taking advantage of computers is key.

Training Administrators

Recent graduates of hospital or business administration programs usually have the experience and mindset which predispose them to use personal computing tools. In contrast, administrators who have been in the field for a number of years may have had little opportunity or inclination to explore personal computers.

Training someone who has already been exposed to similar tools is significantly easier than training a first time user because the basic understanding of how to use these tools has already been formed. Nonetheless, recent entrants to the profession will continue to need training throughout their careers. When they assume positions at different hospitals, they most likely will need to use new software applications as well as differently configured hardware and local area networks.

Training administrators unfamiliar with personal computers is a more formidable task. A person with no personal computing experience whatsoever must learn to activate the hardware and software and to assimilate a new vocabulary with terms like DOS and "booting up." Once new users can initiate a software package, they must begin to learn the mechanics of using it. The new user must learn the types of software packages that are available. With experience, the new user will gain insight into when a software package can be employed to advantage and when it may be most efficient not to use the computer at all.

The person seeking a concentrated dose of education about personal computing may choose to take courses, either those offered by the hospital or by outside organizations. Courses range from introductory classes to advanced seminars focused on specific software packages. Once such classes are completed, students must put what they have learned to use.

Although courses can give users a headstart, developing a working knowledge of personal computing in general or of a specific software package will come only through hands on use of the computer. True, learning comes from doing. Administrators should seriously consider having computers in their offices for easy access and even at home if opportunities to learn are hard to come by during the workday.

No matter what an administrator knows about computing, there is always an opportunity and often the need to learn more. Both hardware and software packages are enhanced and updated. New packages come to market. The hospital changes what it uses, or the administrator moves to another hospital that uses different applications. The administrator needs to assimilate these changes by hands on use of the personal computer.

Whatever the name—keyboard psychosis, PC phobia, computer anxiety, technostress, cyberphobia—it is real. The extraordinary power of desktop and laptop computers offers enormous potential for change. Change is always difficult, and it should come as no surprise that individuals are uncomfortable with something about which they have limited knowledge. Seasoned administrators may also perceive a threat to their self esteem, especially when junior members of the management team have grown up with computers and can move easily from one software program to another.

Most administrators acknowledge that personal computers are here to stay—and on their desktops. Increasing in number and ease of use, computers offer the administrator powerful tools. Mastering the basics is key.

In addition to coursework and self study, administrators may find their peers to be of great assistance, able to offer practical and creative solutions to common problems. Some administrators may search their own organizations for an expert user to act as tutor. To be effective, any tutor must be able to address matters on an introductory level and not intimidate the administrator with advanced concepts or condescension.

Courses on personal computing are offered by vendors and by educational institutions, including adult education programs, community colleges, and universities. The decision to take courses, either introductory or advanced, should consider factors such as motivation, time constraints, political needs, and budget.

Some administrators may prefer to learn by doing, seeking knowledge through self directed, hands on experience at hours of their own choosing. Others may find that a structured educational program offers needed discipline. Individuals reluctant to reveal their lack of computing knowledge to others within their organization may prefer find the anonymity of training outside the hospital.

However, if several hospital personnel need training in the same area, it is prudent to determine whether it is most cost effective to send them all to an external seminar, hire an outside instructor to teach a program inhouse, or tap an expert user from within the hospital to teach a seminar. Administrators need to remember, however, that external education is no substitute for hands on work with the personal computer.

Computer Literacy as a Competitive Advantage

Personal computer literacy offers several competitive advantages to the hospital administrator. Managers plan for the future and chart the organization's direction. The ability to effectively utilize tools such as spreadsheets is essential in arriving at the best possible decisions. Spreadsheets can be used to build complex financial models which, if constructed properly, can rapidly perform massive recalculations based on a change without the fear of introducing errors into the tedious and time consuming manual recalculation process. The benefits to budgeting and financial forecasting are enormous.

To do their jobs well, managers must be able to react quickly to unexpected events. Developments may occur late in the day after secretarial help has gone home, suddenly creating the need for a table, chart, or document for a meeting that evening or early the next morning. Being computer literate gives managers tools to accomplish tasks efficiently and effectively—tools that are not at the disposal of managers who have not mastered computers.

The manager who can be flexible and deliver the product on time clearly has a competitive advantage over those managers who are not able to respond. People take notice of results. The subordinate who is able to deliver information or documents on short notice will gain the notice and appreciation of superiors.

Computer literacy may not be noticed, but the ability to deliver surely will be.

Computer Tools

Most administrators are aware of microcomputer based tools, notably word processing, spreadsheets, databases, and electronic mail. A variety of introductory books offer advice on buying and using personal computers. Their advantages readily become apparent to the practicing administrator.

Word processing makes it possible for the administrator to dash off a late night document for the next morning's meeting. The administrator can draft a document on the home computer, rather than on paper, and run it through the spell checker. The document can then go on diskette to the secretary for subsequent revision, eliminating the need to transcribe dictation or decipher handwriting.

Database programs assist the administrator in storing, retrieving, and manipulating data, sorting it according to specific parameters. For example, with a database of medical staff, the administrator can query for orthopedists, or physicians on active staff, or physicians on staff for more than 20 years, or obstetricians who perform ten or more deliveries a month, or any combination of the above mentioned parameters.

In addition to helping the administrator avoid telephone tag and communicate with people with conflicting schedules, electronic mail systems can transmit documents across local area networks for collaborative review and revision.

Clearly, electronic mail is no substitute for face to face contact and realtime discussion, but it provides administrators with a valuable tool in a sometimes frantic environment.

Decision Support

Administrators stand to gain most notably from spreadsheet support for decision making. Granted, computers cannot make decisions, but mathematical modeling allows managers to perform a series of "what if" scenarios, assisting in analysis of possible outcomes and refinement of financial projections.

Spreadsheet modeling facilitates sensitivity analysis, allowing the rapid recalculation of the bottomline resulting from a 10 percent increase or decrease in volume, a 15 percent increase or decrease in variable expenses, or any other value. Given that projections are quite simply a best guess, the decision making process must assess the implications of deviations from that best guess. Spreadsheet based sensitivity analysis is extremely helpful. The rapidity with which spreadsheets allow for recalculation of a financial model is also of use with the iterations and recalculations required to reach the most likely scenario.

Financial models are often recalculated multiple times based on different interest rates for the loan to finance a project. The variety of interest rates may reflect refinements in the cost of borrowing during negotiation with a potential lender or market fluctuations in interest rates during the period prior to locking in a rate to finance the project in question.

Other iterations of the financial model can reflect a better understanding of the cost structure associated with a proposed program or a refinement in the expected volume.

Impact

In the future as in the past, senior level hospital administrators will gather information, analyze situations based on this information, formulate and review options, and make decisions based on this analysis and review. In completing these tasks, they will use the new tools now at their disposal, an array of off the shelf hardware and software tools that actually augment intellectual capabilities.

Clearly, these tools cannot think for the administrator, but they can furnish more, better, and timelier information that can make perceptions more accurate, deliberations more incisive, and decisions more correct.

Questions

1. Explain how a hospital manager might utilize each of the four major types of software popularly available for personal computers.

2. What advantages does the computer literate manager have that a manager without these skills does not?

3. How can personal computers be of assistance in the decision making process?

4. How can personal computers be best employed to enhance communication? What is the downside of communicating by personal computer?

2
Methods and Models for Planning Strategically

James I. Penrod

Many forces of change will transform the healthcare system in the United States in the 1990s. These include an aging population, sophisticated consumers, pressures for cost containment, a pluralistic healthcare system, new medical technologies, excess physician supply and hospital capacity, increased demand for healthcare, and government's role (Selbert 1989).

The stimuli for change in organizations come from one of three sources (Keller 1983): a major crisis, the exertion of pressure from the outside, or a vigorous, farsighted (often newly arrived) leader. Few departments within the healthcare setting are as impacted by these stimuli as are departments of computing and communications. Coupled with rapid acceptance and escalating demand, technological advances produce crises for information managers. Pressures are generated within as well as by board members and by institutional competitors. Changes in leadership result from management turnover and shuffling.

Dealing with change is a constant in the life of any computing and communications professional. Some sort of planning is a given. It may be formal or informal; short or long range; strategic, tactical, or operational. The real question is what type of planning is best.

Strategic Planning Defined

Long range planning optimizes for tomorrow the trends of today. In contrast, strategic planning exploits the opportunities of tomorrow while minimizing the negative aspects of inevitable or unexpected challenges. Strategic planning goes hand in hand with strategic management and is the activity through which major strategic decisions are confronted, decisions which

- Define the institution's relationship to its environment

- Generally take the whole organization as the unit of analysis

- Depend on inputs from a variety of functional areas

- Provide direction for and constraints on administrative and operational activities throughout the entire institution (Shirley 1982)

Strategic planning differs from long range planning. Its focus on issues makes strategic planning more appropriate for politicized circumstances. Typically, strategic planning summons forth an idealized vision of the organization, while long range planning does linear extrapolations of the present. Strategic planning identifies decisions and actions relating to a range of possible futures identified through environmental assessments while long range planning tends to get locked into a single stream of decisions and actions leading to a most likely future (Bryson 1988).

As defined by Cope (1987), strategic planning is "a proactive problem solving behavior which uses an open systems approach. Its purpose is "to achieve success with mission while linking the institution's future to anticipated changes in the environment in such a way that the acquisition of resources is faster than the depletion of resources."

Strategic planning can result in many benefits:

- A clear and inspiring strategic vision

- Increased external support

- Increased certainty in the lives of organizational members

- A context for resource allocation and reallocation

- An improved image for the organization

- Enhanced expertise and teamwork in the organization

Strategic Planning Models

Healthcare organizations vary immensely in size, complexity, governance structure, and decision paths; their leaders differ in management style. According, planners must analyze their organization and tailor a strategic planning process to fit (Keller 1983).

The first steps an institution should take in choosing a model are to analyze what has led to the adoption of a planning process and to examine its institutional history, including

- Style and context of the organization

- Relative power of external and internal forces shaping decision making

- Nature and success of planning in the past

- Biases and prejudices against planning and their relative strength

- Supporters and detractors of planning and their power to obstruct the process

The resulting insights should be reflected in the charge to plan and the model itself. The model must adapt to accommodate these insights in order for the planning process to become integrated in the decision making and governance of the institution (Norris and Poulton 1987).

In selecting a planning model, certain elements must be considered. According to Moynihan (1988), planning for computing and communications should:

- Be ongoing, regardless of the level of technology used

- Be eclectic

- Be broad but bounded in scope

- Be driven by institutional problems and opportunities, not by technical developments

- Involve a formal process, have the support of senior management, use up to date planning methods, and result in documented output

- Involve senior managers, major users, and information systems staff

- Include a review of the mission and organization of the computing and communication function

- Involve the identification of potentially important technology developments

- Address the computing and communications organization's technical and managerial competence

- Formalize an organizational architecture that addresses medical system, hospital, and departmental levels

- Result in an organization wide technical architecture and vendor policy

- Formulate an organization wide application system architecture

- Develop an organization wide tool architecture

- Yield an organization wide architecture for voice, data, and image networks

Initiating a strategic planning process for computing and communications is not a trivial undertaking. It cannot produce positive results overnight, but takes time to evolve and to be assimilated into the organizational culture. However, certain factors will lead to success if the institution seeks persistently and patiently to ensure their presence:

- *Top Level Support.* First and perhaps most important, the process should have the support of the board and the chief executive officer (CEO).

- *Identifiable Outcomes.* Planning processes should focus on identifiable outcomes which directly support the mission of the healthcare unit; these will serve as criteria for measuring success.

- *Participatory Ownership.* The planning committee membership should be carefully selected and given an active role through the process to ensure that healthcare professionals, managers, and organizational staff have a sense of ownership in the goals which drive the planning process.

- *Formalized Process.* The planning process should be consciously and formally organized, assigning planning responsibilities to both management and support staff.

- *Accountability.* Staff should be held accountable for support of the planning process, pulling together what is needed for decision points and maintaining the flexibility required.

- *Comprehensiveness.* The planning process must be comprehensive in scope and participation, responding to critical issues or involving significant segments of the organization.

- *Incorporation.* Strategic planning must be incorporated into policy, procedures, and operating decisions (including budgets and resource allocation) which in turn produce institutional change.

A Proposed Model

The elements of the planning model described below are primarily taken from the work of Robert Shirley and John Bryson. Shirley's work has evolved from classical business oriented strategic planning models and focuses on higher education. Bryson's model was developed for use in public and nonprofit organizations. Merging these methodologies and tailoring the model for particular circumstances allow for adaptation to most healthcare settings; the author of this article has in fact utilized the model in an academic health center.

Figure 1 depicts the planning model that has been postulated. The figure shows the interrelationship between the various steps and illustrates potential feedback loops used in modifying ongoing cycles. The advice which follows draws upon Shirley and Bryson and the experience of this author. The steps below reflect their recommendations for the strategic planning process; tailoring the process to the specific environment remains critical in any adoption of these recommendations.

Step 1: Establish Planning Parameters

Document and clarify the initial agreement, including purpose; steps; form and timing of reports; role, functions, and membership of the coordinating committee and of the team to write and implement the plan; commitment of resources in support of planning; and specific documents or requirements to be incorporated into the process (Bryson 1988a,b).

Step 2: Assess the Environment

In an external environmental analysis, identify and assess major forces in the economic, social, technological, political/legal, demographic, and competitive areas presenting specific opportunities, threats, and constraints. In an internal environmental assessment, identify organizational strengths and weaknesses, using the elements of a simple systems model. This latter assessment should focus on outputs and might include a stakeholder analysis.

Step 3: Determine Values

Systematically identify the values of primary stakeholders or constituencies and integrate those findings into the process. This requires a sensitivity to institutional cultures and should result in a vision statement that articulates a philosophy for managing the organization. It may be helpful to have managers within the organization develop vision statements for their individual units (Block 1987).

Step 4: Specify Areas for Strategic Decisions

Develop a blueprint for the future. Address the decision areas below, acknowledging interactions and interdependencies and revising across all areas before making final determinations.

Organizational Mission and Purpose. In an extended mission statement, describe:

- Fundamental purposes of the organization

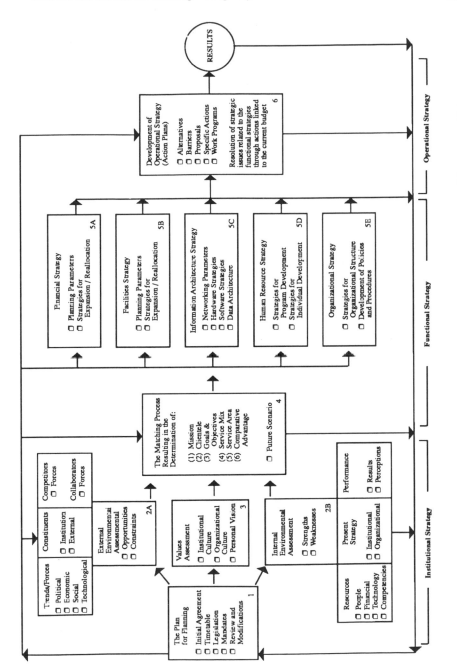

Figure 1. A Strategic Planning Model for Information Resources in Healthcare Facilities

- Characteristics that distinguish the organization from other units

- Obligations assumed by the organization with respect to its clientele

- Types of units and nature and role of support services offered by the organization

- Relative emphasis on areas such as patient care, education, research, and administration; computing, voice, video, and data networks; centralized and distributed facilities; institutional and external services

- Major stakeholders to be served

- Style of governance and decision making structures that the organization employs

- Philosophy of the organization related to effective/efficient use of resources, including human resources

Clientele to Be Served. Identify the audience of clientele being targeted. Define organizational stakeholders in sufficient depth to set expectations and to evaluate whether they are being met.

Goals and Outcomes. Develop goals that state the desired outcomes and accomplishments. Develop a futures scenario to use as the vision of success. Establish goals with five to ten year horizons; identify time bounded, measurable, behaviorally oriented objectives related to the accomplishment of specific goals, and linked to a budget cycle.

Service Mix. To define service mix, develop a mechanism for reviewing organizational units and support services offered during the time covered by the strategic plan. This may involve considering whether an information resources management approach or a chief information officer function is viable within the institutional culture. Also develop a means for establishing priorities among the service mix and a process outlining how new services will evolve.

Geographic Service Area. Identify the primary service area of the computing and communications organization. If responsibility and resources for computing and communications are assigned to different segments of the institution, clarify organizational guidelines for the respective service mix and service areas (Heterick 1988).

Comparative Advantage. Identify features which differentiate the computing and communications unit from other institutional units and from the computing and communications organizations of competing hospitals and clinics.

Step 5: Form Functional Strategies

Develop strategies which address fundamental policy questions affecting the computing and communications mandates, mission, services, clients, financing, management, and structural design. Because strategic decisions almost invariably involve conflict, pose the issue as a question that the organization can address, list the factors that make it strategic, and state the consequences of failure to address the issue.

Group strategic issues by area, including financial, facilities, architecture (network, hardware, software, data design), human resource development, and organization. Formulate strategies, establishing timelines and operational parameters and linking the strategies to a broad based, multiyear budget.

Step 6: Develop Action Plans

Develop operational strategies to deal with issues identified. These action plans may be within organizational units or other hospital units; they may span part or all of the computing and communications organization or of the entire institution. Regardless of where they are to be carried out, relate action plans directly to functional parameters (financial, facilities, architecture, etc.) to ensure appropriate trade offs, integrated action plans, and respected institutional bounds.

Evaluate the Planning Process

Formal and informal processes should measure effectiveness (doing the right things) and efficiency (doing things right). Regular reviews by management should determine whether the process produces decisions and which parts of the process work.

Because determining strategy requires a blend of rational and economic analysis, political maneuvering, and psychological interplay, the process must be highly tolerant of controversy (Keller 1983). The key is to identify those components of the process that need not be participatory and can be centrally directed, while subtly but firmly providing direction to those areas where participation and consensus are critical. The planning structure must achieve a balance between top down and bottom up planning. Moreover, it should (Shirley 1987):

- Evidence top management support

- Involve appropriate constituents meaningfully and in an ongoing way

- Concentrate on substance rather than on form and paperwork

- Provide for continuity of involvement by key individuals and from one cycle to the next

- Employ the appropriate quality and quantity of data and analysis in decision making

- Work to culminate deliberation with decision making (Shirley 1987)

Methods of Evaluation

As those ultimately responsible, senior management should evaluate the decisions emerging from the computing and communications planning process. Questions of interest to senior management, which might be answered in an executive summary of the annual report (Below et al. 1987), include the following:

- How is computing and communications performing in relation to the milestones outlined in the strategic plan?

- What are the key computing and communications budget items for the organization and the institution over the planning period?

- What are the critical strategic issues that will affect the hospital's performance? The performance of the computing and communications organization? Why?

- Why are the strategies identified in the plan appropriate to the institution?

- What are the critical success factors necessary for successful implementation of the plan?

Evaluation tasks vary in difficulty. The evaluation of decisions probably requires the most judgment. However, perceptions of decisional results can be collected and quantified in fairly straightforward ways. The evaluation of data and process is usually easier and may be accomplished through the accumulation of periodic analyses throughout the planning cycle. Appropriately written action plans and behavioral objectives provide a strong platform for analysis (Shirley 1982).

Hospitals or medical centers belonging to larger systems may be assigned specific criteria and report formats by their system planning office. When possible, criteria for the system and the institution should be meshed so unnecessary duplication is avoided. It may prove useful to enlist a consultant who can bring an unbiased perspective and lend credibility to the evaluation effort.

Summary

Computing and communications are being increasingly used in patient care, research, education, and management, at every level of the institution and in every medical discipline. The growing importance of strategic planning for resources in these areas gave rise to this attempt to develop a generic guide to strategic thought and action. Clearly, those who become planners must be careful in adapting strategic planning concepts. Every situation is different, and planning can be effective only if tailored to a specific situation. To be successful, a strategic planning process must fit the environment of the organization and institution where it is implemented. Above all, planning requires political astuteness and a solid understanding of the culture of the place and time.

Experience shows that a clearly defined strategic vision can help generate support from both internal and external groups, develop coherent future oriented decision making, assist in resource allocation, improve the organizational and institutional image, and encourage organizational teamwork while creating smoother relations between units. Surely, over the long term, healthcare institutions will find that the benefits of planning make commitment to the process worthwhile.

Questions

1. How does strategic planning differ from long range planning?

2. Select a specific healthcare organization and write an idealized planning charge for the information resources unit. Would this charge, if carried out, lead to a changed decision making structure? Why or why not?

3. Develop six to eight succinct sentences which taken together would constitute a vision statement for the information resources unit in question two. How do you feel the user community would respond to this statement?

4. Who in the organization described in questions two and three would be involved in review (buy off) at the institutional strategy level? At the functional strategy level? At the operational strategy level?

5. Briefly outline an evaluation process for an information resources unit. Who in the unit would be responsible for each element of the process?

References

Below, P. L., G. L. Morrisey, and B. L. Acomb. 1987. *The executive guide to strategic planning*. San Francisco: Jossey-Bass.
Block, P. 1987. *The empowered manager*. San Francisco: Jossey-Bass.
Bryson, J. M. 1988a. A strategic planning process for public and non-profit

organizations. *Long Range Planning* 21:78.

Bryson, J. M. 1988b. *Strategic planning for public and non-profit organizations*. San Francisco: Jossey-Bass.

Cope, R. G. 1987. Opportunity from strength: Strategic planning clarified with case examples. Report 8, no. 3. Washington, D.C.: Association for the Study of Higher Education.

Heterick, R. C. 1988. An information systems strategy. CAUSE Professional Paper, 9-10. Boulder, Colo.: CAUSE.

Keller, G. 1983. *Academic strategy: The management revolution in American higher education*. Baltimore: Johns Hopkins University Press, 164.

Moynihan, J. 1988. Propositions for building an effective process. *Journal of Information Systems Management* 5:61-4.

Norris, D. M. and L. Poulton. 1987. A guide for new planners. Ann Arbor, Mich.: Society for College and University Planning, 16-7.

Selbert, R. 1989. The health care future. *Future Scan* 1:624.

Shirley, R. C. 1982. Limiting the scope of strategy: A decision based approach. *Academy of Management Review* 2:262-8.

Shirley, R. C. 1987. *Evaluating institutional planning*, 16-8. Evaluating Administrative Services and Programs: New Directions for Institutional Research, no. 56. San Francisco: Jossey-Bass.

Select Bibliography

Freund, Y. P. 1988. Planner's guide: Critical success factors. *Planning Review* 16:20.

Langly, A. 1988. The roles of formal strategic planning. *Long Range Planning* 21:47-48.

Lelong, D. and R. C. Shirley. 1984. Planning: Identifying the focal points for action. *Planning for Higher Education* 12:4.

Morrison, J. L., W. C. Renfro, and W. I. Boucher. 1984. Futures research and the strategic planning process, report no. 9, 8. Washington, D.C.: Association for the Study of Higher Education.

Shirley, R. C. 1983. Identifying the levels of strategy for a college or university. *Long Range Planning* 16:9-10.

Shirley, R. C. 1988. Strategic planning: An overview. *Successful Strategic Planning: Case Studies, New Directions for Higher Education* 64:11-12.

Strategic and Operational Planning for Information Systems. 1985. Chantico Series. Wellesley, Mass.: QED Information Sciences. 1985.

Wallace, R. E. 1986. Why strategic planning? *Journal of Information Systems Management* 3:51.

3
Organizational Change and Technological Innovation

John Melvin and Michael McLoone

The development of informatics systems, more commonly known as hospital information systems (HIS), is one of the most challenging tasks facing hospitals today. Automated systems affect the daily routines and activities of all hospital staff, including doctors, nurses, paramedical staff, and financial and administrative staff. No group of staff is unaffected. Information technology offers enormous potential at affordable prices. The staggering rate of development means that concepts like the electronic medical record can begin to become a reality today.

Information technology is of particular significance in hospitals, where the communications flow is truly information intensive, even when compared to industries commonly identified as information intensive, such as airlines and banks. However, unlike those industries, hospitals in particular and healthcare in general are characterized by the slow adoption of information technology.

The traditional concept of information systems as understood in information technology circles involves the processing of data, whether by manual or computerized methods. The concept is evolving to incorporate the concepts of information and information systems as they function in decision making. This expanded concept of information systems has significant consequences for the future of healthcare information systems.

The Beaumont Hospital Experience

The analysis and conclusions related in the text below are based upon the experiences of the Beaumont Hospital in Dublin, Ireland, as it developed and implemented the various modules of a hospital information system. A 700 bed tertiary care facility, Beaumont has a large volume of outpatient and emergency care activities. As a facility in a country where managed healthcare is a reality, it may serve as a guide to facilities of like size in the United States as they enter the 1990s and are required to meet growing demands for controls on costs and quality. Smaller hospitals, it should be noted, may need to modify the methodology described here to meet their particular requirements.

Development Methodology

There are many excellent information technology methodologies available in the marketplace today. Beaumont Hospital adapted these methodologies and followed a model with four phases, moving from planning and selection to design and implementation. Each phase is described below.

Planning. The long range plan developed for information technology at Beaumont Hospital has a five year horizon, with several components extending farther out. Given the rapidity of change, this would be equivalent to a much longer timeframe in more mature technologies. However, the plan is revisited every year and updated as necessary.

The planning phase adapted by Beaumont required that the planning team:

- Identify objectives for information technology (e.g., electronic medical record, cost reduction, improved quality of care)

- Review current information technology services (strengths, weaknesses, skill sets, key issues, etc.)

- Analyze the hospital's long term and strategic plan to ensure that information technology development could support the hospital's objectives and strategies (e.g., new organizational structures and processes, such as nursing care planning)

- Outline management information needs and transaction requirements

- Analyze data flows and the relationship between data and "business" functions to help construct its target information environment

- Identify the target systems environment and key strategies to achieve this environment

- Identify the target information technology (hardware and telecommunications) environment to support the systems environment and associated key strategies

- Analyze the impact of these environments on hospital processes, personnel, and role definitions

- Identify the target information technology department environment

- Outline the steps/actions, sequencing timeframes, associated responsibilities and resources (including financial) to achieve the target environments

- Report to management/board, including cost/benefit

The resulting plan is comprehensive in scope and addresses the integration of the HIS and the core information technology environment with office automation systems (including word processing and electronic mail), telecommunications, and systems for management, transactions, and clinical information. The plan also included a component which addresses the initial and ongoing training of personnel. Training assumes added significance in a teaching hospital like Beaumont.

For the Beaumont Hospital, a major outcome of planning was the realization that information technology was in fact underresourced. For Beaumont, achievement of their information technology objectives would require a significant infusion or redeployment of resources. Beaumont was not unusual in this regard; many hospitals are in the same position.

Selection. Like most hospitals, Beaumont opted to purchase packaged software to address the majority of their computing requirements and identified the software selection process as vital to the success of their information technology plan. In this process, Beaumont recognized two options: (1) develop their individual (departmental) systems first, i.e., on a standalone basis, and later consolidate the systems at the overall hospital level, and (2) develop individual (departmental) systems into an integrated hospital information system from the outset.

Beaumont decided against the first strategy. Aware that problems might arise later on, it elected to avoid the risk of finding themselves caught in a web of proprietary systems. Although commercial standards such as OSI, MEDIX, or HL7 are now becoming available, these solutions are still only partial. Thus, Beaumont Hospital opted for the second strategy, to plan an integrated system from the onset.

To create an integrated information technology environment, Beaumont focused on the selection of core HIS modules, including admission, discharge, and transfer; outpatient management, including emergency; resource scheduling; order communications; and results reporting. This development strategy identified the electronic medical record as the base for the integration of systems. Financial and insurance data (and systems) would be derived from the basic clinical data, along with data for management systems.

The selection process for Beaumont Hospital operated within the framework defined by the European Community. Steps included the identification of requirements, development of a request for proposal (RFP), issuance of the RFP to vendors, and selection of the successful vendor. Beaumont emphasized the development of selection criteria and a scoring system. Believing that, in the past, too much attention had been given to the application functionality of the software concerned, Beaumont elected to take a more comprehensive approach to evaluation, starting with the hardware platform. It is worth noting that, for Beaumont, hardware accounted for over half the total costs of its system solution.

Beaumont Hospital focused on selecting a system appropriate for the present and future, one capable of linking various departmental systems into an integrated system. Evaluation of core HIS modules and the environment involved a skilled project team whose capability encompassed the entire range of hospital functions. The selection process could then be identified for individual departmental systems, enabling departmental users major input in the development of their own particular system within an overall "corporate" framework.

Design. The design phase started once the core HIS and information technology environment were identified. Although the design phase for a totally customized HIS would differ from that described below, we understand that such custom systems are rare in a hospital environment. The costs of developing what is offered today in the form of packaged software are estimated as exceeding $50 million.

The HIS modules were grouped into systems areas and assigned to specialist project teams, in the areas of finance, administration, order communication, and so on. The purpose was to incorporate hospital specific requirements into the packaged software. This activity also involved identifying customization requirements.

The effort involved in design approximated one quarter of the total development process. By separating the design work from the implementation phase, the hospital ensured that its requirements could be implemented using the package selected. This also ensured that hospital staff were appropriately involved in the development of "their" system.

The main steps in the design phase included:

- Installation of the packaged software in its "vanilla" form for prototyping

- Definition of hospital specific reports; screens, dialogues, and control/security features; forms

- Definition of interface requirements

- Specification of changes in hospital work and the decision making structure; implementation approach; software, parameters and table requirements

- Definition of processing requirements

- Confirmation of workload volumes

- Definition of implementation workplans; system acceptance testing; data conversion plan; training approach

- Update of the cost/benefit analysis

In both design and implementation, the approach was to stress cooperative efforts with the software vendor.

Implementation. Although the implementation involved maximum effort by the hospital staff, it carried minimum risk due to the approach in previous phases of work. Project management was critical, because systems implementation affected the practices and procedures of nearly every staff member. Beaumont advises other hospitals to enter into the process of addressing key hospital issues, such as the frequently undefined relationship between medical staff and other staff.

Other areas addressed include work descriptions, decision making structures, procedural documentation, custom programming and testing (where necessary), system testing, data conversion, training of hospital personnel, and system cutover.

One final point to note: once the installation is completed, the hospital's policy states that there should be no changes made for a period of time, e.g., six months. This means that the system is allowed to "bed down" before a post-implementation review determines whether the system complies with requirements and is effective in its fullest organizational sense. The review should also focus on documentation and potential changes and enhancements, and confirm cost/benefit. The hospital strongly recommends that this post-implementation review be carried out, especially if benefits are to be realized.

Project Management

Much of the information technology work in any hospital is project oriented. In healthcare as elsewhere, the information technology function acts as a key agent of change, particularly in relation to processes, procedures, and management. With the advent of clinical information systems, information technology is becoming an increasingly integral part of the process of diagnosing and treating patients. These clinical systems will grow as the use of expert systems and artificial intelligence in hospitals increases. HIS can help hospital management progress from a general administrative to a more professional role, using information technology as a key mechanism in achieving this process.

Project management should use a team approach, with the composition of project teams varying for different phases, as shown in Table 1. Information technology planning and core HIS and information technology environment selections are strategic hospital projects. The responsible project teams should report directly to the chief executive officer (CEO) on a regular basis and be managed on a day to day basis by the chief information officer (CIO). Project teams responsible for the selection of departmental systems and implementation projects should report to the line manager or "custodian" of the system

Table 1. Project Committee Membership

Information Technology Plan and Core HIS and Information Technology Environment Selection

- Chief information officer (CIO)
- Senior clinical analyst (i.e., analyst who understands the medical processes of the hospital)
- Senior financial analyst
- Senior administrative analyst
- Senior departmental analyst (nursing or laboratories)
- Senior information technology analyst (high level technical expertise)

Departmental Systems Selection

- CIO
- Departmental manager
- Departmental analyst
- Information technology analyst

Design and Implementation

- Full time project manager where possible
- Information technology analyst
- User analysts from the systems area(s) involved

or the steering committee of line managers for the system(s) concerned. The project teams should also have a functional reporting relationship to the CIO. Other hospital personnel may be assigned to the project teams as needed.

Hospitals should also consider retaining a management consultant for the planning or system selection phases, to bring not only an independent viewpoint to the processes, but also industry knowledge and wide experience with like assignments. One caveat, however: the hospital should act to ensure the accountability of any consultant retained. Experience demonstrates, for example, that a vendor should not be retained to make a selection from a field that includes that vendor's own software. Nor should a consultant be allowed to construct unrealistic demands for either the vendor or any other consultant to be involved in subsequent phases of an acquisition and/or installation.

Project management is key to the success of information technology work. Management requires the subdivision of the project into a number of tasks, with each task defined in terms of its end product, or deliverable. Other success factors include the commitment of senior management to the project, specific terms of reference/scoping of each project, the appropriate involvement of users and user management, and the skill level of project team members.

Information and Decision Making

Organizational Structure and Development Issues

Defining the Issues. It is difficult to determine the effects a computerized information system will have on the way in which a given hospital is organized and run. No single concept or set of concepts in the information or social sciences defines the issues involved. Because there are no universally accepted definitions for terms such as organization, information systems, accountability, or even manager, perceptions of what is meant by an organizational problem or what is meant by an information need vary widely. As yet, there is no accepted scientific methodology for analyzing the issues involved in organizing hospitals requisitely to use information.

Observation and a review of the literature suggest a diversity of views about the purpose of information technology, its organizational implications, and its costs and benefits. Organizations often express some disappointment in the benefits of information technology following installation. Although such perceptions may not be justified, depending on the criteria upon which such judgments were made, questions arise as to why the perceptions are negative.

Is information technology not all it is trumped up to be as a solution to such problems in healthcare management as cost containment, accurate and timely billing, excessive paperwork, or too much administrative work for professional staff? Or are hospitals so poorly organized and ineffectively managed that information technology compounds existing problems, adds further capital and revenue costs, and releases only "soft" benefits described in qualitative or intangible terms?

How then does one begin to construct an analysis of the failure of information technology to impact the healthcare market? What tools are available to construct an analysis?

Identifying Outcomes. Although outcomes of an information technology installation are often described in monetary terms, it is difficult to demonstrate how claimed savings were accomplished and to isolate the role of information technology in achieving those savings.

As a rule, computing technology will benefit hospitals by reducing the time required of staff and patients in admissions and in record creation and retrieval (from patient record to nursing chart). Other benefits will accrue from error reduction (for drugs, pathology tests, or x-rays) and billing efficiencies (lost charges reduction). By automating a variety of tasks, computing technology can save labor costs by reducing the number of personnel in different departments.

With the help of the information technology department or outside consultants, individual departments can plan, design, and install automated systems. Organizational consequences can be contained within the individual departments by adjusting staff or work assignments with appropriate training or redefinition to include tasks associated with automated data collection, coding, entry, and validation.

Moving From Automated Skills to Information Systems

Automating hospital functions offers many benefits without using the automated system as an information system. The distinction between these two types of systems is critical, however. Information technology (i.e., automation) cannot generate information or make decisions. It is humans who convert data from either manual or automated systems to information. In sum, an information system is a function of the people who convert data to the information they require to deal with the complexity of work/decisions for which they are responsible (Table 3).

To be meaningful, any discussion of information systems requires, as a precondition, descriptions of the work being done in the hospital and the decision making structure required for its efficient operation, including its continuous strategic development and transformation.

An Integrated Management Framework

The decision to move beyond automation to integrated hospital information systems requires a fundamental analysis of the nature of information needs in a hospital and the management structure responsible for all levels of decision making.

The analytical and conceptual tasks considered fundamental in developing the methodology are found in Jacques' seminal work, *Requisite Organization* (1989), and are illustrated diagrammatically there in Annex 2. For a self contained hospital like Beaumont, this methodology clarifies the linkages throughout the system, from the work of the board to the operational tasks at the ward level. This process also involves the independent clinical consultants

Table 3. Transforming Data
from Automated Systems into an Integrated Information System

- Data are captured and classified according to diagnostic related grouping (DRG) or operative procedure type

- Along with associated information, internal and external to the hospital, this information is used

By medical records	To encode for billing patients or insurance companies
By financial officers	To price services and raise charges
By clinicians	To determine diagnosis or treatment modalities
By nursing managers	To plan changes in nursing systems or training programs
By planners	To decide the future balance of specialty work in the hospital

A stratum specific system like this shown in Table 3 is characterized by the fact that the higher levels of decision making require higher levels of human interpretation. Hence, computerized information retrieval has more limited use at the higher levels of decision making.

and specialty groups associated with the hospital in articulating the hospital's mission in realistic terms that fit within the board's future strategy. The direction and level of their clinical work shape the future pattern of support services, including, but not limited to, nursing, laboratory, radiology, facilities, and administrative and control functions in finance and information.

The requisite structure through which accountability and authority are to be exercised, including the critically important relationship of clinical consultants to the board/president or chief executive, can be recreated or redesigned to establish the information needs related to the level of work and decision making throughout the structure. The starting point for establishing the requisite structure depends on the current state of organizational development and information use in the hospital. Success will depend on the involvement of the board and the chief executive in setting the corporate strategy consistent with the hospital's values, culture, and objectives. This strategy is critical to creating a context for full participation of all staff in the hospital.

This integrated framework is designed to ensure that organizational structure and development work is appropriately tied into information technology development. When applied, these concepts can assist the hospital as it moves from an automated system to an integrated information system, through a design and development process. By merging organizational and information technology development processes, and implementing them as a single project, the hospital can create an information system which is directly related to the level of work and decision making. An integrated system, in which the hospital's organizational structure supports the effective handling of information, serves the work of the hospital. It is not installed as simply another piece of new equipment.

Without an organization that can manage work effectively, there is no reality in the concept that information can be generated and used to run hospitals. No matter what the computer software vendors promise, information is the creation of hospital managers and clinicians. Information technology does no more or no less than manage data that are converted into information at different levels of abstraction to solve problems at different levels of complexity. An information system can exist only in the minds of people who create and use it to make decisions.

Questions

1. Has your hospital adopted an appropriate information technology methodology for the development of systems?

2. How has the hospital gone about integrating the management framework with the information technology development process?

3. Does your hospital have an information technology plan, and how has it gone about selecting, in particular, the core HIS modules and general information technology environment?

4. What kinds of resources and skill sets are dedicated to information technology in your hospital? How do these compare to those in commercial organizations?

Reference

Jacques, E. 1989. *Requisite organization: The CEO's guide to creative structure and leadership*. Arlington, Va.: Cason Hall & Co.

4
Information Systems: A Competitive Advantage for Managing Healthcare

James M. Gabler

The term "competitive advantage" is increasingly used to describe business initiatives in healthcare and elsewhere. Yet only history can judge whether in fact an initiative did make a difference. Time must pass before the competitive impact of a particular product or service can be appropriately evaluated. Moreover, an apparent competitive advantage is difficult to sustain since it is limited by *time* until

- a competitor matches or exceeds the advantage

- a competitor's advantage is matched or exceeded

- an advantage is regained

Competitive Advantage in an Information Society

Sustaining a competitive advantage in an information oriented society requires a strategic, communication based architecture which can quickly adjust its content and presentation as customers change. The architecture for information delivery must be in place before any product or service can consistently utilize timely information. This delivery mechanism is more critical to sustaining a competitive advantage than are the key information components required for specific products or services.

Furthermore, this advantage is enhanced for the early investors since market saturation and/or costs can limit or prevent duplicate delivery mechanisms later. For example, when banking was deregulated, most banks focused on new products and services; only a few banks developed networks of automated teller machines (ATMs). Today, those *few* ATM networks dominate as national delivery vehicles across the banking industry.

Information is as critical a resource as people and money. Today more people work with information than produce manufactured goods, making our post-industrial society an information society (Naisbitt 1982). White collar work is almost all information intensive, using the brain rather than muscles. Like money, information even has a time value.

Timely information can create a competitive advantage. The retailing and textile industries have sophisticated processes which capture daily purchasing patterns and turn that information into marketing advantages, such as altering distribution and production plans to optimize anticipated sales. These loosely integrated networks tie together separate, independent businesses to reduce information float which can often return more benefits than reducing monetary float.

The Airline Industry Example

The airlines offer striking examples of information as competitive advantage (Keen 1986). When airlines were deregulated, most airlines competed for market share through fare wars; only a few airlines invested heavily in reservation systems. Today those *few* systems dominate the industry as national and international delivery mechanisms.

In 1984, Delta Airlines admitted it suffered for failing to invest early in reservation systems. Currently, American Airlines generates more income by selling its reservation system to travel agents than by flying passengers.

Timely information served as a basis for offering new services and extending established ones. Through its frequent flyer program, American Airlines captured not only market share but also information on the flying public, which they combined with hotel and car rental information. The resulting service differentiation and target marketing improved customer ties while generating additional revenue through custom tailored travel packages.

The loosely integrated, strategically interconnected design of American's travel agency services gives competitive information advantages over other airlines' reservation and frequent flyer information systems. The same is true for United Airlines. It is clear that timely integrated information has optimized existing resources and enhanced services.

A Competitive Advantage of Information in Healthcare

In healthcare, information systems can provide a competitive advantage for management if the systems are implemented as part of a communication architecture rather than strictly as support for specific functions, such as billing, registration, cost accounting, and lab. Given the pressures of competition and limited resources, healthcare providers must be able to add, drop, or change information system components as quickly as they can adjust programs and services provided to patients. Whereas investing in a monolithic system tends to limit options, investing in a communication architecture can protect against being locked in to one vendor, frustrated by different priorities and incompatible alternatives.

In fact, the specialization and diversity within a hospital require an interconnectivity foundation to effectively address both financial and quality care issues. If a hospital is integrated by an information delivery mechanism which funnels information through the organization, extending that structure to key relationships outside the hospital is relatively simple with existing technology.

This new integration model opens up opportunities for business relationships and joint ventures inside and outside the organization—opportunities limited or excluded by centralized storage models which depend heavily on ownership and/or direct control. The critical difference is the design, not the technology.

The Role of Information Professionals

With their ongoing contact with all departments in the organization, information professionals can develop a unique perspective on how all the pieces fit together. This perspective should be utilized to make money for the organization, not just save money. It should add value, not just reduce costs. Executive management should view information system expenditures as an investment, and the information professionals should justify this perspective with verifiable results. This requires that executive management and the organization as a whole develop an information perspective and a strategic communication vision.

Information systems are most effective when their top manager becomes an active participant on the executive management team. That team can then pursue opportunities to use information to gain a competitive edge. Since any contact with the healthcare buying public is an opportunity to capture strategic information, it is imperative that the information linkage (the delivery mechanism) be considered from the origination of every program or service offered by the organization. Information oriented leadership must find opportunities and turn them into competitive advantages by preparing a strategic platform, recognizing industry trends, and seizing opportunities when they arise.

To create a competitive advantage, executive management must value the capture of information and its flow through the organization. Otherwise, the information resource will eventually be utilized by their competitors (and their successors).

All managers must recognize that information integrity originates at the information source and degenerates as manual handling increases prior to its capture in an information system. If the personnel capturing the information can use it at its source, they will be motivated to ensure its quality and timeliness. If the information is perceived as benefiting only upper management, it will be less reliable, regardless of any management edicts.

This updated form of the original GIGO principle (garbage in, garbage out) has implications that can be effectively and efficiently addressed by information architecture. Disruptions in the information chain, like the food chain, tend to have a much larger overall impact than would initially appear to be the case.

The Information Architecture

According to Porter (1985), "Interrelationships among business units are the principal means by which a diversified firm creates value, and thus provide the underpinnings for corporate strategy." In healthcare, competitive advantage must come from diverse and specialized departments in the form of better, faster, more productive departmental information solutions and enhanced interrelationships among the departments. The ability to capture and later provide meaningful information within and across these departments can bring added value to healthcare services. Because functions within healthcare are highly specialized, and because medical technology and knowledge are expanding rapidly, the healthcare industry will likely be the forerunner of a new information architecture.

Design Approaches

This new architecture represents the latest generation in information designs, moving beyond the process oriented designs of the 1970s and the database oriented designs of the 1980s, as shown in Figures 1 and 2. The systems of the 1990s will be flow oriented, characterized by data movement and multisystem designs, as shown in Figure 3. The capture process can be moved to the source at which data are generated, thus eliminating errors associated with manual data capture and its subsequent entry. As in earlier systems, output can be used in various ways. What is new is a design which uses output in summary form as input to another system.

For example, systems A and B in Figure 3 could be lab and pharmacy summarizing charge events to patient accounting represented by system C. System D could be general ledger which receives summarized journal entries from patient accounting, system C. This model could be extended right to include a separate cost accounting system, or left to include the registration system.

Connectivity difficulties are being overcome with new tools such as local area networks (LANs) and standards for moving summarized data. However, the dominant technical expertise continues to overlay these new technical tools with single database concepts, and the resulting designs minimize the potential for modularity. Information flow creates different architectural and control issues, but the new flow oriented designs can be much more sensitive to the capture, accuracy, control, usage, and relevance of information from a functional perspective (i.e., more people oriented). The technology is available, but more than technical expertise is needed. An information architect is critically necessary.

Due to the prevalent database orientation, most available systems tend to combine multiple functions. Although separation may not seem easy or natural due to familiarity with combined designs, functional system separation can be realized with commercially available information systems. These separate functional systems can then be architecturally combined and recombined as needed or desired. The integration of these modular systems occurs on the

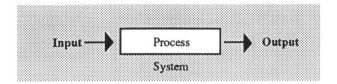

Figure 1. Process Oriented Designs

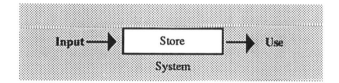

Figure 2. Database Oriented Designs

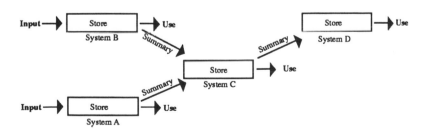

Figure 3. Flow Oriented Designs

network rather than on a single database; this integration is the most distinguishing characteristic of flow oriented designs. Other characteristics are as follows:

Single Entry. Information can be entered once and reused without reentry when appropriate summary information is moved between systems. These summary flows may be immediate; but if immediacy is not necessary, periodic batch flows remain simpler and more reliable. A single official source for each information item and a cohesive flow can ensure that information is reconcilable, i.e., balances between systems.

Operational Accountability. Information can be captured at the source as part of the tool used to perform detailed tasks (i.e., developed from the line workers' viewpoint). Job performance accountability can ensure detailed accuracy, allowing accurate summary information to be quickly extracted as a byproduct.

Functional Modularity. Each system module can focus on a functional work unit's similar usage patterns and performance criteria. The resulting modules generally reflect the organizational entities at or below the department level. This direct relationship to function allows management to determine a system's value to the organization relative to costs and priorities. Accountability is also clear.

Open Architecture. This design can accommodate modular, incremental changes resulting from growth and replacement. Because few limits if any are placed on hardware or software options, functional areas have freedom in system selection and require very few departmental productivity compromises. The open design allows each module to simply plug in to the integrated architecture, with standards such as HL7, MEDIX, ASTM, ANSI X.12, ACR/NEMA, etc., facilitating and accelerating the process. Furthermore, this approach favors off the shelf, turnkey systems which minimize development time, learning curves, and costs.

Information Architect. This design requires a new and critical role. An information architect, rather than a technician, is needed to define the scope and boundaries of each functional system and to maintain the integrated structure. By defining an official source for each information item, the architect can control the synchronization and reconciliation of information flows. By limiting the summarized information to be transferred, duplicate information can be minimized. Synchronization is best controlled by avoiding two-way transfers and using one to one transfers rather than one to many transfers (e.g., striving for an assembly line model). Communications must also be standardized. Information flows must be logically defined and monitored to ensure information integrity between systems. The architect must ensure that the information is suitable for the receiving system and must control architectural cohesiveness through veto power over system connectivity and flows.

Benefits

To justify an architectural design change of this magnitude, there must be significant benefits over existing database designs. Clearly, such benefits do exist and have in fact been demonstrated in early installations of integrated systems utilizing local area network technology. These benefits include the following:

Operational Productivity. Since functions are separated, there is a clear accountability for the productivity of the system, and the relationship between functional areas can be clearly defined.

Understandable Systems. Open architecture of the type described here focuses on the functional roles of individual systems rather than the technical details. (One does not need to understand copier technology to understand the role and value of a copier.) It is easier to identify the role and value of a single functional system than to determine the role and the value of one function of a large, multifunction system.

Organizational Adaptability. This architectural structure is readily adaptable to organizational requirements. Its decentralized technical structure can support either centralized or decentralized controls, whereas a centralized technical structure is not amenable to decentralized control.

Management Control. This structure offers management a high degree of control. In response to changing business priorities and resources, management can control *timing* since modular components can be added, replaced, or deleted relatively independently of the rest of the architecture. Management can control *costs* based on the relative value of the system to the organization, ensuring that value exceeds cost as business sense requires. Given that value based on operational and/or strategic impact can be subjective and hard to quantify, it is upper management's responsibility to determine the relative value of each area for system priorities. Middle and lower management must sell their information system's value in terms of upper management's criteria rather than from their own point of view.

With this architecture, management can control the *benefits realization* process. Measurable commitments should be made by the functional area's managers during the approval process (e.g., workload levels, personnel allocations, expenses, etc.). Line managers should then be held accountable for the delivery of those commitments. Management can also focus on the productivity issues enhanced by each information system.

System statistics can be used to measure productivity and pinpoint areas of greatest gain. Detailed analysis of these statistics can optimize resources; with an objective and highly precise tool for evaluation, creative managers can discover new efficiencies.

For example, some hospitals have reduced their length of stay by changing the dates when hip replacements are performed relative to the start of physical therapy. Meaningful information capture and feedback facilitate this type of analysis.

Decreased Risk. Because of its lower costs, both initially and incrementally, this architecture involves less risk. Risk is further decreased by narrowing the focus for each system, or individual target area, and providing a single focus for accountability, functionality, costs, and benefits. This architecture also encourages the use of turnkey systems which eliminate system development costs and time, thus placing the focus on implementation and production.

Departmental Commitment. A department, freely choosing and having its own system, experiences pride of ownership. Control of its own tools makes the department logically accountable for its own job performance. This accountability reflects a recognized role for the functional area within the organization.

The clarity of role in turn generates a synergistic environment and encourages the mutual resolution of problems. Areas with their own resources are more likely to collaborate with one another in resolving working level problems.

Economies. Multiple, smaller systems generally have both lower initial and incremental costs and a lower total cost than do the typical single, large systems in the marketplace. Additional economies accrue over time as a result of continued vendor competition since the organization is not locked in to one vendor. This generally yields continuing economies up to twice as great as typical large volume purchasing discounts.

Further economies result from the continued focus on departmental usage and productivity rather than on technical development, maintenance, and enhancement.

Natural Redundancy. By design, this architecture has no single point of total failure. A single system failure primarily affects only that functional area. Other areas may lose access to the failed system, but can continue to serve their own areas. Additional and/or special hardware is not generally required, but management can selectively apply non-stop technology to areas where it is determined that a functional role is sufficiently critical to justify the additional expense.

Strategic Structure. Because network adjustments can be made quickly and relatively easily, the organization can more quickly take advantage of opportunities that arise. The only requirement is that the information linkage is part of the initial decision/planning process. With the growing focus on quality of care, the ability to address clinical issues will become increasingly critical. The new architecture empowers management to control the technology rather than vice versa.

Strategic Value

Sustaining quality customer service is the competitive edge in any business, and especially in healthcare. Internally, this means efficiently providing the best patient care; externally, it means maintaining and expanding the customer base served. Maintaining a competitive edge in the 1990s will require the strategic architecture described above. With this structure in place, management can control costs by

- relating the value for functionality to specific expenses

- increasing accountability for productivity

Healthcare providers can then strengthen their customer relationships by linking patients, physicians, and payors. With easier access and added value, utilization patterns can be encouraged rather than forced through such tactics as ownership, control, etc.

Timing is paramount and flexibility is critical, but this strategic architecture can be created with limited financial resources. Overall costs can be reduced if all planning strategically includes linkages to the information architecture from inception rather than added as an afterthought. Although there are always constraints on the resources available, an information perspective must guide the decision process.

Information systems should be measured by their effectiveness in meeting business objectives, not by their utilization of sophisticated technology. With a strategic information vision and the architecture described above, healthcare institutions can take a giant step toward creating and sustaining a competitive advantage.

Questions

1. How does an information perspective affect management decisions?

2. How can patient demographics be used for target marketing?

3. How can information systems encourage physician usage? What role does timeliness of information play in encouraging this physician usage? In what ways can services be most easily accessed inside and outside the facility?

4. How can timely information be used to enhance patient and visitor contact?

5. How does the communication architecture allow true clinical care applications to be more economical and justifiable?

6. Contrast the three design approaches described in this chapter. (Hint: Categorize a familiar system and note strengths/deficiencies.)

References

Keen, P. 1986. *Competing in Time.* Cambridge, Mass.: Ballinger Publishing.
Naisbitt, J. 1982. *Megatrends.* New York: Warner Books.
Porter, M. 1985. *Competitive Advantage.* New York: Free Press.

Select Bibliography

Freedman, D. 1989. Cancelled Flights. *CIO* 2(7):48-54.
Porter, M. 1980. *Competitive Strategy.* New York: Free Press.

5
Financial Systems: Trends and Strategies

Douglas A. Ryckman

"No money, no mission."

This phrase, often repeated in hospitals with religious affiliations, is indicative of the challenge facing the healthcare industry. As economics have tightened and competition has increased, healthcare providers have sought new ways to use financial information systems for competitive advantage.

Scope of Current Financial Systems

The scope of healthcare financial systems varies based on interpretations of where financial, clinical, or administrative systems begin and end. Figure 1 provides an application level schematic which will be used in this chapter. The applications, which are defined as financial systems, are highlighted in the figure and briefly described in the text that follows.

General Accounting

General accounting systems incorporate the following applications:

- General Ledger/Financial Reporting
- Budgeting
- Accounts Payable
- Payroll

General accounting systems provide the basic transaction level support to record, classify, and report financial information. These systems are typically present in all healthcare organizations. With a few exceptions, they resemble their counterparts in non-healthcare settings. One exception is the growing trend to report actual costs on a product line as well as traditional line or-

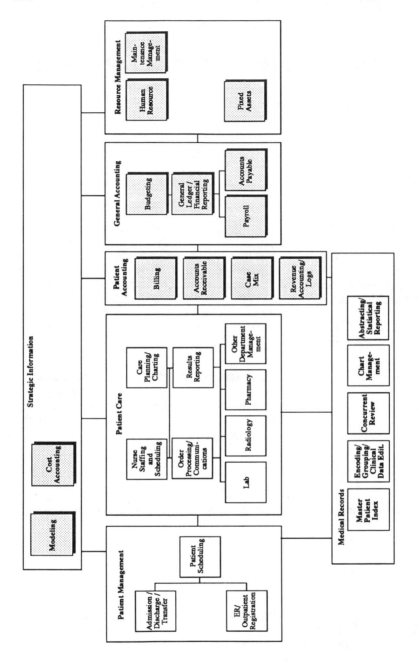

Figure 1. Application Schematic—Hospital Information System

ganization structures. This can require significant additional segregation of information within the chart of accounts, as well as additional complexities if product lines are changed over time. Another distinguishing feature in the healthcare area is in the variety of payroll arrangements which must be accommodated in terms of shift differentials, eight versus 12 hour shifts, and overtime payment calculations.

Resource Management

Resource management systems incorporate the following applications:

- Human Resource Management
- Materials Management
- Fixed Assets

These systems build upon the transaction level information present in general accounting systems. These systems are present in most larger healthcare organizations, and provide information directed at operating management rather than financial/accounting personnel. Both human resource and materials management systems have become increasingly important as profitability pressures have increased. Since labor costs typically represent 50 to 60 percent of hospital expenditures, healthcare organizations are investing more heavily in human resource systems which provide position control, labor cost reporting, and hiring and retention data. Significant future changes to the materials management area will also take place through the development of electronic data interchange (EDI) linkages to suppliers. These are discussed later in this chapter.

Patient Accounting

Patient accounting systems have gone through a significant evolution over the past 10 years, with further changes to be expected. The basic elements of patient accounting remain in terms of accumulating charges, billing appropriate third parties or the patient, and collecting and recording reimbursements. However, the capabilities required to maximize profitability have significantly changed. With the advent of DRG based payments for Medicare and contracted rates for many other payors, patient accounting systems capabilities have changed as shown in Table 1.

Strategic Systems

The final area, strategic systems, currently focuses on two major types of capabilities: modeling and cost accounting. Both of these capabilities are at relatively primitive levels and should evolve over the coming years. In the modeling area, systems have supported "what if" analysis, particularly in the area of budget projection and analysis of changes in activity levels. Cost

Table 1. Major Changes to Patient Accounting System Requirements

Area	Prior to Prospective Payment Payment System (1983) and Increased 3rd Party Contracting	Current
Change Accumulation	Charge capture was critical since virtually all claims were based on detailed bills	Charge capture is critical for remaining charge-based business (usually less than 30% of total)
	Rate setting was critical since many payors paid based on charges or ratios of cost to charges.	Rate setting is also critical only for the remaining charge-based business.
	A billing diagnosis (often inaccurate) was used to send out bills, but had no direct impact on payment amount	Diagnosis is a critical factor in accurate grouping of patients into correct product line (DRG)
		Payments are dependent upon product line
	Limited relationship between billing and medical records	Documentation in Medical Records becomes critical to support grouping decision
	Manual (paper) claims generally submitted	Electronic submission of claims and receipt of payments for Medicare and many third parties
Accounts Receivable/ Collections	Interim (PIP) payments were available from the Federal Government-no immediate penalty for receivables problems	No interim payments-need to track and resolve problems to get paid
Case Mix	Not relevant	Used to adjust payments based on severity of case mix
Revenue Accounting/ 3rd Party Logs	Medicare reimbursement based on detailed log of services, and Cost Report of allocated costs	Logs kept for all payors to serve as basis for contract negotiation
		Medicare Cost Report is less important

accounting capabilities have often been limited due to microcomputer technology on which early systems have been built. Future changes in these systems are discussed in the next section.

In summary, current financial systems provide information to financial personnel and, in some cases, to operating (middle) management. As we predict developments throughout the 1990s, the major changes will involve moving up the information hierarchy to provide better information to top management.

Significant Changes and Issues

"The key to forecasting well...is to forecast often."

Over the next several years, a number of factors will influence the direction of financial systems in the healthcare industry. Four factors which may have a significant impact on systems requirements are

- Increased contracting and financial risk assumption by providers

- Quality as a competitive differentiator

- Relationships between healthcare and other industries with the proliferation of electronic data interchange (EDI) linkages between providers, payors, and suppliers

- Emphasis on strategic information and the executive information system

Each of these factors is discussed below in conjunction with its potential systems implications.

Trend 1: Increased Contracting and Financial Risk Assumption by Providers

The United States currently outspends virtually every other industrialized country on healthcare in terms of percentage of gross national product, per capita expenditures, and almost any other measure. Both the government and private employers are searching for ways to limit their future commitments. Providers will increasingly be asked to assume risk based contracts in which payments are made on some fixed (per case or per capita) basis. Under these systems, several factors will be critical:

- Verification of medical need and the care setting required

- Control over utilization (units of service required)

- Control over efficiency (cost per unit of service delivered)

To respond effectively, healthcare organizations will need systems with enhanced capabilities in the areas of certification, utilization management, and cost accounting.

Certification Systems. These systems will help clinicians to assess whether a patient's symptoms meet the criteria for treatment and whether this intervention requires hospitalization versus outpatient or home settings. While this certification software will not be practical in all situations, high cost diagnostic or therapeutic procedures will be precertified. These types of systems are currently used on a limited basis by HMOs and large employers and often use rule based concepts (also known as artificial intelligence) to evaluate the need for expensive or elective procedures. They will become important as providers accept capitated types of payment engagements.

Utilization Management Systems. Software which evaluates utilization versus best demonstrated protocols will also become important. These protocols will come from a variety of sources, primarily from preeminent institutions or professional groups.

This utilization software will be most effective when used on a concurrent basis as services are ordered. Experimental systems currently exist which perform order checking at the time of order entry. These systems also use rule based logic to establish warnings to clinicians if ordering patterns are dangerous or inefficient. Other software, discussed later in this chapter, which does utilization analysis retrospectively, can be used to weigh cost versus quality. It will be discussed later in this chapter.

Cost Accounting Systems. Finally, more sophisticated cost accounting systems will be required to assist management. These systems should have the capability to:

- Assist in building cost standards, developing relatively precise standards for activities which are significant cost drivers and higher level (RVU-type) standards for less significant activities

- Produce volume based budgets each period

- Use department and product line variance reporting to compare actual expenses and revenues to standard costs and expected revenues

- Provide responsibility reporting of cost variances, with roll up of cost variances to line and product line managers

Trend 2: Quality as a Competitive Differentiator

As pressures on costs increase, institutions and regulators have already begun looking to quality as a competitive point of differentiation. In its initiative for change, the Joint Commission on Accreditation of Healthcare Organizations (JCAHO) is clearly focused on ensuring a base level of quality as a condition for accreditation. To compete effectively, healthcare organizations will have to stake out their positions along the quality/cost continuum.

Systems Implications. Information systems can play a major role in helping executives and medical staff to manage cost/quality tradeoffs. A new breed of systems which integrates cost and quality data will be required. Running in large part on a retrospective basis, this cost/quality management system will need to:

- Record services provided for each patient, with the capability to roll up utilization patterns by DRG, physician practitioner, or other product line definition

- Compare utilization patterns against protocols for best demonstrated practice or against utilization patterns in peer providers. Comparison across providers will be critical in establishing and refining protocols

- Monitor outcome indicators which serve as proxies of quality care, including items such as mortality and co-morbidity/complication indicators

- Adjust data for severity among institutions so reasonable, valid comparisons are possible. This will require the continued development of severity measures with an acceptable level of sensitivity as well as realistic data collection requirements.

The protocols defined from the retrospective evaluations will be used by the concurrent utilization management software discussed in Trend 1.

Trend 3: Proliferation of Electronic Data Interchange (EDI) Linkages

As healthcare has become a larger portion of the nation's business, other industries have become increasingly interested in establishing linkages with healthcare providers. Many of these linkages are currently manual, but will be subject to increasing automation in the future. As these linkages are built, electronic data interchange (EDI) networks will be developed among providers, payors, and suppliers. Systems implications of these linkages fall into four areas:

Electronic Claims/Reimbursement Processing. Providers already use electronic linkages to transmit claims and receive payments from Medicare, Medicaid, and major commercial insurers. An electronic claims clearing house was established in the mid 1980s to facilitate the transmission of claims between providers and commercial insurance companies. This trend will continue, replacing paper processing with the electronic transfer of most funds between financial institutions representing payors and providers.

Financial Service Company Brokering of Accounts Receivable. Major financial services companies such as American Express and Visa may enter into the claims processing arena, taking over a provider's entire billing and accounts receivable management process. The same types of credit verification, credit financing, and product marketing services provided to retailers could be extended to healthcare. The recent acquisition of healthcare software vendors by these financial services companies suggests the beginning of this trend.

Electronic Ordering and Inventory Management. Linkages between providers and suppliers are growing. The concentration of medical/surgical supplies and pharmaceutical products within a limited number of manufacturers creates an opportunity for electronic ordering and inventory mangement. Already established by many large companies, this capability will be enhanced in the coming years.

Preferred Provider/Employer Linkages. As an increasing number of employers become self insured, employers will be motivated to establish electronic linkages with leading providers. These preferred provider organization (PPO) linkages will require both parties to control utilization and cost through the use of cost/quality management systems.

Trend 4: Increasing Emphasis on Strategic Information

As the healthcare industry becomes more cost and quality competitive, the providers with the best information will be the winners. Creating meaningful information from the abundance of available data will be a key challenge. Information systems developers must remember that executives within healthcare organizations are user professionals, not professional users. Because of executives' limited keyboard skills and natural wariness about computers, systems will be redesigned to respond to their needs.

Improved Executive Interfaces. Software will be redesigned to present information in graphic, color oriented formats. Information will be arranged so that executives can view summary trends and "drill down" to locate additional detail. Executives will be able to navigate using mouse or touchscreen capabilities. All information will be available online, with hard copy reports produced on demand. These tools are already available through software on timesharing executive information systems (EIS). Similar presentation tools are also being developed to operate on intelligent workstations and inhouse computers.

Integration of Internal and External Information. Healthcare executives will combine data from a number of different sources, increasingly using external databases to complement internal information. For example, an assistant administrator who is developing a geriatric medicine program might draw information from:

- An external demographics/marketing database to identify population trends by age, sex, and service area

- An external statistical analysis package to calculate potential service demand

- External data available from a state rate setting commission to evaluate the extent to which competing institutions are already providing this service

- Internal information regarding reimbursement experience and cost levels to forecast the new program's profit/loss

The information from these internal and external sources will be combined into decision support databases capable of being accessed by executive information tools.

Strategies for Managing the Successful Introduction of the New Technology

The four trends discussed above will add new dimensions to existing financial systems. To return to our original application schematic, these trends will provide new applications in the areas highlighted in Figure 2. These applications surround existing transaction systems and have the potential to add significant value. Several implementation related strategies will be important to a healthcare organization's ability to realize this value.

Multidisciplinary Project Teams. Most of the new application areas will require participation and cooperation among personnel from financial, clinical, and administrative areas. Particularly in applications such as utilization and cost/quality management, the involvement of medical staff leadership will be essential. In some cases, the sponsors of the financial systems outlined in this chapter may be nonfinancial personnel.

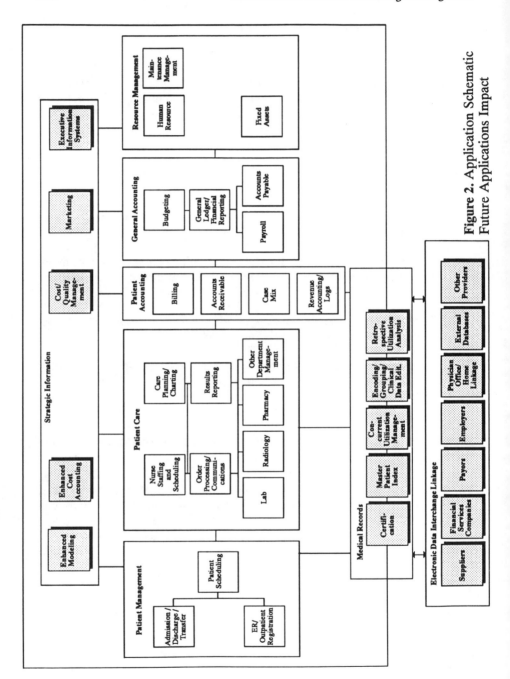

Figure 2. Application Schematic
Future Applications Impact

No Apple Polishing. In the past, information systems personnel have had a tendency to redo existing transaction systems rather than pushing into new strategic systems areas. Systems professionals will have to move outside their traditional comfort zone in the coming years. Successful organizations will be the ones which have the creativity and courage to address new challenges rather than fine tuning old accomplishments.

Open Architecture Technical Standards to Facilitate Systems Improvements. Significant progress is occurring regarding the development of technical systems integration standards. These open systems standards should allow providers to be able to replace applications more easily as richer systems options become available. Providers who are looking ahead will begin to incorporate these integration standards into their system. This will provide important flexibility as the pace of change accelerates.

Emphasis on Change Management. Organizational rather than technical solutions will be required as healthcare providers move into the 1990s. The structure, workflow, and basic ways of thinking will need to change. The organizational re-engineering, training, and benefits realization components of new systems will become more important than their technical characteristics. Personnel working with systems will need to become true change managers. As is shown in Figure 3, these implementation considerations become more important as providers focus higher on the systems pyramid.

The Future

Financial systems will evolve significantly in the coming years as the healthcare industry undergoes a similar degree of change. Systems must grow from an internal focus, directed primarily at finance personnel, to a broader mission of dealing with cost/quality relationships and other CEO level concerns.

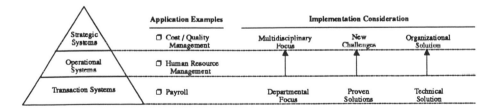

Figure 3. The Systems Pyramid

Questions

1. What are the major systems areas and applications included in current healthcare financial systems?

2. What are some of the ways in which the patient accounting application area has changed since the introduction of the prospective payment system?

3. Discuss some of the factors causing healthcare providers to develop new cost, quality, and utilization management systems.

4. Describe at least three examples of the potential use of electronic data interchange (EDI) linkages by healthcare providers.

5. How will future executive information systems (EIS) differ from systems currently available?

6. What are some key implementation strategies which should be considered as providers put in place new financial systems for the 1990s?

6
Cost Justifying Information Systems

Brian T. Malec

With information systems technology expanding into all areas of healthcare, the cost justification of information systems is a major issue. Managers are being forced to justify expenditures based on the potential return on investment (ROI) for a particular alternative. Despite the difficulty of measuring benefits, decision makers will be pressured to cost justify potential purchases of advanced healthcare technologies, including information systems.

In the 1980s, information systems technology advanced faster than its potential impact could be assessed. The invasion of the microcomputer and other information technologies created organizational stress as healthcare struggled to cope with their implications. Healthcare computing can anticipate still more advances, including interactive voice technology, megastorage capabilities like compact disk (CD) technology, the application of artificial intelligence, high resolution television, standardized information protocols (open architecture), digital imaging networks, holograms, and robotics.

Some of the pressures on organizations will be to replace or update information systems purchased in prior times. The move from the earlier dominance on financial systems to rapid growth in clinical systems at the end of the 1980s has created a market for system upgrades and for information system infrastructures that can support both clinical and administrative decision making.

Management support systems, including decision support systems (DSS) and executive information systems (EIS), that began to develop in the 1980s will become common.

All these information systems technologies will have to be cost justified as healthcare organizations face increasing economic constraints. The impact of these technologies will vary as a function of an organization's information systems infrastructure and strategic mission. Decision makers must be familiar with the theory and practice of assessing costs and benefits of information systems and able to communicate that information to hospital boards.

Basic Economic and Information Systems Definitions

Cost Benefit Analysis

A firm's decision to make an investment, whether to purchase an information system or build an office complex for physicians, is traditionally characterized by four major steps (Stiglitz 1988): (1) Identify various alternatives which will achieve the desired goal; (2) identify the full range of expected costs and outcomes (benefits) for each of the alternatives; (3) determine a monetary value for the expected costs and benefits for each alternative; and (4) apply a decision rule such as which alternative has the greatest profitability (benefits over costs) or which alternative has the highest ratio of benefits to costs (Stiglitz 1988).

When cost benefit analysis is related to healthcare computing technology, costs are defined as "the total expense associated with the acquisition of a computer system or with the use of computer resources, plus all other project-related noncomputer costs." Benefits "refer to the dollar value of all resources created or freed up by the project" (Covvey et al. 1985). Cost benefit analysis considers tangible and intangible economic impacts of a set of alternatives. The method of calculation for cost benefit analysis can be found in any finance or economic textbook. Although the structure of the analysis is clear, there may be debate regarding the conceptualization of the model used to determine the costs and benefits associated with the proposed system.

The estimated future stream of both costs and benefits for an alternative must be discounted to determine a net economic impact of a project based on the current or present value of these future events. Discounting protects against undervaluing an alternative that may not realize its anticipated benefits for several years or that has high costs in the first few years only. Discounting future costs and benefits to a value in present dollars enables an organization to compare resource use among alternatives based on a common reference point.

A final step in cost benefit analysis is to apply a decision rule to the costs and benefits valued in monetary terms. One method determines which alternative has the greatest benefits over cost (B-C). A second method establishes which alternative has the highest ratio of benefits to costs (B/C). The first method favors large projects that have both high costs and high benefits. The second method allows smaller projects to be evaluated on the basis of benefits per dollar of cost. A critical concept in cost benefit studies acknowledges the possibility that no alternative is profitable or has a favorable ratio of benefits to costs and that the best choice may be to make no investment at all.

Cost Effectiveness Analysis

An alternative to cost benefit analysis is cost effectiveness analysis. This method of analysis is appropriate when benefits of a particular project are hard to evaluate in monetary terms. The objective, or outcome, of the project is then taken as a given; and the question becomes what is the most effective way to achieve this objective.

Cost effectiveness analysis is used when the benefits involve issues of mortality or morbidity; alternatives are evaluated on the cost per incremental change in some target statistic, e.g., cost for bone marrow transplants per leukemia patient saved. If the goal is determined as worth doing by other than economic means, then cost effectiveness analysis can be used to find the alternative which uses the fewest economic resources to achieve the stated goal.

Economic Efficiency versus Managerial Effectiveness

The cost justification of information systems must consider both economic efficiency and managerial effectiveness. Although an efficient information system may perform tasks cheaply and may appear to be a good value (printouts arrive on schedule), decision makers should not overlook issues of managerial effectiveness (the printouts actually help the manager perform a task). This may increase the project's costs, due to a greater effort put into systems design, but will generate more effective decisions which contribute to an organization's bottom line.

The key to resolving this issue lies in carefully balancing system design costs against the resulting increase in managerial effectiveness. In these terms, installing an executive information system may result in a more effective CEO; the question becomes how much this is worth to the organization.

Hierarchy of Information Systems

Healthcare information systems can be categorized to help in conceptualizing their function and assumed benefits. Figure 1 shows a pyramid approach often used to illustrate the building process in designing information systems. At the base of the pyramid are transaction oriented systems, or operations functions, which are the engine that drives the patient care and financial systems. Building upon these are the management functions, or management control systems, which support areas like departmental management, DRG analysis, product line analysis, and other tactically oriented management decisions. The next level consists of planning functions, or decision support systems, including strategic planning models, feasibility studies, and market analysis models. An area of emerging potential are executive or information support systems (ESS or EIS), of use in setting policy, choosing objectives, and keeping the CEO informed of internal and external trends that affect the organization. This hierarchy of systems reflects the costs and benefits associated with the various levels and should be considered in cost justifying any information system.

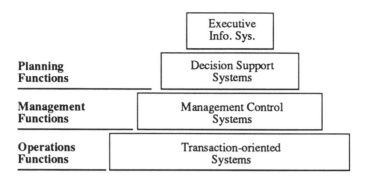

Figure 1. Hierarchy of Healthcare Information Systems

Structured versus Unstructured Decision Making

Costs and benefits are closely tied to the intended outcome of a proposed system and its use in decision making. At the management control level in an organization, tactical decision are made which require information systems capable of supporting semistructured types of inquiry. Departmental and other midlevel managers often use information generated by operational systems to support decisions which, for example, might involve the price sensitivity of a new product or service. Decision models can be developed which use the same data each time the decision is needed. Ad hoc inquiries can be developed to fit into a decision model created for a special purpose. Information systems at this level support the day to day tactical decisions of the organization and may focus on departmental issues as well as institutional profitability.

Decision support systems (DSS) are information systems capable of providing input for the planning functions of an organization. While simple DSS applications may be used at various levels in the information system hierarchy, at the upper levels DSS tend to support decisions that are unstructured in nature. Strategic decision which focus on planning, marketing, or policy fall into this category. A specialized subset of DSS, executive information systems (EIS), are highly unstructured and allow the CEO to look across the organization for trends and to relate factors in a way that may possibly not interest other managers. DSS can be used to address a variety of questions (Buckland 1988):

- Where is performance weakest? Strongest?

- How am I doing in relation to the plan?

- What will happen if conditions change?

- What would a purposed merger do to profitability and market share?

- How do these external trends look as compared to internal conditions?

The costs and benefits of an information system must be directly related to its level in the hierarchy of systems applications and the types of decisions which will result from its operation. In moving from structured to unstructured decision making within an organization, benefits become harder to quantify, as outcomes support management effectiveness rather than economic efficiency. Failure to value increased management effectiveness can result in undervaluing a new system's potential. Investment decisions will suffer.

End User Computing

An expanding trend in healthcare information systems development is increased end user computing. Buckland (1988) defines this trend as the "individual use, or group use, of computer equipment, separate from the organization's computer center, to perform such tasks as: manipulate data; perform analysis; establish local files; and generate reports." This trend accelerated in the 1980s with the spread of personal computers and local area networks. Its potential benefits (Buckland 1988) to an organization are increases and/or improvements in:

- Productivity of management and healthcare professionals
- Direct support to managers and executives
- Competitive advantage in the marketplace
- Effectiveness as well as profitability of the organization
- Management support for a relatively low price
- Communication through electronic mail and teleconferencing

Organizations should develop policies and strategies to maximize the benefits of end user computing. Failure to do so may result in undervaluing a new system or in unplanned and ineffective growth in end user computing.

Determining the Costs and Benefits of Information Systems

In listing factors affecting the cost benefit analysis of a proposed information system, Flaatten (1989) suggests both guidelines and questions.

Guidelines to Be Followed

- A successful cost benefit analysis requires at least two alternative proposals.

- All costs and benefits should be stated conservatively.

- Standard organizational assumptions should be used in addressing inflation, risk factors, and methods of calculating costs and benefits.

- The expected intangible benefits of the proposed project should be discussed as thoroughly as costs.

Questions to Be Answered

- What is the cost of operating the present system?

- Is the proposed information system part of a larger development project? How will future phases affect the costs and benefits of this project?

- How will the costs and benefits change over time due to such factors as inflation and volume increases?

- What risks are associated with either doing or not doing the project?

If an organization uses only a business perspective in calculating costs and benefits, it may undervalue alternatives which have public or social costs and/or benefits. Focus on its mission can help the organization determine how to establish the economic value of alternatives. It is undeniably difficult to place monetary value on benefits and/or costs such as improved patient well being, reduced waiting time, increased community goodwill, or reduced community mortality or morbidity. Hence, organizations may choose to factor out from analysis costs and/or benefits which they cannot charge for or realize monetarily, even though those costs and/or benefits do accrue to the community.

This choice does have the potential to realize private goals, given the current stress on profitability and cost containment. However, it fails to maximize society's goals. An example might be a hospital's decision, based upon a cost benefit analysis, to stop participating in a local trauma network. The decision to withdraw may be supported by costs far exceeding financial benefits for the individual hospital, but costs to the community and to trauma victims will likely increase. Few projects in the healthcare field can be assumed to be asocial or devoid of significant external effects which impact patient care and/or society.

Economic benefits of information systems can be difficult to measure. Some remain intangible because no monetary value has been assigned to the outcome. Information systems which make a manager more effective or simply provide information in a new context may be assumed to have no direct payoff. However, these systems may contribute to increased managerial control of costs and changed managerial and staff attitudes toward information as a corporate asset. At higher levels in the systems hierarchy, information can have direct economic benefits when it affects decisions in the areas of marketing, planning, strategic goal setting, and reimbursement.

Costs and Benefits within the Hierarchy of Information Systems

Whether a proposed information system is designed for operations, management control, or decision support, the tools of cost benefit analysis are similar. The differences generally come within the context of intangible benefits or as a result of misspecification of costs.

Operational Level (Structured Decisions). Transaction oriented systems, which form the base of the information systems hierarchy, are among the most common and most expensive systems in healthcare. Large patient care systems, clinical systems, and administrative systems form the base structure upon the other levels in the hierarchy rest. Covvey (1985) lists the more common costs and benefits associated with these healthcare information systems:

> *Costs:*   Hardware
> Software
> Maintenance (both hardware and software)
> Personnel and staff
> Supplies
> Environmental and construction costs
> Inflation and other external economic costs
> Training
> Documentation

> *Benefits:* Decreasing personnel and staff
> Increasing staff efficiency
> Reducing turnover rate
> Saving supplies
> Increasing collections
> Decreasing the use of more expensive methods
> Reducing or avoiding cost increases
> Making information available earlier to decision makers

Estimates of costs associated with the present system will normally be calculated during an intensive systems analysis. The expected costs and benefits of the proposed new system will be generated during the system design phases of development. If an organization chooses to rely on vendor companies to identify the costs and cost savings (benefits) of their products, that organization must take due care. It should carefully research all vendor claims and extensively interview other clients of the vendor to determine whether the proposed costs and/or benefits are what should be expected given their organization's characteristics and present information systems infrastructure. For example, reduced personnel costs may never materialize due to volume changes and external economic conditions. Freeing personnel from paperwork may appear to result in savings, yet time savings may not produce economic benefits unless they are redirected.

The realization of benefits can be enhanced through project management which has the end user department detail the functional requirements for the proposed system, stating each requirement in measurable terms and specifying the estimated economic benefit in achieving it. Project management should also hold the end user department accountable for achieving the stated benefits after implementation. These management practices will combine to produce conservative but realizable economic benefits from any new information system.

Management Control Level (Semi-Structured Decisions). Most transaction oriented systems produce management reports for the control and monitoring of those systems. At the next level in the hierarchy, that of management control systems, costs are affected by system design, vendor selection criteria, and the organization's capacity for inhouse design. In cost justifying these systems, an organization must determine whether the proposed system will be a separate standalone system, a byproduct of an existing system (such as patient accounting), or the result of a centralized database designed for ad hoc inquiry. Each design alternative has its own array of costs and benefits which must be factored into the analysis. Once the design approach is determined, a major portion of costs is determined by the functional requirements specified for the proposed system.

On the benefit side of the analysis, management control systems provide both tangible and intangible outcomes. Generally, the goal of the management control system is greater efficiency or lower operating costs for transaction oriented systems. These savings can be projected if the functional requirements are specified in monetary terms.

Decision Support Level (Unstructured Decisions). Information systems designed for decision support can cost from a few hundred dollars for a spreadsheet program to well over $200,000 for an executive information system. The range in cost is associated with both the system's intended use and the organization's ability to support end user computer assisted decision making. Packaged programs can assist senior management in market analysis, financial feasibility studies, trend analysis, and decision simulations.

In developing the capability to use a DSS, an organization will incur costs associated with:

- The information system infrastructure
- Staffing an information support center
- Purchase and maintenance of a personal computer networks
- Training of upper management to use DSS effectively
- Software design
- Subscription services to external databases

The benefits of a DSS will generally tend toward the intangible, including such items as :

- More effective organizational decision making
- Better communication among senior management
- More timely decisions
- Intensified focus on critical factors for overall organizational success
- Improved problem identification

To be effective, DSS must be compatible with management style and organizational culture. The concept of knowledge engineering refers, in part, to the careful matching of the computer aided decision support system to an individual's management and decision style. The benefits of DSS can be enhanced with attention to this concept, but the costs of such systems increase as details of the system design increase.

Introducing DSS to an organization invariably involves disruptions to both formal and informal communication and reporting relationships. Increased knowledge and use of computer assisted decision capability may be either the cause or the effect of changes in organizational structures and corporate culture. Though intangible, these impacts must be considered in the cost justification for a decision support system.

Summary

Information systems will continue be critically important in the healthcare industry. Economic constraints will demand a balance between controlling expenditures and providing information systems which contribute to greater efficiency and effectiveness. In the search for efficiency, institutions run the risk of overfunding transaction oriented systems with easily measured benefits, while underfunding higher level systems which have intangible benefits.

As vendors build in more features, management control systems will become more sophisticated. Increasingly, middle and upper management will consider decision support systems and executive information systems as a natural extension of their management style. Cost benefit analysis will continue to require detailed estimates of the tangible attributes of proposed systems. The greatest need, however, is to accurately value intangible attributes of information systems—a task increasingly more complicated at the upper levels of the hierarchy of healthcare information systems.

Questions

1. Using a local healthcare facility as an example, and using the analytical structure described in Figure 1, Hierarchy of Healthcare Information Systems:

   a. Prepare an executive summary of the major information systems currently being used at the transaction level and the principal vendors

b. Give specific examples of management control systems and describe how the resulting reports support the management functions

c. Describe and give specific examples of decision support systems which support the strategic functions of the organization

2. Using a local healthcare facility as an example, survey the institution to determine the current extent of end user computing activities and describe any institutional policies which either encourage or constrain the development of end user computing skills.

3. Select a management control system used in a local healthcare facility, and develop the general structure of a cost-benefit model specifying the tangible and intangible elements of the model in monetary terms. For example: a DRG analysis software package; nursing staffing software; or other departmental control system.

4. Interview a healthcare administrator. List and describe some of the decisions he/she makes on a routine basis in terms of the degree of structure and the sources of information the administrators use to make the decisions.

5. Compile an annotated bibliography of recent articles which discuss techniques for assessing the potential benefits, both tangible and intangible, of healthcare information systems.

Acknowledgments

The author would like to thank Stuart Boxerman from Washington University, Judith Douglas, co-editor and Executive Assistant to the Associate Vice President of Information Resources at the University of Maryland at Baltimore, and Richard Peterson of Andersen Consulting, Arthur Andersen & Co. for their comments and suggestions.

References

Buckland, J. A. 1988. *Management support systems: executive support, decision support, operational support.* Carrollton, Tex.: FTP Technical Library.
Covvey, H. D., N. H. Craven, and N. H. McAlister. 1985. *Concepts and issues in health care computing.* St. Louis, Mo.: C.V. Mosby Company.
Flaatten, P. O. and Andersen Consulting, Arthur Andersen & Co. 1989. *Foundations of business systems.* Chicago: Dryden Press.
Stiglitz, J. E. 1988. *Economics of the public sector.* New York: W.W. Norton & Company.

Select Bibliography

Austin, C. A. 1988. *Information systems for health services administration.* Ann Arbor, Mich.: Health Administration Press.

Bologna, J. S. and R. Ziaee. 1990. Measuring the effectiveness of management engineering and information systems—are you worth your weight in gold? In *Proceedings of the 1990 Annual Health Care Information & Management Systems Conference,* American Hospital Association.

Cash, J. I., Jr., F. W. McFarlen, and J. L. McKenney. 1988. *Corporate information systems management: The issues facing senior executives.* Homewood, Ill.: Irwin.

Eastaugh, S. R. 1987. *Financing health care: Economic efficiency and equity.* Dover, Mass.: Auburn House Publishing Company.

Kennedy, O. G. and S. Collignon. 1988. Selecting patient accounting systems: What are the key criteria? *Healthcare Financial Management* 3.

Malec, B. T. and C. J. Austin, eds. 1990. Special issue: Information systems education for future health services administrators, *The Journal of Health Administration Education* 1.

Peterson, R. and S. Hume. 1989. The hospital of the here and now. *Health Progress.*

Priest, S. L. 1989. *Understanding computer resources: A healthcare perspective.* Owings Mills, Md.: National Health Publishing.

Remmlinger, E. 1990. The new realities of justifying clinical information systems. In *Proceedings of the 1990 Annual Health Care Information & Management Systems Conference,* American Hospital Association.

Rochart, J. F. and D. W. DeLong. 1988. *Executive support systems: The emergence of top management computer use.* Homewood, Ill.: Dow Jones-Irwin.

Section 2–Managing the Institution

Unit 2—New Visions of Technological Leadership

Unit Introduction

Technology today enables healthcare institutions to transfer information across all levels of their organizations and to external locations as well. This revolutionary capability necessitates a leader to plan, coordinate, and control information flow throughout the organization. In order to do so, a leader must be positioned to effect decisions and to deploy financial personnel resources. This unit offers different vantage points of the evolving chief information officer (CIO) position.

Active in healthcare information management and current president of a national professional association, Correll joins with healthcare economist Malec to report on a national survey of healthcare CIOs and discuss their evolving role. Hersher, a healthcare consultant and recruiter, characterizes the CIO organizational view. Trained as a health administrator and now an executive search consultant, Plemmons lays out strategies for recruiting a CIO. Vice president for information systems at a university with a medical center, Barone and her colleague, Chickadonz, dean and professor of nursing, discuss how information technology affects hospital organizational structures and propose a matrix approach to organizational design.

It is no accident that the chief information officer is sitting at the right hand of the chief executive officer. Information is power.

1

The Chief Information Officer as a New Administrator

Richard A. Correll and Brian T. Malec

The chief information officer (CIO) is new in healthcare compared to other industries. By October 1986, *Business Week* reported that over half of the Fortune 500 companies had a CIO position. They went on to forecast that the position would proliferate further, especially in the service industry sector. That prophecy has since been borne out in the information intensive service industry of healthcare, where the position has flourished over the past few years.

The Healthcare CIO

A national survey of healthcare CIOs in 1987 revealed the following characteristics of this new position:

CIOs report to CEO/COO. While the information systems function originated under the responsibility of the finance area, the information management function is independent from the finance area. CIOs indicated that they generally report to either the chief executive officer (CEO) or chief operating officer (COO) of the institution.

CIOs are members of the executive cabinet. The majority of CIOs surveyed consider themselves to be part of the executive cabinet along with the CEO, COO, and chief financial officer (CFO). A new management triumvirate of the CIO, COO, and CFO has direct line responsibilities to the chief executive officer.

CIOs attend board meetings. As a reflection of their upgraded management status, CIOs reported they are invited to attend the board meetings. Recent reports indicated some CIOs have been made actual voting members of their institutional boards of directors.

CIOs manage three primary functions. The departments most frequently cited as reporting to CIOs are information systems, management engineering, and telecommunications. Also reporting to CIOs, though less frequently, are medical records, admitting, and materials management.

CIOs have increasing budget responsibilities. While information systems budgets comprise only 2.8 percent of the hospital's overall budget compared to 5 percent for manufacturing and 7 percent for banking, the CIOs surveyed reported average increases of 16 percent per year to their budgets.

Background

Although 55 percent of the CIOs surveyed named information systems as their primary background, the remaining 45 percent indicated their background was in other areas, such as general healthcare administration, management engineering, and finance. This parallels findings in other industries, where CIOs are more likely to have a generalist background than a technical one. This background reflects the nature of the CIO position which, unlike the position of director of information systems, emphasizes strategic and managerial functions.

Vital Responsibilities

Consistent with this orientation, the highest ranked responsibility among the CIOs surveyed was strategic planning. Leadership ability, vision, and imagination were ranked as the most important critical attributes of CIOs, while technical skills were ranked low. It has been said that CIOs need to be "snowproof" in order to understand the requests of their subordinates. Most critical, however, to the CIOs is the ability to comprehend the strategic use of information systems to support institutional business needs.

Salaries

CIOs in multi-institutions reported salaries and bonuses on a level consistent with their high stature within the organization. (In 1987, salaries averaged

$85,000 and bonuses $10,000.) Perks and benefits pushed total compensation well into the six-figure level. Even in times marked by hospital downsizing and curtailment of expenses, CEOs apparently are recognizing the need to invest in the critical function of information management. Their determination is demonstrated by the fact they are bringing CIOs on board as high level, highly paid executives.

Future Trends

Survey respondents agreed that the CIO position will continue to develop toward the strategic role. A majority suggested that the CIO will become more influential in working with top executives to determine business direction and competitive strategies, emphasizing cost benefits realization along with strategic systems direction.

Despite the tendency for CIOs to assume more and more managerial responsibilities, those who want to maintain an emphasis on a strategic and advisory role may well pass up such opportunities, lest they become managerially overburdened.

The CIO Title

Initially, though a number of hospitals created CIO positions, there seemed to be some hesitancy in utilizing the CIO title itself. As the 1980s ended, however, use of the title appeared to be increasing. Although the original survey revealed that only 6 percent of functioning CIOs had the CIO title, preliminary indications from the 1989 update of the survey reveal a significant increase in the title itself.

Expectations, Education, and Other Issues

The ever changing technological environment of healthcare and health administration places considerable demands on the emerging CIO. The educational background and career development of individuals seeking the position must be enhanced if the CIO position is to gain importance and stature within the healthcare organization.

Based on the 1987 HIMSS survey, 68 percent of all respondents had an advanced degree, either MBA, MHA, PhD, MD, or other master's degree. Combined with an average age of 50 and a primary functional background in information systems, this gives the picture of a successful, experienced, and educated data processing manager evolving into the CIO role. The fact that only 18 percent of the respondents listed administration as their primary functional background suggests that current CIOs may be technically based rather than strategically oriented. The point is that the individuals who have obtained the position of CIO in healthcare may not necessarily be the role model for future CIOs. The current distribution of CIOs is what would be expected from the growth and evolution of this position in healthcare.

The CIO of the future will be an individual with a different educational background as well as a different career path. Additionally, he or she will be the executive to assume responsibilities now nonexistent or held by others in the organization. The challenge is to provide continuing education for practitioners who seek to become CIOs and to retool the graduate programs which will produce the future CIOs.

An Evolving Role

The CIO role is a relatively new issue for the healthcare industry to address. The American Hospital Association (1988) characterizes the role as requiring technical, operational, and managerial expertise. The CIO must understand the computer market, know the healthcare institution's organizational structure and product lines, and be an effective manager of resources and personnel. Critical attributes of the CIO include personal communication skills and the ability to work effectively with senior management and boards. These roles are in part driven by the need for the healthcare institution to compete in a restrictive and often hostile marketplace.

Despite a relatively short history of considering information as a strategic asset, healthcare organizations are seeking to assess and to integrate into their environment those technologies which produce quality products. However, the lack of information systems sophistication on the part of healthcare institutions has not been lost on the highly profitable computer vendor industry. According to Kerr and Jelinek (1990),

> The healthcare industry is for the first time under tremendous pressure to become competitive and to take advantage of whatever can improve efficiency and effectiveness. Because of the size of the healthcare industry and the lack of incentives in the past to apply some of these technologies, the opportunities for growth of information systems (products and vendors) are tremendous and probably greater than in any other industry.

Given the rapid advances in information systems technology in the 1980s, it is not surprising that the primary focus of the current generation of CIOs is data processing. Technical competence is vital to the CIO's role and performance. However, the greater emphasis is on and will continue to be on management skills and abilities. Technical competence is necessary to manage highly technical professionals and to be able to understand the limits of the technology, whether developed inhouse or purchased. Since the CIO will most likely be managing such areas as information systems, telecommunication, management engineering, and other specialized technical areas, the effectiveness of the CIO will in part depend on the respect of these professionals.

However, the attribute that will in the long run determine a CIO's success within an organization is the effectiveness of that CIO's strategic management skills. While technical competence assists with management activities down the organization, strategic management skills are needed to effectively communicate up the organization to the CEO and board and laterally to other senior managers like the chief operating and financial officers (Bell and Malec 1990).

A vital role of the CIO is and will be the responsibility to educate the board and senior management in several key areas:

- The importance of information to the success of the organization

- The kinds of information needed for institutional planning and development

- Information systems procurement and contract negotiation techniques

- The use of consultants in planning and installing information systems

- Managing the use of computers in health services organizations

- The state of the art of clinical, administrative, and decision support systems (Boxerman 1990)

The CIO also provides the CEO with information in a timely and effective manner. To accomplish this, the CIO must work with a number of individuals to develop decision support systems and other infrastructures, at both the departmental and institutional level. Effectiveness in decision making requires the technology to support the decision making process and the knowledge to use the technology.

Career Paths

Leadership expectations, the educational role, and the management role of the CIO have put demands on this emerging position—a position which has yet to be fully accepted in the corporate boardroom or the individual facility. How should an individual prepare for a career path leading to the CIO position?

As in any field, exceptional individuals will emerge who on paper do not possess what might be considered desired characteristics. There is always some natural selection involved. The balance of technical competence, management effectiveness, and personality forms an equation that is impossible to solve. Future CIOs may come from three principal backgrounds: other industries; technical areas like information systems, management engineering, medical records, or other allied health professions; and general administration. Each career path has its particular educational needs.

The lack of a large pool of CIO candidates in the healthcare industry has prompted personnel raids on other industries. The individuals recruited have unique experiences and abilities, but are often surprised at the lack of product identification in healthcare and the lack of sophistication of the information users. A continuing education program for this group must focus on the role and functions of healthcare professionals, such as doctors, and provide an orientation to the strategic issues in healthcare. To gain knowledge of the healthcare industry and its issues, these individuals should participate in such healthcare professional organizations as the Health Information Management Systems Society (HIMSS) and the American Council of Healthcare Executives (ACHE).

Healthcare professionals with data processing backgrounds often seek the CIO position as a logical career path. While possessing technical competence, they often have had limited exposure to institutional strategic issues and a management view of the whole institution. A degree in health administration or advanced management courses would strengthen these individuals' career paths. However, they also will have to overcome the stereotyping associated with technical professionals.

Non-data processing healthcare professionals who seek the CIO career path have educational needs which may include both management skills and technical competence in information systems. In addition to appropriate advanced degrees, individuals should seek continuing education within professional organizations such as HIMSS and ACHE.

The generalist health administrator will be the fastest growing component of the CIO career path. Individuals with a master's in health administration (MHA) or a master's in business administration (MBA) have already observed the career growth opportunities associated with the CIO position. Individuals with backgrounds in operations and planning will be in demand for the CIO position. Educationally, the generalist tends to be thin in the technical areas of information systems, but strong in strategic management experience. In response to the changing employment market, MHA and MBA graduate programs have begun to develop information systems sequences for the generalist.

The Challenge

The CIO position is creating challenges both for healthcare institutions to understand the CIO's contribution to the organizational structure and for individuals who seek a career path leading toward the CIO. Institutions must assess their competitive environment and adopt a perspective that information is an asset and its effective management is vital to the future of the organization. Individuals must assess their strengths and weaknesses in terms of technical competence, experience, management abilities and style, and educational background before embarking on the CIO career path.

Questions

1. Survey several non-healthcare industries in your local area to determine the following:

   a. Do they have a CIO?

   b. How long have they had a CIO?

   c. What is the academic and practical background of the CIO?

   d. Where does the CIO fit within the organizational structure? Develop a brief organizational chart.

2. Survey several local healthcare facilities to determine the same information as in the question above. What similarities and differences did you discover?

3. Compile an annotated bibliography of recent articles which discuss the organizational impact of the CIO in healthcare.

4. In what areas of strategic planning should the CIO be involved?

5. What steps must a CIO take in order to remain current, and what is happening within the computer healthcare industry?

References

American Hospital Association. 1988. *Guide to effective health care information management and the role of the chief information officer.* Chicago: American Hospital Association.
Bell, R., and B. Malec. 1990. The CIO's location in the organizational structure: Implications for health administration education. *Journal of Health Administration Education* 8(1).
Boxerman, S., et al. 1990. Continuing education needs of board members, administrators and health care personnel. *Journal of Health Administration Education* 8(1).

Kerr, J. K. and R. Jelinek. 1990 Impact of technology in health care and health administration: Hospitals and alternative care delivery systems. *Journal of Health Administration Education* 8(1).

Select Bibliography

Bock, G., K. Carpenter, and J. Davis. 1986. Management's newest star—meet the chief information officer. *Business Week*, October 13, 160-72.

2

The Evolution of the Chief Information Officer

Betsy S. Hersher

The need for senior global executives in response to the sudden shifts and challenges within the healthcare industry has touched every function in the hospital.

The Chief Information Officer

The chief information officer (CIO) role in healthcare enterprises has evolved as a result of the 1982 TEFRA regulations and reporting requirements. As hospitals fought to remain viable and competitive, they began to view information as a key corporate resource—a drastic change from their previously rather laissez faire attitude.

Medicine was advancing rapidly, but traditional healthcare information systems were not supporting that growth. For a systems industry that was started in 1967, the progress made by 1982 was not sufficient to put information directly into the hands of the users, particularly the clinical users.

Data processing directors found it difficult to meet these new needs. The reporting structure in which they were placed was not supportive of relationships with key users, and the level of their positions within the organization did not provide the power or authority to effect change. Many data processing directors were technical by training and territorial and controlling in approach.

Defining the CIO Role

The CIO role has had a multitude of definitions that are different for each setting. There were, and still are, critics who hold that the concept represents nothing more than data processing directors pursuing advanced titles or chief executive officers (CEOs) seeking to hire or promote CIOs in the hopes of magically solving their information requirements. As this backlash to the position made clear, the concept of control of information was a factor, a factor exacerbated by the lack of understanding and a clear vision of the CIO role. The we/they attitude persisted between the information systems organization and the growing number of physicians who were solving their information needs through departmental computerization.

As the dust settles, however, the key indicators and factors for the success of a CIO function remain clear:

The corporation

- Is committed to information as a key corporate resource

- Views the CIO as a key senior executive

The CIO

- Reports to the highest level possible, either Chairman, CEO, or Chief Operating Officer (COO)

- Has oversight of all the corporation's technology, hardware, and software

- Is key contributor to the overall architecture plan for the organization

- Concentrates on strategic information and long term strategy rather than day to day operations

- Champions a strategic information plan that is synergistic with the corporate long range strategic plan

The last two years have seen a sudden shift in the information systems industry, one directly paralleled in healthcare. Today both are responding to rapidly emerging technology and the communication and networking requirements of the users. As Donovan (1988) points out in "Beyond Chief Information Officer to Network Manager," "Decentralized computing is sweeping business...network managers won't just accept decentralized computing. They will encourage it."

CIOs are restructuring their organizations to support this decentralization and the technology that makes it possible. They are restructuring to support the use of networks and clinical information systems, to respond to user needs through the provision of client services and training. They are looking to satisfy requirements for physician systems, research and development, and advanced technology.

The role of the CIO in healthcare has evolved rapidly in response to the acceptance and requirement for information as a key corporate resource, widespread decentralized computing power, and users who are quickly growing comfortable with technology. The CIO has become a change agent in the role of providing access to data, and is no longer solely the implementor of systems, but the architect of the overall plan for systems integration and connectivity. The decreasing costs of technology and the availability of powerful departmental tools dictate that someone must orchestrate the flow of information, foster the integration of systems, ensure the integrity of data, and monitor for redundancy. The CIO must have the vision to view these issues from a senior executive perspective, to match business and organizational needs to the appropriate information and technology platforms. The emergence of clinical systems and sophisticated connectivity tools points to the role of architect/leader, not controller, of information resources. The successful CIO requires sound technical resources and acts as a consultant to the sophisticated users in the organization.

As the party responsible for setting standards and procedures in support of the growth of technology and maximizing the benefits of the technology investment, the CIO must be able to deal with the abstract and monitor, but not necessarily directly manage, all the departmental resources. This involves dealing with many new issues today: benefits realization, executive information requirements, clinical workstations, the automated medical record, data administration, and quality of care, to mention only a few.

Successful Reporting Structures

In a single entity, the CIO needs to report to the highest executive level possible with the highest title appropriate for that organization and must sit on the senior executive council. A shift in structure, with the CIO reporting to the senior vice president of finance, can occasionally be seen. Generally, this tends to occur in organizations where the CEO is new, has too many vice presidents reporting directly, or is not able to champion the CIO position. In most cases, this is successful if the senior vice president of finance is as global an executive as the CIO is expected to be. The reporting structure should be evaluated carefully by an incoming CIO. It requires the confidence of not only the CIO, but also the clinical community.

The corporate CIO is a relatively new role and a variety of reporting structures are operative across the country. In a corporate setting, the CIO should be on the same level as the senior financial officer.

Emerging enterprises and turf issues have resulted in a variety of gymnastics in defining reporting relationships. Ultimately, the most successful structure for individual entity vice presidents of information systems (VPIS) is to report directly to a corporate CIO. The survival of corporate CIOs without this reporting structure is at risk. The question must be asked whether the overall information needs of the corporation are being met with an indirect reporting structure. The CIO needs access to the major information systems resources within the corporation. This does not mean that the director of laboratory computing in hospital A should report directly to the hospital VPIS or to the corporate CIO. Clearly, the hospital VPIS should report directly to the corporate CIO while acknowledging the CEO of the individual hospital as his/her major client.

The organizational charts shown in Figures 1 and 2 represent a corporate CIO organization and the CIO reporting structure within the corporation.

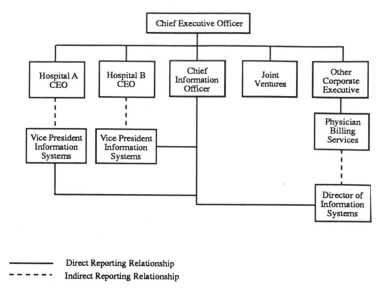

Direct Reporting Relationship
Indirect Reporting Relationship

Figure 1. Corporate Entity

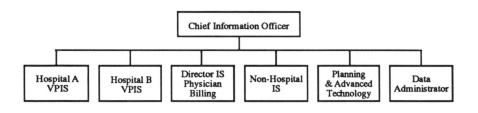

Figure 2. Corporate Chief Information Officer Organization

Emergence of Clinical Systems and the Role of the Physician

For years, there has been a struggle between the clinicians and the data processing director. When the data processing director was under the control of finance, the clinicians felt their needs were not being met. Minicomputers and excellent new departmental system vendors allowed clinical departments to begin their own computerization efforts. Once computerized, they did not want their systems under the control of the data processing director. Generally, they did their own thing, without consulting or getting help from data processing. Issues of redundancy and lack of integration began to grow with so little communication between clinician and data processing director.

As the CIO concept has matured, many forces have contributed to the growing effort to work closely with physicians and satisfy their critical data needs. Reporting requirements and the need for clinical and physician auditing forced the industry to focus more attention on clinical systems. Administrators and physicians alike need quick access to data for reporting and decision support. With connectivity tools allowing users easier access to data and technology, CIOs and physicians are working together to provide timely, accurate information. In the past, the relationship between clinicians and data processing directors has been marked by struggle, on occasion intensified by some administrators' attitudes about "computer savvy docs" and data processing. Today, the emerging role of clinical and medical information manager requires the cooperation and support of the CIO in a joint effort to support decentralized computing. The role is also effective in involving physicians in the implementation of hospital wide systems.

A New Organizational View

In an environment marked by an explosion of technology issues and increasing user demands, the senior information systems executive cannot do it all and must rely upon the support of others. The CIO needs to hire excellent people in specific areas of expertise to be able to manage strategically. The organizational chart shown in Figure 3 is a composite of what is currently happening around the country and what the consultants and CIOs contributing to this article suggest will be future trends. The functions are described below.

Data Administration. This function addresses the overall planning, control, and management of data and databases as a corporate resource, with special attention to

- Support of the mission and business objectives of the organization

- Development and administration of data policies, standards, and procedures to define ongoing projects and effectively utilize data

- Coordination and development of the database and other data structures to minimize redundancy and maximize the realization of the data

Client Services/User Support. There is an increased demand for responsiveness to the users. This function can encompass the following:

- Information center
- Benefits realization
- Education and training
- Decision support systems
- Office automation
- System implementation and support
- Help desk
- User liaisons

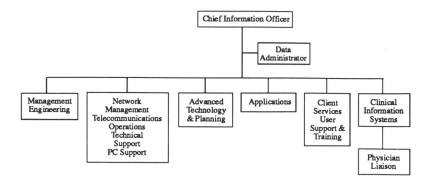

Figure 3. A New Chief Information Officer Organizational View

Network and Technology Management. This function and the individual meeting it will fast fill one of the most critical roles in the CIO's organization. This will be the key technical guru who should be responsible for the following functions:

- Network management
- Operations
- Technical support
- Telecommunications
- Education
- Help desk

This function will have a significant impact on a complex multisite organization and be responsible for the continuity between systems internally and effective communications between external sites.

Together with the data administrator, the network and technology manager will have a significant impact on the CIO's organization in the future. They hold the key to connectivity and data repositories, as they work together to address these questions:

- Who has the data?
- What are the data?
- What form are the data in?
- How are the data extracted for use?

Clinical Information Management. This function can encompass but not necessarily control systems in the following clinical areas:

- Laboratory
- Radiology
- Pathology

- Pharmacy
- Nursing

*Physician Liaison.*This role can report separately to the CIO or be included as part of clinical information management. The key success factor is that the individual filling this role assume a consultative attitude to departmental users. The role may be well served by a clinician, such as an inhouse physician who is "computer savvy" and has excellent rapport with the rest of the clinicians and medical personnel. For the clinician to succeed in this role, the CEO, CIO, and clinical information manager need to share an exact understanding of the function and be clearly non-territorial in their approach.

Advanced Technology/Planning/Research and Development. Frosting on the cake? Perhaps not. This function can keep up with regulatory issues and their impact on technology and healthcare trends as well as leading edge application development and emerging technology research. This is an excellent place to have the users explore some of their ideas.

Future Requirements for the CIO

The past two years have seen an incredible advancement of the CIO concept within the healthcare arena. The CIO position is becoming an understood and necessary function for the advancement of a healthcare enterprise. Successful CIOs have responded to the changed requirements and are learning how to make the most of sophisticated users and the trend toward decentralization.

Among the skills CIOs need for continued growth are great flexibility and the executive ability to manage and support information flow without absolute control of decentralized systems. The CIO will need to have the strategic vision to set the overall architectural platform for the organization and function as a change agent and risk taker. Leadership, communication, and political skills will be paramount. The CIO must be able to ensure the continuity and integration of systems, thereby supporting the future growth of the enterprise without controlling all resources.

The CIO will need to be a great negotiator, building long term business relationships. Business sense and the ability to communicate ideas and support solutions will be important for success. The CIO will have to be a survivor and be viewed as absolutely credible in order to set standards and procedures for the organization.

The CIO will have to be action oriented and welcome other experts into the information systems organization. Strategic planning has become a key component of the CIO's job, not something to do when the fires are put out.

The skills required for success in the 1990s will be the same for the CIO as for the COO and CEO. In the last 18 months, the CIO role has become established in healthcare. At this point, with the growing demand for information and exploding technology, this role will continue to grow with individuals who have the right skills.

Questions

1. How should the CIO report within the overall hospital organization?

2. Contrast the role of the CIO as a strategic planner rather than as an implementer of systems. Are the systems the CIO will be involved with strictly computer systems?

3. How must the CIO relate to the physicians practicing within the hospital?

4. What new skills will be required of the CIO in the future?

Reference

Donovan, J. 1988. Beyond chief information officer to network manager. *Harvard Business Review.* 66(5):134-40.

3
Replacing a Chief Information Officer

Patrick F. Plemmons

Nothing is more important to the success of an organization than leadership. No matter how large or strong an organization is, no matter how much money and equipment, or how many people it commands, the one and only factor that can bring together and best employ those resources is leadership. In any field, the right person at the right time makes the difference between success and failure. Leadership is especially important in information management because the field tends to be perceived as technical and cold.

Although the departure of a leader may be regarded as a setback, an organization can take strategic advantage of such a major change if the replacement process is handled correctly. This chapter describes how to replace an information resources director, with or without the use of an executive search firm, from the resignation of the incumbent up through the orientation and corporate assimilation of the new hire.

Reacting to the Resignation

When an announcement is received that a chief information officer (CIO) or other highly placed information resources manager is resigning to accept a new position, the CEO's reactions can range from anger or panic to resignation. To ensure that the hospital survives the loss, the CEO should immediately begin planning for the replacement process.

Within several days of the announcement, the CEO may want to make a strong attempt at retention, if the individual leaving is a valued employee. It is easier and less expensive in the long run to retain a valued employee than to recruit and hire a new employee with all the attendant costs and risks, especially if the salary, job title, and responsibilities are increased when the position is refilled.

At a separately called meeting with the CIO, the CEO should discuss the reasons why the CIO is leaving. If the CIO has an opportunity for career advancement, there is little to do but accept the departure. If, as is often the

251

case, the decision to leave is not irrevocable, and the departing employee is feeling unappreciated, underutilized, or misunderstood, the CEO may choose to explore what would make the job more attractive. Although more common in the business world than in hospitals, a counteroffer may be an appropriate and viable option and should carry no stigma.

In the event that the counteroffer fails, as often happens, a thorough exit interview with the CIO should focus on how the position can be improved and what type of person (or even specific people) should be considered for the position. The departing CIO's recommendations should not be taken at face value, however, since individuals frequently tend to recommend successors less qualified than themselves.

Planning for the Replacement

At this point, the CEO should evaluate the information management department and assess the critical information issues facing the organization in the near and long term. Replacing the CIO gives the CEO the opportunity to reevaluate and, if necessary, to change information management strategies. Different individuals have different strengths, and the organization may have been constrained from achieving its objectives in the past by the limitations of its CIO.

The CEO should also examine organizational philosophies about hiring and determine whether the organization is committed to a recruitment process which will find the very best candidate. This determination has direct implications for the search in terms of timing, compensation, and benefits.

A commitment to finding excellence means paying the market rate, tailoring the position to suit the wishes of the desired candidate, and potentially spending many months to find, woo, and land the perfect CIO. It may also mean that top management, including the president or CEO and board members, will have to be intimately involved in the search and spend considerable time romancing candidates, especially during the final negotiations.

Organizations are not always willing to put this level of commitment into a recruitment. Frequently, organizations set tight salary parameters and job descriptions, and then try to find the person who will fit within those limits. How aggressive the organization wants to be in recruitment is actually a function of how critical a role it perceives the CIO position to play. Although the organization's cost benefit structure for the CIO position will determine the type of recruitment done, the smart organization is always willing to deviate from the tight constraints of job positions and salary ranges to attract the best talent when it is available.

An old adage says, "If you don't know where you're going, any road will take you there." Translated to the recruitment process, this means simply that the organization needs to know what it is looking for before it begins to look. The CIO sought will vary with the organization, its needs and strategies, and the involvement of other key individuals in information management, especially the CEO.

Describing the Position Requirements

In organizations where the CEO is closely involved with information management, other managers tend to be knowledgeable and involved. In organizations where the CEO asks the CIO to serve a standalone staff function, other managers tend to remain uninvolved and look to information management to supply a repository of knowledge. Because of this variability, there is no perfect CIO. Generic job descriptions can be good starting points, but the individual organization always needs to tailor the position description to its own needs.

Two issues always come up in a healthcare CIO recruitment: the importance of healthcare/hospital experience and of technical skills. Experience shows that CIOs from other backgrounds can switch into the healthcare field and be excellent performers. Nonetheless, there are good reasons to require healthcare experience of CIO candidates. The CIO who fully understands the business, the marketplace, and the forces acting upon it will be quickly accepted and able to contribute strategically within the healthcare organization. On the other hand, healthcare tends to be somewhat inbred, and looking outside the field can yield a larger applicant pool and bring in new ideas and new solutions.

The technical skills issue reflects the prevailing view in healthcare that information resources is a technical discipline, narrowly focused on maintaining hardware and software. In reality, the information resources function cuts across the total organization and has strategic significance. Thus, the highest priority in recruiting a new CIO should be top management skills—among them the ability to plan, delegate, manage, and implement as well as to contribute to the overall strategy and general management of the organization. Although the CIO should be solidly grounded in technical disciplines and theory, the hiring organization should be careful not to fall into the trap of recruiting a technician. Above all, the CIO needs to be able to work with people and get things done through them.

Before beginning the recruitment, all the support which the CIO will use should be identified and, preferably, in place. This includes office space, administrative support, and budgetary and departmental support. Superior candidates will easily discern any major gaps in the package. Also critical is the timing of any other important recruitments. If the organization is recruiting for the position to which the CIO will report, that individual should be selected and on board to personally manage the recruitment of the CIO.

Conducting the Search

There are two ways to replace a CIO. The healthcare organization can do the search on its own or hire an executive search firm. Either way, it is the responsibility of the hiring organization to complete the hire and to integrate the new CIO into the management team. The decision whether to use an executive search firm to find the new CIO is not simple. An organization may choose not to retain such a firm because of the fee involved, yet will neglect to tally up the expenses, less obvious but still very real, of conducting the search inhouse. Among the expenses easily overlooked is the investment of management time.

An organization conducting the search itself typically uses a vice president or director of human resources to conduct the intake phase of the search. A search committee made up of hospital managers then reviews the resumes and interviews the candidates. This arrangement overlooks the difficulty the human resources officer may encounter in trying to be a consultant to top management; suggestions may be overruled or ignored, and good candidates may drop (or be dropped) from the pool. In addition, using a committee in the difficult task of evaluating individual candidates magnifies the problems involved in managing any committee.

Besides involving considerable time and expense, the approach is essentially passive. With little or no control over the applicant pool, the organization frequently finds that the candidates do not meet the qualifications, even though they fancy themselves ready for the job or think that they would like to have it.

An executive search firm uses a much more proactive approach. They identify superior candidates already known to them or found through searching and original research, who meet the specifications. They approach these candidates directly, tell them about the job, and evaluate whether there is a good fit. At this point, search firms generally contact references to verify the candidate's situation and good standing. Then, and only then, is the candidate presented to an employer for consideration.

The search firm thus saves hospital personnel a significant amount of time, by eliminating marginal candidates and identifying those most qualified. Moreover, search firms handle candidates expeditiously. When inquiring regarding a search and their own status, candidates often find contact with a search professional more personal, immediate, and occurring at a higher level than direct contact with a human resources department.

With many other functions to perform, the human resources officer may not have time to devote to an executive search. The same is true for the chief executive officer and other senior managers. Although the organization which devotes top management time to an executive search can do as good a job as any executive search firm, few employers are willing to commit the time or resources required. This is especially true if the goal is to hire the best talent available.

There are, however, times when an employer may elect to fill a position rather than seek the best talent. This tends to be the case when there are no pressing needs in the information management department and the road to the future appears smooth. This may also be the case in organizations that do not put a high value on the information management function. Whatever the circumstances, these organizations should probably advertise and do their own recruitment. Clearly, for the employer who deems the information management department critical to the overall success of the organization and who wants the best CIO possible, the executive search is a viable option.

Once committed to secure the best, an employer must be ready to "go the extra mile" necessary. Top CIOs in the country are not eager to leave their jobs. To attract them, an employer must offer them more responsibility, increased scope, more money, more benefits, or all of the above. Location is important as well; compensation, benefits, or other job aspects may vary according to the candidate's perceptions of the employer's location.

Table 1. Going It Alone

Agree on Objectives

Probably the most important part of the search is the initial planning. Try to reach general agreement on the kind of person you are seeking, the responsibilities of the position, and the overall strategy of the search. The embodiment of agreement on objectives is the position specification. This will state in writing the responsibilities of the position and the experience and qualifications that successful candidates should possess. If this document is done correctly, it can also become a very valuable sales tool during the search.

Advertise Widely

The next step in the recruitment is to place advertisements in appropriate journals, newspapers, and other media that will most effectively reach your desired candidates. If the search is national, you will want to use *The Wall Street Journal;* major metropolitan newspapers across the country, especially within your region; hospital trade journals, such as *Hospitals and Modern Healthcare*; and specific MIS publications. It can also be helpful to touch base with professional societies, selected university departments of MIS, and similar interest organizations.

Involve Top Management

Most likely, the search will be conducted day to day by human resources personnel, but it is critical to involve top management in every step of the process. Time and again, it has been shown that managers make moves not necessarily because of more money or more responsibility, but because they perceive they are wanted and needed in a new organization. If you want to be successful in hiring the best information managers, make sure top management is personally involved in dealing with outstanding candidates, particularly when it comes to making and negotiating offers.

Give References the Importance They Deserve

Probably the biggest mistake employers make when doing searches themselves is not to do adequate referencing. Interviews are important, but references are far more important because you get a better feel for a candidate's work habits, personal quirks, and strengths and weaknesses.

Be Timely

A serious error in recruiting is to drag out the process so that candidates become disillusioned and uninterested. In every aspect of the search, especially interviewing, be timely, follow up and, above all, make decisions quickly. If the search drags on, candidates will begin to imagine all kinds of dire consequences, usually that you have lost interest in them, especially if they are looking at other things, and this can cause the best of them to drop out.

Anticipate Counteroffers

The ideal candidate is not in the job market. He/she is well employed and probably highly valued by the current employer. Even if you have made a fantastic offer and the candidate has accepted that offer, do not think that is the end. The smart employer will make a counteroffer when a valued employee is leaving. You can anticipate this and blunt its effect by letting the candidate know that a counteroffer may be coming and having them think through in advance how they will deal with it. You might also keep in reserve some more money, perquisites, or the like to sweeten your offer if need be at the last moment.

Table 2. Using a Search Firm

Stay Involved

Remember that an executive search professional is not a substitute for you or your own effort and judgment in a recruitment. You probably need to work just as hard and stay just as involved in the project as you would if you were doing it on your own. The only difference is that the executive search firm will bring you "pre-qualified" candidates and free you from the onerous task of advertising, screening, and pre-interviewing.

Work with the Candidates

Do not expect the headhunter to bring the perfect candidate who is immediately ready to accept your offer and move to your organization. If your executive search firm is doing its job, the candidates will be highly qualified and will be the best available at any given point. But you still need to work with the candidates and convince them to make the move.

Avail Yourself of the Firm's Consultant Skills

Remember that a good executive search firm acts as a consultant. Ultimately, the most important contribution they can make to a recruitment is their experience and informed judgment. Do not treat executive search professionals as hired hands. Seek their input and counsel at all milestones in the recruitment, and you will be rewarded with a better hire.

Use the Full Services of the Search Firm

In addition to bringing in outstanding candidates, any good executive search firm should assist you in the following areas by:

- Verifying each candidate's formal education and degrees

- Extensively evaluating candidates' references, both before and after they are presented to the client

- Assisting in presenting an offer to the chosen candidate and in serving as a go between in any ensuing negotiations

- Smoothing the candidate's transition from the previous organization to the client's

Depending on how demanding the specifications are, the average search today takes about 120 working days, if scheduling is not complicated by Christmas and summer vacations. Spring is a popular time for searches, because of the ease of moving children into new schools. However, timing is not nearly as important as making the right hire. Organizations should not be stampeded into filling a position just to complete a search within 120 days. A long search will not adversely affect the morale of an organization if the status of a recruitment is reported often.

Choosing a Search Firm

There are two major types of executive search firms: contingent and retained. A contingent executive search firm usually works on a non-exclusive contract and does not receive final payment until a candidate has been hired. A retained search firm, on the other hand, receives a set fee for the work whether or not any placement is made, although in almost every case there is a hire.

While a contingent search may appear less costly, the professional fees for both contingent and retained firms typically are one third of the first year's cash compensation for the person hired. In addition, direct and indirect expenses associated with the search are charged to the client. The main difference is in the timing of the fees. Although no payment is due a contingent firm if no placement is made, the client has still invested time in the process and lacks a CIO. A retained firm, on the other hand, does not quit working until a placement is made; its main advantage is that the search professional serves as a consultant to the client organization. As conducted by the retained firm, a search includes personal and indepth interviews, detailed documentation, and extensive referencing—these features are not characteristic of most contingent searches.

Damon Runyon supposedly once said, "The battle is not always to the strong nor the race to the swift, but that's the way to bet." A superior track record in recruiting CIOs is probably the single most important variable to look for when choosing a search firm.

Large firms do CIO recruitments in addition to other types of management work. Some small firms and individuals specialize in CIO searches, and there are firms that specialize in healthcare searches. A rule of thumb is to hire a company large enough to have the necessary resources, but small enough to give personalized service.

Executive search firms are invariably a collection of individuals, very much like other independent professionals such as doctors, lawyers, or accountants. Their only real product is the skill, intelligence, and dedication of the professional who services the client's needs.

To ensure the full attention of a seasoned and senior professional, the potential client should interview search firms to determine exactly who will be doing the work and what that individual's track record is in doing the type of search the client has in mind. The practice in many companies, especially the larger firms, is to have "senior business developers" sell searches and then have junior associates actually do the work.

Before contracting with a search firm, the client should require references and check them with former clients, candidates, and placements. It is unwise to rely on the recommendation of a single advisor, who may have personal reasons rather than the best interests of the client organization in mind. Clients should always do their own homework.

The very best executive searches are carried out as a team effort between the search firm and the client organization. If all parties are working together, the search will be efficient, timely, and ultimately successful.

Integrating the New CIO into the Organization

For the hiring organization, the most demanding task begins once the selected candidate has been recruited. To be effective, a new CIO needs wide ranging support, including help with relocation. The employer should never underestimate the importance of bringing the family into the overall organizational life as well. The "trailing spouse," be it wife or husband, influences the candidate's decision to move and contributes to (or detracts from) the CIO's long term effectiveness.

The individual to whom the CIO reports should give the new employee extensive support during the first few months. Every organization has its corporate culture, and it is only fair to acquaint the new executive with it as quickly as possible.

Regular progress meetings between the boss and new hire in the early period will also pay dividends. Goals and objectives should be crystal clear so the new CIO knows where to place the most emphasis.

To become truly integrated into a new organization and to become fully effective takes a new manager one to two years' time. During this period, timely counseling and corrective action should address any problem areas or, in the worst case, set the stage for a termination.

Should termination become necessary during the first year, a reputable search firm will usually redo the executive search for expenses only. This can be a valuable insurance policy, especially with highly paid executives.

Looking into the Future

Today there is a shortage of highly qualified candidates for the chief information officer position in hospitals. Most likely, the supply will increase as the CIO position itself matures and as information technology continues to proliferate in the hospital industry.

Hospitals will contribute to the increased supply by developing more junior information management executives and giving them the opportunity to grow into the CIO role. However, the supply probably will remain inadequate to the demand, and hospitals will continue to seek CIOs from industries outside of healthcare.

To prepare for the future, CIOs need to become generalists, better able to blend seamlessly into the overall top management group of hospitals. Hospital managers need to become better acquainted with information technology.

Reliance on executive search firms will probably increase as the CIO role becomes more visible and top candidates more highly sought after. In the future, there will probably be fewer and larger search firms as industry consolidation continues with an emphasis on creating large international firms.

Flexibility in fee structure also seems to be increasing as the search industry becomes more competitive. For instance, more and more firms are willing to depart from the usual formula and to fix fees at an agreed upon rate based on the effort expended on the search. Although this could result in a search for a highly specialized information resources manager costing more than a search for a higher ranking CIO, the client organization would know exactly what the fee would be and would not have to worry about the motives of the search firm in presenting highly paid candidates.

There is also a trend among executive search firms to link fees to the long term success of placed executives. In public companies, this takes the form of payment by stock or by tying the fee to some agreed upon financial results in the future. Client organizations should be ready and willing to sit down with search firms in the future and structure any creative fee arrangement that may benefit both parties.

Questions

1. What are the costs/benefits of attempting to do the "perfect search" as opposed to simply filling a position?

2. How can the loss of a chief information officer be turned into a major strategic opportunity for the organization?

3. What are the pros and cons of bringing in a chief information officer from outside the healthcare industry as opposed to only considering candidates with hospital or healthcare experience?

4. When might it be more appropriate to hire an excellent technician rather than an accomplished manager in the chief information officer slot? Or vice versa?

5. What are the benefits of an organization conducting its own executive search as opposed to hiring an outside firm? What are the drawbacks?

6. What is the real function of a search firm? Is it responsible for producing exactly the right candidate to fill a given position or is it only responsible for presenting a broad slate of possible candidates?

7. What types of managers are likely to be the CIOs of the future?

4

Organizational Transformation: Responding to Technological Innovation

Carole A. Barone and Grace H. Chickadonz

Information technology forces organizations to consider their structures because it heightens concerns about structural impediments to information flow and access. In many instances, hospitals commit to an infusion of information technology in anticipation of the benefits of better and more efficient care and administration. However, information technology is costly and constantly changing. To realize its benefits, hospitals must also commit to major and continuous change and to the associated investment of energy in creating and sustaining a new and flexible organizational climate focused on the relationship between information and the outcome goals for patient care and the organization.

Hospitals need to examine their governance patterns and organizational structures and to consider how these organizational forms affect their ability to utilize, to their strategic advantage, the enormous amount of information they generate. Bolstered by appropriate organizational forms, information technology is capable of transforming the way hospitals administer themselves and deliver medical services. This transformation is likely to be the base on which financial viability rests.

Information as a Resource

Early computing applications automated discrete functions, such as payroll, admissions, and purchasing. Concerns about the impact of automation on the organization, if they arose at all, were confined within each functional unit's delineated territory. There was little need to worry about the new system's effect on other units or to involve other units in systems planning and design. Indeed, analysts employed by the computing center did most of the systems planning and design and implemented systems to achieve efficiencies or to provide better service. The heads of most functional areas remained aloof from such activities and the resulting impact on their departments.

The objective of the current generation of systems, however, is to make better decisions. For example, fourth generation software products and personal computers allow unit heads and administrators to create and access databases stored both on personal computers and central mainframes. As cost containment efforts force fiscal as well as clinical accountability to occur at the unit level, hospital administrations embrace these developments in information technology because they facilitate the flow of information to the locus of decision making.

Today, hospital organization charts routinely include information centers, usually located in the computing center, established to assist medical and administrative units in their efforts to create and use databases as decision making tools. Information centers provide training; consult with clients on the design of microcomputer based systems; produce downloads, file extracts, and flat files of data stored on a mainframe for analysis by the client on a microcomputer. Some offer programming services.

Management theorists now claim that information technology is sufficiently mature to be used by organizations to attain strategic advantage. The management of information as a strategic resource of the organization, just as cash or supplies or people are considered resources, requires an integrated vision of the entire organization. This radical shift in the way information is viewed causes the entire organization to become caught up in its pursuit. Organizations become introspective; they change in fundamental ways. Not only do their structures change, but organizations also perceive the purpose of structural forms and design—and the process of change itself—differently.

Ethical Concerns

The number of ethical and professional practice issues will skyrocket in this new information rich environment. For example, it would be possible to have an application at the unit level which connects each patient's diagnosis on admission (DRG) to the amount of money the institution will receive and allocate to care for that client. The expenditures for care could be monitored daily, showing the resources required to care for each patient and the total unit costs against the resources allocated to clinical care. The impact on decisions about clinical care and financial viability would be enormous and not necessarily all beneficial. Moreover, the information produced by the new generation of technology may be more powerful than the people who are expected to use the system are prepared to handle.

Changes in Information Use

The most recent developments in technology and software require far more intense and sustained involvement of the heads of functional units in systems design and information management than in the past. If design is left to computing center staff or to staff members with limited or no scope of responsibility, projects risk delays while policy matters are referred to the appropriate decision level. Chiefs of service, head nurses, directors, and vice presidents must participate in systems planning and design. In addition to ensuring that policy decisions related to the project are reached expeditiously, these people must have a vision of what they desire the system to accomplish, i.e., how they expect information technology to change and improve decision making and the delivery of services. Otherwise, there is a further, and perhaps worse, exposure. The resulting system may automate individual functions, be overly complex, and perhaps remain as burdensome as the unautomated function.

A nurse staffing module automates a function and produces certain efficiencies. Hospitals view and manage this application system as an important hospital resource. However, for such a system to help in achieving strategic advantage, it must be far more sophisticated about incorporating patient acuity and goals for patient care, variables which affect nurse staffing requirements. Designed as an expert system with patient acuity information and care goals integrated into the database, it becomes a powerful knowledge based system with the potential of changing the way physicians, hospitals, and nurses interact in the provision of patient care. To create such a system requires the formation of a project team composed of physicians, nurses, computing center staff, and administrators, interacting as coequal members of the team.

The information used in knowledge based systems transcends organizational and professional boundaries. It will no longer make sense to have separate medical and nursing care plans and patient progress records. Logic will demand their integration. Knowledge based systems will call attention to the need for change in traditional styles of interaction among groups responsible for the delivery of medical care. Hospital organizational structures affect the speed and ease with which such systems arise; and efforts to deal with information as a hospital resource, in turn, create direction for change in hospital organizational structures.

Hospital Organizational Structures

Hospitals resemble universities in their organizational structures and in their need to operate with limited resources. Both organizations include cadres of self governing professionals with administrative support furnished by staff members who, except at the highest levels, ordinarily are not physicians or faculty members. Hospital and university organizational structures depart from the rigidly hierarchical chain of command and narrow spans of control typical of business and industry (Drucker 1988).

Some aspects of hospital organizational structures manifest, at least on the surface, the ingredients that are critical to organizations that know how to obtain, integrate, and use accurate and timely information in many different decision making centers. Because of their dependence on information to deliver their services, hospitals understand its enormous power. Hospital organization charts tend to show flatter organizations and depict on the formal chart management councils, coordinating bodies such as joint conference and planning committees or patient care councils, and medical specialist groups

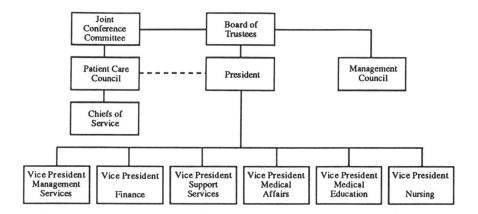

Figure 1. Hospital Organizational Structure

not found on traditional business organization charts. The manner in which the hospital represents its organization on paper is an important reflection of its culture.

Hospital Culture and the Decision Making Process

An organization's culture is reflected in the way it operates, in its vision, its goals, and its values. The flat structures and coordinating mechanisms found on hospital organization charts reflect a culture that engages in joint planning and decision making at the institutional level. This flatness further suggests decentralized decision making with accountability pushed down to the clinical care unit level.

The team approach to the delivery of healthcare at the unit level is another indication of a culture that supports collective decision making and one that knows the importance of integrating information from many different expert and dispersed sources to make the best patient care decisions.

However, the hospital culture also retains vestiges of authoritarianism and centralized decision making that are antithetical to the creation of the kinds of knowledge based information systems that will cause a transformation in the delivery of medical services. Hospital culture tends to be authoritarian in terms of the physician's relationship with the caregiving team and in the hospital's relationship with the staff. Accountability for patient care and fiscal management rests with the clinical care unit, but discretionary authority remains structurally centralized or limited to physicians. Certain groups, such as nurses, are often left out of the process of designing patient care but retain responsibility for 24 hour care of the patient and have enormous influence on the quality of service provided and the speed of the patient's recovery.

This expression of hospital culture impedes the free and informal exchange of ideas and the mutual respect for each project team member's viewpoint that are central to the collective decision making process required to design and implement an integrated information system. As a result, a great deal of time and energy is invested in designing nursing care plans, but this aspect of computerization is more likely to be at the first level of development, i.e., as a discrete function, rather than as a part of an overall patient information system focused on designated outcomes.

New Roles

Hospital information systems must meet diverse needs. In earlier eras of information technology the task was to manage the system. The current objective is to design systems to create and utilize a hospital database that serves as a decision making resource to produce better, more cost effective patient care and better information to hospital administrators and planners. The attainment of these goals requires the adoption of new roles by professionals in the medical environment.

As noted earlier in this chapter, high level administrators, physicians, and nurses must become involved in systems design in order to ensure that the system will generate the data required to make better medical and administrative decisions more quickly. To function effectively as a project team, these individuals must acquire some knowledge of information technology and systems design tools and techniques. Similarly, computing center staff must develop strong people skills in order to work effectively with the professional staff and administrators involved in the project.

With changes in information technology, the working relationship between the computing staff and those in the administrative units has become much closer. There are few traces of the former "we/they" mentality. Computing staff spend much more time in the administrative units. In some cases computing center staff regularly work in an administrative unit in order to understand the mission and priorities and interactions of the unit with its clients. Managers of computing staff look for interpersonal as well as technical skills in prospective employees. Programmers and analysts are learning how to negotiate and to deal with ambiguity. New positions are being created to reduce the complexity of the database for administrators and professional staff who are becoming more and more proficient at accessing and manipulating the data stored in these databases.

Clinical and administrative units find themselves engaged in new activities when they treat information as a resource, and they demand different services from the computing center. Some staff members in administrative units assume quasi-data processing positions; they perform security and data coordinating functions, such as authorizing access to systems, scheduling, programming reports, performing data analyses, and monitoring system maintenance and revision. The line of demarcation between the administrative unit and the computing center has become wavy and blurred. In many instances positions are being moved from the central computing staff into the administrative units. At the same time the computing center is reorganizing to provide support to the client units doing their own systems design and programming. The information center is an example of such support. Changes in technology and software are the impetus for structural changes within both administrative units and central computing services.

Within an administrative or clinical unit, the effects of the introduction of the information technology that permits access to databases, perhaps via a network, will have subtle but often far reaching consequences. When people assume new functional responsibilities, such as those described in this section, the status quo changes. "People think, work, and interact differently...schedules and routines change. Expectations...about staff performance change" (Barone 1988). Some positions need to be redesigned and redefined to accommodate the new information environment.

At the very outset of the design phase, people in management positions should have a vision of the desired state of the functional unit once the project is completed. The unit will have to reorganize in order to garner the full range of benefits of the new system.

Matrix Organizational Design

Hospital staff, perhaps more than those from most other types of service organizations, are accustomed to the formation of teams to accomplish a task. This organizational form is often called a matrix organization or matrix management. In a matrix structure the designation of a project leader depends on the nature of the project, not on profession or status. For example, when a system, such as a staffing module, is being designed, the vice presidents for nursing, finance, management services, and personnel and a representative of the patient care council must collaborate on policy and design matters, participate in the project decision making process with the applications manager from the computing center, and negotiate data definitions with the database administrator.

Staff members from various levels of the administrative hierarchy, representing several professional groups, must work together as coequals on the project. Project team members are responsible both to their formal line officer and to the project leader for its success or failure, but they take their direction as members of the project team from the project leader.

The matrix organizational design is especially useful to organizations, such as hospitals and universities, that generate and use massive amounts of information. The matrix design provides a formal structure to accomplish the lateral relationships (Griffin 1984) essential to the successful integration of the information produced and needed throughout the hospital environment. The matrix design lessens the frequency of change in the formal organizational structure and also tends to make the formal structure less complicated because people come together and disperse as projects arise.

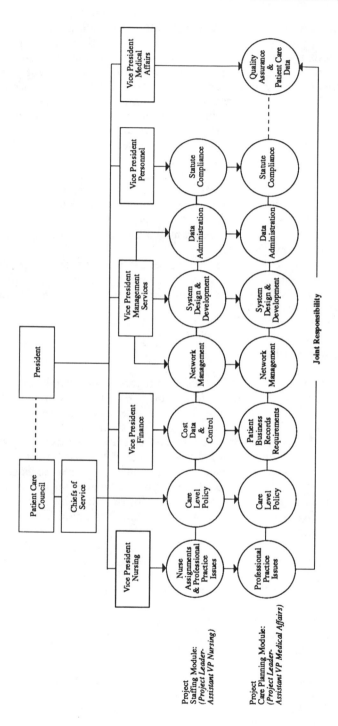

Figure 2. Matrix Organization Chart

Management Style and Politics

Management style and politics play important roles in the information conscious organization. Traditional roles and relationships are threatened in the fast paced, change oriented environment characteristic of an organization that views information as a strategic resource. Owing to the need to have staff members with a variety of skills and perspectives participate on project teams, status and formality are often disregarded in the pursuit of a solution.

Managers in these environments need to relate to their staffs in an informal but attentive manner. Staff members tend to need to check their thinking or perceptions more frequently because past history often does not apply in an environment that relies on matrix management and flexibility. Turf battles, low morale, and indecisiveness arise when people feel threatened by the pace or degree of change or by the disregard of traditional roles and unit boundaries. Managers must feel secure in their positions in order to provide a secure environment for their staffs; they must also be self confident, politically astute, and have good diplomatic skills. Once managers come to the realization that their information requirements will only be met through an integrated database, they will begin to forge the alliances across organizational boundaries necessary to create an information based environment. Those in management positions who fail to adapt their styles to this more team oriented environment will become professionally isolated and will be cut out of the information network.

Networks and the Future

Data communication networks that connect computers at sites throughout the hospital to each other and to a central database allow the sharing of data by all those who require the data. Patient care data collected, and often stored, at widely scattered locations are accessible when needed via the hospital's data network. With the deployment of microcomputers and powerful workstations to the desktops of administrators and medical staff, it is possible to integrate and analyze patient data at the desktop. One might view the data network as the most powerful integrating force in operation in the modern hospital. The desire to access and use the information available via the network could be the catalyst that produces a working integration of the professional groups involved in the delivery of medical care. For example, agreement across functional areas on data definitions is essential to the ability to use this resource. Many computing centers are adding a data administrator position to make certain that shared data elements are properly defined and protected. Often the negotiations among administrative units sharing a common data element take on the trappings of arms reduction treaties as administrators squabble over data ownership.

Networks facilitate the adoption by hospitals of a distributed computing model which fits well with their organizational structures and cultures. Networks foster and support the flattening of organizations by eliminating the need for numerous intervening levels responsible for the collection and transmission of information up the organizational ladder (Drucker 1988a).

The paradigm for computing has changed because of the existence of networks. Initially, organizations depended on central mainframes to store and process data. This was termed the centralized computing model. The appearance of the microcomputer diverted attention from the mainframe to the standalone microcomputer at the site of data collection and utilization, a decentralized model. The appearance of a network connecting microcomputers, minicomputers, and powerful workstations to each other and often to a central mainframe heralds the distributed computing model. The distributed computing model preserves aspects of the autonomy so integral to the hospital culture, yet fosters the sharing of essential information.

The computing center provides the support services required for a robust distributed model. The focus of attention of the computing center is shifting from an emphasis on mainframe computing to the management of a distributed computing environment. The computing center's role in the future will be to furnish a network and promote the standards that will permit self directed users to employ computing resources (Donovan 1988) at their discretion.

A distributed model will also cause hospital decision making to become less centralized. There will be a need for more people to function as boundary spanners and liaisons across the functional units participating in the information based hospital environment (Griffin 1984). New organizational arrangements will likely emerge in which people will be expected to take individual responsibility for nurturing the organizational relationships that facilitate the rapid communication of information to the point of decision making (Drucker 1988b).

The communication made possible and encouraged by the network will cause the rapid breakdown of status barriers because people become less bound by convention when they communicate freely via the network (Kanter l986). The hospital has in place many of the organizational forms that could facilitate a rapid transformation of its culture as an information based organization.

Relationships

Hospitals are the quintessential example of an information-based organization. Information is a resource to be managed toward specific organizational goals and desired outcomes, usually relating to the quality of services and cost of care.

The process of linking information to organizational goals, of viewing information as a resource of the organization, raises the necessity of changes in information management. This calls into question existing organizational structures which typically both facilitate and impede the flow of information.

Hospital organizational structures are already much more decentralized than typical corporations. Specialists in various services manage and deliver their own professional services. However, authoritarianism continues to guide organizational relationships with nurses, for example, who have a substantial impact on the achievement of organizational goals.

New roles and relationships will be essential for achieving information based organizations for the future. These roles will be characterized by egalitarian relationships within a group of patient care professionals, managers and computer experts working together to design and manage information systems. Influence and communication skills will provide more power than traditional hierarchical authority. Data communication networks will draw together everyone "who needs to know" by permitting them to access, contribute to, and utilize the information system. Through these processes, information will be generated and used to guide organizations in attaining their goals and maintaining competitive advantage.

Questions

1. Define information resources management.

2. What is meant by the culture of an organization?

3. What is an information center?
4. Define matrix organizational design.

5. Define a distributed computing model.

6. Why should high level administrators and physicians be involved in systems planning and design?

7. What kind of organizational structure is best suited to an information based organization?

8. What is the role of networks in an information based organization?

9. What is the difference between the centralized, decentralized, and distributed computing models?

References

Barone, C. 1988. Being realistic about technology. *EDUTECH* 4(3).

Donovan, J. J. 1988. Beyond chief information officer to network manager. *Harvard Business Review* 66(5):134-40.

Drucker, P. F. 1988a. The coming of the new organization. *Harvard Business Review* 66(1):45-53.

Drucker, P. F. 1988b. Management and the world's work. *Harvard Business Review* 66(5):65-76.

Griffin, R. W. 1984. *Management.* Boston: Houghton Mifflin Company.

Kanter, R. M. 1986. *The strategic and organizational impact of information technology.* Background Paper, Institute for Information Studies.

Select Bibliography

Ball, M. J., K. J. Hannah, U. G. Jelger, and H. Peterson. 1988. *Nursing informatics.* New York: Springer-Verlag.

Barone, C. 1987. Converging technologies require flexible organizations. *Cause/Effect* 10:20-5.

Section 2–Managing the Institution

Unit 3—Evolution of Information Management: Organization and Technology

Unit Introduction

Different corporate cultures require different organizational structures as well as different computer architectures. Only if corporate culture is accommodated can information transfer technology mesh with everyday operations and optimize effectiveness and efficiency. This unit examines architectural and organizational strategies and their ability to influence change through information technology development.

President of a consulting firm and experienced in technology management and software applications, Hammon adds his insights to those of Pickton, vice president for management systems of a 500 plus bed regional medical center which pioneered a local area network solution to information needs. Recently retired from the positions of assistant vice president for health affairs and information systems at a university medical center and assistant administrator for the hospital, Spraberry discusses the organizational structure of information resources management departments. Wilson, director of information systems for a multi-site medical center, explains how to manage successful implementation projects. Sharrott, who came to healthcare from the telecommunications industry, reports on his experience designing and implementing distributed systems at a large university hospital.

These authors share their successes and failures managing information resources in real healthcare institutions.

1

A Local Area Network Solution to Information Needs: The Moses H. Cone Memorial Hospital Experience

Gary L. Hammon and Robert J. Pickton

In the 1970s, the midsize hospital had the staffing and money concerns of a smaller hospital, but shared the need for technology driven procedures with larger facilities. Administrators had to be managers and leaders, not just caretakers.

In the 1980s, the typical midsize community hospital found itself facing new concerns and/or endeavors, e.g., freestanding surgery centers, decentralized outpatient facilities, physician office interaction, long term care facilities, development and marketing activities, emphasis on quality of patient care, concern over length of patient stay, and additional technology for handling procedures. These new challenges underscored the need for improved and timely management information in order to make informed budgetary, organizational, and personnel decisions.

Computing at Moses Cone

The Moses H. Cone Memorial Hospital fits the picture drawn above. In the 1970s, the hospital was not an active user of automation. A friendly manufacturing company provided basic off-premise accounts receivable processing, and the clinical laboratory had a computer system installed. The remainder of the work was handled in the manual mode. The hospital did not have a person on the staff, other than in the laboratory, with computer systems experience.

In the middle 1970s, the board of the hospital recognized there were potential problems with the operation of the hospital. A team of consultants was engaged to examine the current situation and to make recommendations. The study was completed and the report rendered to the board. The major recommendation was to move away from the manufacturing organization that was the supplier of automation and either establish an inhouse facility or use

273

a shared service from a healthcare oriented provider.

Moses Cone Hospital decided to opt for a shared service from a vendor because it

Reduced risk

- Facilitated meeting administration imposed deadline for start up (critical and immediate)
- Used application systems working and proven in a similar situation
- Supplied documented manual systems to meet automation needs

Controlled costs

- Had lower start up costs than inhouse system
- Could provide same functionality as inhouse system at lower cost

Addressed staffing issues

- Acknowledged lack of trained data processing personnel
    Within the hospital
    Within the geographic area

- Had minimal staffing needs
    Fewer staff required
    New positions primarily clerical
    Programmers not required

- Provided information processing training for existing hospital personnel, stressing
    New work discipline
    Structured working environment

In this same time period, the clinical laboratory decided that their system was reaching the point of saturation and needed to be replaced. A selection team was appointed, and in due course a new system was selected and installed. The hardware component was state of the art technology and would prove to be an excellent selection as the hospital's plans continued to unfold.

Phase One

The hospital went through a selection process and contracted with a prominent shared hospital system provider. A person to run the newly formed department was hired and the staffing begun. Figure 1 is the initial organization chart of the new department of management systems.

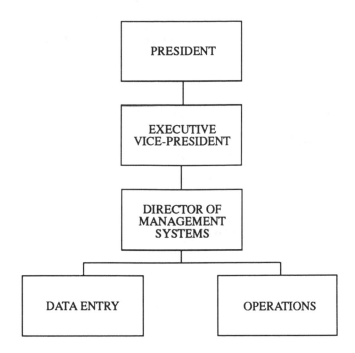

Figure 1. Organization Chart
Department of Management Systems

The on-premise equipment (remote job entry station) for the shared system was installed and the training of the hospital staff initiated. Subsystems were installed for admissions, discharges, and transfers (ADT), patient accounting, and accounts receivable. The hospital administration began to see the benefits of automation as a result of the availability of timely census information, inpatient and outpatient receivables totals, and revenue reports by various components.

Phase Two

Based upon the hospital's experiences using the information provided by the shared system vendor, the administration foresaw the need to move beyond the administrative functions into patient care applications. The hospital's healthcare professionals needed support and assistance.

The administration formed committees of the appropriate staff members to provide direction, suggestions, and comments on the development of a strategic information systems plan. A retreat was organized to initiate this undertaking. Consultants were hired to serve as leaders for the learning and idea generating sessions. The fellowship and informal discussions were most beneficial to future activities. As a result, a strategic plan was developed. A chart of the familiar hospital systems triangle depicts the plans of the hospital, as shown in Figure 2.

A Different Approach

In 1983, the hospital embarked upon a strategy of using local area network (LAN) technology to build a distributed hospital information system, as opposed to using a central computer system to handle all the work. This was to be a pioneering effort.

The design objectives for this new technology approach at Moses Cone Hospital were to

- Make summary data readily available

- Minimize duplicate data

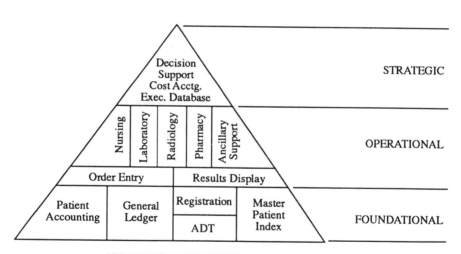

HIS SYSTEMS OVERVIEW

Figure 2. Moses H. Cone Information Plan
HIS Systems Overview

- Minimize immediate data transfers

- Localize processing

- Standardize communications

- Establish an architect/custodian

The organizational benefits the Moses Cone Hospital hoped to derive from this approach were

- Management control
    Adaptable to the organization
    More easily understood
    Decreased risk through modularity
    Pride of ownership

- Management flexibility
    Freedom in selection
    Freedom to change
    Natural redundancy

- Economic savings
    Cost competition among vendors
    Lower initial and incremental costs
    Lower total cost

The shared hospital system was to continue to be utilized, while the major thrust was to be into the patient care areas. The two systems, administrative and patient care, would exchange information via the LAN. There was a potential problem to be faced with this planned strategy, i.e., the question of interface (shared system) and integration (remainder of the system).

During the course of the effort, it was determined that the ADT portion of the shared system needed to be replaced with a more responsive system. The interface was cumbersome and slow, and not responsive to the demands of the LAN based system. A microbased system was selected and attached to the LAN.

One of the key points in the plan concerned the involvement of the potential users of distributed systems. The plan called for nominations of departments to be automated. The selection of the hardware and software for the systems was to be user driven. The management systems department would serve as the inhouse expert and consultant to the users embarking upon a selection process. In addition, the department would be responsible for monitoring the interface specifications for attachment to the LAN and for exchange of data between operating system software and application programs. This has proved to be a popular and effective strategy.

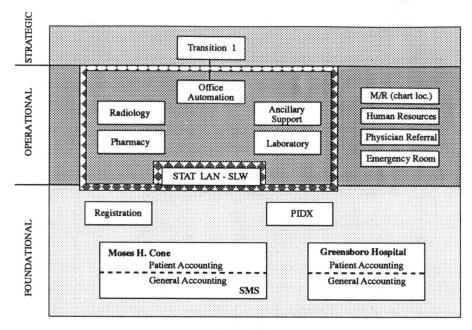

Current Systems

Figure 3. Moses H. Cone Information Plan
Current Systems

Current Status

As of March 1989, the hospital had installed an operational LAN and microbased shared application systems, as shown in Figure 3. In addition to the original hospital entity, Moses Cone Hospital, a new facility was acquired, Greensboro Hospital, and is included in the system picture.

As would be expected, the organizational structure of the management system department has changed over the time period of the planning and implementation of the LAN based systems. The current structure is shown in Figure 4.

The Future

The hospital plans to replace the installed shared hospital system within the next two years. The hospital is doing so because it

- Has no sense of control (expertise resides in vendor, not the hospital)

- Finds vendor slow to respond to needed changes

- Finds service expensive (large discounts gained only when complaints are lodged)

- Has difficulty interfacing the system to newly acquired systems

- Wants freer access to data, including different stages of summary throughout the month (not just month end)

- Finds the existing system inflexible

The hospital has a planning document and a work plan for the continued evolution of the distributed system. Figure 5 shows the hospital's view of the strategic systems. The administration, physicians, nurses, staff, and the management systems department are talking and actively reviewing the progress and removing obstacles as they occur. It appears that the hard work, achieving a consensus as to the proper course of action, is behind them. The fun is ahead—the selection of technology and integration into the existing system.

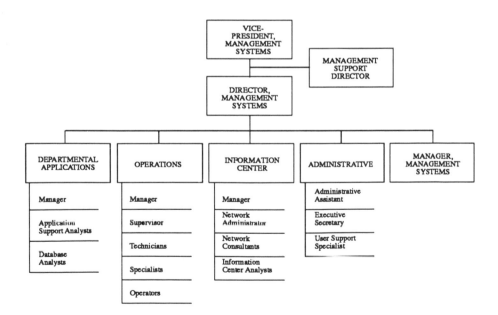

Figure 4. Moses H. Cone Current Organizational Structure

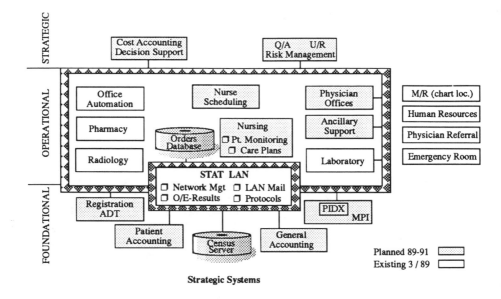

Figure 5. Moses H. Cone Information Plan
Strategic Systems

The story of Moses Cone Hospital is typical and atypical at the same time. The difficulties and problems associated with lack of automated systems were common in the 1970s. Also, the initial selection of a shared vendor was typical for this size community hospital. However, the selection of the LAN technology, using distributed processing, was atypical. Today the hospital is still far ahead of the field in the use of this technology. They have taken the role of a flagship institution as their model in the use of automation.

The Moses H. Cone Memorial Hospital is looking at a bright future in the use of information technology to support the physicians, nurses, paramedical staff, and administration.

Questions

1. What are the advantages and disadvantages of selecting a shared hospital system vendor?

2. What are the factors that would determine if a hospital would benefit from using a shared vendor?

3. What are the factors, tangible and intangible, that enter into a decision to either use the central computer/mainframe concept or the LAN/micro-based distributed systems approach?

4. If the reader were to be responsible for starting a new automation project or directing the expansion of the existing technology in a healthcare institution, what are the steps to be taken or the tasks initiated for the following: administration, physicians, nursing staff, paramedical, administrative staff, and information resources department?

Select Bibliography

Ball, M. J. 1988. Integrating information systems in health care. In *Towards New Hospital Information Systems, Proceedings of the IFIP-IMIA Working Conference,* ed. A. R. Bakker, M. J. Ball, J. R. Scherrer, and J. L. Willems, 39-44. Amsterdam: Elsevier Science Publishers.

Bodenbender, J. 1989. Integration vs interface. *U.S. Healthcare* 6:22-6.

Donovan, J. J. 1988. Beyond chief information officer to network manager. *Harvard Business Review* 66(5):134-40.

Gabler, J. M., and R. J. Pickton. 1988. Integrating distributed data processing. *Computers in Healthcare* 32-4.

Gabler, J. M., and R. J. Pickton. 1988. A new definition for integration. *Computers in Healthcare* 20-2.

Glass, B. 1989. "Smart hubs" handle network problems. *Infoworld* 11:14.

Howe, R. C., and V. Oestreicher. 1988. Corporate strategies: Organizational structure. *Computers in Healthcare* 24-7.

Moses H. Cone Memorial Hospital. 1989. *Information Systems Plan.* Greensboro, N.C.

Peterson, R.O. 1989. The best of both worlds, *Computerworld* 23:87-93.

Simmons, A. Connectivity is key to communication highways, *Government Technology* 2:6-7.

Sullivan-Trainor, M. 1989. Sharing the wealth: Data becomes community property. *Computerworld* 23:71-6.

Waters, S. 1989. 15 questions to ask before you buy your LAN. *Infoworld* 11:S7-S8.

Suggested Serial Publications

Monthly Journals

U.S. Healthcare

Healthcare Financial Management

Computers in Healthcare

Datamation

PC Resources

PC Computing

Hospitals

Weekly News Publications

Computerworld

InfoWorld

2
Organizational Structure in a University Teaching Hospital

Mary Nell Spraberry

Information Resources Management (IRM)

The past few years have seen rapid growth in the use of information systems technology due in part to advancements in computer technology, reduction of cost of hardware, widespread availability of personal workstations, and a growing familiarity with the use of the technology. Like other service industries, hospitals have experienced dramatically increased demands to incorporate emerging technologies into their work environments, for varied levels and types of staff.

In a time of technical change, it is important to have organizational structures that can adapt quickly in response to new opportunities. Computing organizations in large financial and other service industries have evolved to accommodate the convergence of the emerging technologies that support distributed systems, decision support systems, telecommunications, and fully integrated networks.

However, according to Barone (1987), "Many traditional computing organizations are structured and populated in ways that resist change and, indeed, are often muddled and strangled by it." The hierarchical and fixed organizational structure characteristic of hospitals is often reflected by the status, structure, and roles assigned to their information resources management (IRM) departments. Hospitals, which have traditionally placed IRM under the control of the finance office, with its focus on the development and implementation of financial or administrative systems, have lagged behind in developing and implementing cost effective information systems technology. In point of fact, hospital IRM departments have rarely been involved in the institutional planning process, even though IRM is critical to the successful implementation of strategic and operational goals. If recognized in the planning process for its ability to cross departmental boundaries, IRM can have a significant, positive impact on organizational effectiveness and efficiency.

283

In the late 1980s, many large hospitals recognized the strategic importance of information systems technology to the future success of the hospital. As hospital administrators began to understand more clearly the role of information systems and communications technology in the implementation of strategic business opportunities, the director of IRM was increasingly recognized as an individual who should participate with senior management in developing strategic objectives for the hospital. As this occurred, hospitals created a position referred to as the chief information officer (CIO), which reported to the chief executive officer (CEO) or the chief operations officer (COO).

This chapter addresses the issues related to the current organizational management of IRM departments by describing a typical organization in a large hospital and by suggesting future requirements for such organizations.

The Mission of IRM

The primary mission of the IRM department is defined as providing professional and cost effective systems solutions to satisfy information requirements of the hospital and related organizations. In support of its mission, the department (Penrod and Dolence 1987) acts as a repository of information and

- Provides technical resources and leadership for all elements of automation
- Promotes coordination, standardization, and compatibility in the storage of information
- Provides increased awareness, understanding, and effective use of information
- Provides mechanisms to allow access to information at the least possible cost
- Recommends and implements policies and plans to ensure meeting the overall objectives of the hospital

IRM within the Hospital Organizational Structure

In most hospitals during the past three decades, information systems had departmental status like that of ancillary services, administrative services, and support services departments. Even as information resources management (IRM) departments evolve, organizational reporting structures often reflect their earlier role and status.

The chief executive officer of a large hospital not owned by or affiliated with an academic institution generally reports to a board of trustees. In academic medical centers, there is usually a direct link between the CEO of

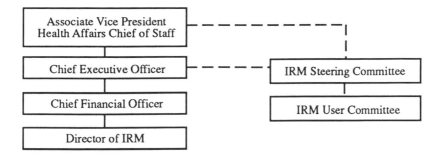

Figure 1. Organizational Structure of Information Resources Management within a Large Hospital

the hospital and a senior level physician who may have any one of a variety of titles. In one such case, as shown in Figure 1, the latter position is titled associate vice president for health affairs and chief of the medical staff. As is typical, the director of the IRM department reports to the chief financial officer (CFO).

Decision Making in Relation to Organizational Structure

The scope of service, staffing, and budget for the IRM department is determined by the director of IRM and the CFO with concurrence by the CEO. Policy issues, large scale systems development projects, and major software and hardware capital expenditures are reviewed and approved by an IRM steering committee. This committee is composed of a select group of clinicians, nurses, and key individuals in hospital management. Its major tasks are to formulate and enforce policy, approve the acquisition of major hardware or software systems, and determine the priorities of specific projects.

The steering committee is assisted by an IRM user committee composed of physicians, nurses, and hospital department representatives. This user committee is responsible for overseeing IRM work requests, conducting cost benefit analyses of proposed projects, recommending acceptance or rejection of projects, and otherwise assisting in the setting of priorities and the tracking of project development cycles. It also advises the steering committee on the appropriate use of IRM resources and provides progress reports on active projects. The IRM department is represented on both committees, with the chairman of the user committee and the IRM director usually also serving as members of the IRM steering committee. IRM management and staff also work with other hospital personnel to ensure that the IRM department plans, monitors, and executes its assigned mission in an acceptable manner.

The decision to develop and support software applications is the responsibility of the hospital administration through the IRM steering and user committees. The approval of all information systems projects, the allocation of resources, and the setting of priorities are ultimately the responsibility of the CEO with concurrence of the IRM steering committee. Proposals for computer applications are submitted to the IRM steering committee for review and approval by way of the IRM user committee and IRM management.

Following acquisition or development, applications software must be certified by the technical support staff in IRM for the purposes of quality assurance, data security, and documentation before the applications can be placed into production. In like manner, acquisition of computer hardware, including office automation systems, must be approved by IRM management and the hospital administration. Standards established by IRM and approved by the steering committee, such as requirements for data transmission compatibility and uniformity of data element definition, are critical to the integration of multiple systems in a networking environment.

Impact of Organizational Structure

Due to the vertical integration of hierarchically structured organizations, information passes through multiple layers where it is interpreted by managers with limited authority over narrowly focused areas of activity (Penrod and Dolence 1987). Such a structure creates limited spans of control with limited opportunity to initiate change. The position of IRM in the organization determines its opportunity to identify and implement improvements in functional or operational effectiveness (Penrod and Dolence 1987; Robinson 1988). Hierarchical organizational structures tend to be bureaucratic, rigid, tightly controlled, and frequently inefficient as a result of narrow spans of control. Decision making is obstructed or slowed as information flows up or down the chain of command.

The flow of a service request may begin with a hospital department submitting a request for service for information systems support. The IRM department logs in the request, assigns a project number to the request, and then submits it to the IRM user committee. As is typical of such groups, the IRM user committee meets periodically (usually monthly) to review new requests, review cost benefit analyses on proposed projects, prioritize approved projects, and track the progress of projects not yet completed. New requests may be assigned to a subcommittee for further study.

Internal Organizational Structure of IRM

The IRM department typically is organized with four major divisions called systems and programming, information center, data center, and planning and staff services, as shown in Figure 2. The manager of each of these divisions may have the title of manager or assistant director of IRM.

Systems and Programming Division. Staffed with systems analysts, programmer analysts, and programmers, the systems and programming division installs, develops, and supports application software.

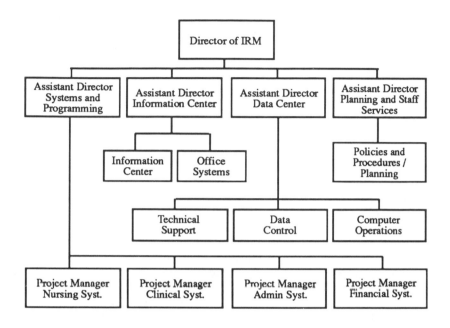

Figure 2. Organizational Structure of Information Resources Management within the IRM Department

Information Center Division. The information center division provides a large range of services to the staff in hospital departments including training and use of hospital applications, consultation on office systems, microprocessor configurations, installation of personal computer equipment and software including local area networks, support and training in the use of high level languages, and generation of ad hoc management reports using high level languages. This division is staffed with consultants, programmers, micro-processor hardware and software specialists, and local area network specialists.

Data Center Division. The data center division is responsible for the operation of the mainframe computers, maintains the communications network, the operating system software, the security system, the large databases, manages and controls the program libraries, data libraries, report distribution, and maintains a service desk in response to the emergency needs of a user of the network or the mainframe applications. The data center is staffed with systems programmers, database analysts, telecommunications specialists and coor-dinators, librarians, and computer operators.

Planning and Staff Services Division. The planning and staff services division may or may not be found in large hospitals; however, when this division does not exist, the activities of this group are handled by staff from one or more of the other three divisions. The planning and staff services division performs a variety of support functions for the IRM department, including long and short range planning and the development of requests for information (RFIs) or requests for proposals (RFPs) for acquiring computer hardware or applications software. Staffed with analysts and technical writers, this division also prepares department activity reports, develops standards and procedures manuals, assists in capacity planning, defines staff educational needs, coordinates activities with outside consultants, and performs or coordinates any special projects for the department.

Centralized vs. Decentralized Organizational Structures

The rapid emergence of end user information technology and its adaptation in the workplace has made centralized management of technology resources increasingly difficult. The proliferation of minicomputers and microcomputers has rendered policies instituted in centralized systems no longer appropriate (Donovan 1988). Professional workstations in hospital departments spread so widely and so rapidly that IRM departments were unprepared to manage or control the de facto decentralization of computing resources. In the foreseeable future, large hospitals will continue to require large computers to support all hospital wide systems. These systems will require a staff of information systems professionals under centralized management to handle computer operating systems, database administration and management, communications and network management, and security.

The centralized, hierarchical structure of most large IRM departments tends to be inflexible in responding to the needs of hospital departments. The levels of bureaucracy associated with the processing of requests for information systems services has driven hospital departments to become self sufficient in solving information systems problems. User departments have found that most of their needs can be met by vendor developed applications software running on minicomputers or powerful, inexpensive microcomputers. Information systems activities and responsibilities have been transferred from the centralized IRM department to the user departments where they have control over their own systems (Hughes 1989). This shift in responsibilities makes it necessary to redefine the IRM department's organizational structure in support of decentralization.

Large hospitals have begun to move toward a three-tiered computing and communications strategy that incorporates the integration of microprocessor professional workstations, minicomputer departmental systems, and large mainframe corporate systems. The integration or networking of these three levels of computing requires changes in the role of information systems and communications managers from one of control to one of strategic planning, coordination, and management of networks, consultation, and service (Donovan 1988).

Technological innovation has been the driving force pushing decentralization of computing resources. Hospital departments have learned that tightly controlled and centralized information is inefficient (McLaughlin et al. 1987). Decentralization of computing resources in large hospitals is well established; there is no turning back to the management styles of the previous decades. Changes are required in the organizational structure that will support the development of policies and procedures to ensure the appropriate use of information technology to achieve the operational and strategic goals of the institution.

Future Developments in the Management of IRM

In the turbulent healthcare environment, hospital management must address the use of the emerging information technology to improve operational effectiveness. Despite financial constraints, the demand to invest in information technology increases as users see its benefits demonstrated. For the hospital to compete for its marketshare in the healthcare delivery system, department managers must understand the uses of information technology.

To successfully implement information technology and information networks, hospitals must empower the IRM organization to develop strategic plans compatible with the hospital's business plans. The senior information executive should become a member of the executive governing body of the hospital and a major advisor in planning, implementing, and managing change to achieve operational effectiveness (Robinson 1988). This information officer should have equal status with the chief operations officer and chief financial officer and share the responsibility for determining and realizing the strategic directions established by the organization (Penrod 1987).

Updating the senior information officer position, Donovan (1988) advocates the concept of network manager, responsible for building and maintaining the communications network that links the computing resources of the institution. Linking the three tiers of computing, namely professional workstations, departmental computers, and corporate mainframe systems, requires connectivity at three levels:

- Communication software systems

- Application software systems

- Physical, i.e., wire, fiber, or other media (Donovan 1988)

Only then can patient, departmental, and institutional information be effectively shared.

The network manager would encourage the decentralization of computing from the institutional level to the departmental or personal level. Department managers would assume the day to day responsibilities for managing the computing resources of their own department. Although the IRM department would retain the responsibility for managing the corporate mainframe systems,

most of the systems and programming staff would be found in the departments supporting the departmental systems.

The network manager or the CIO of the future must develop a strategy
that will allow integration of multi-vendor products, both hardware and
software, across an institutional network that supports voice, data, graphics,
imaging, and text. As the network expands to support multiple distributed
systems, the management of security systems will become a major issue.
Security policies governing access to information and control of institutional
databases must be developed and enforced at the institutional level.

Davenport et al. (1989) have suggested that executives can shape their
organizations' information systems through the development of principles
which clearly state how the institution wants to use information technology to
accomplish its goals over time. These principles would be used as a guide by
department managers to make technology decisions. He suggests the
development of five or six principles for each of the following technology
divisions:

- Types of computers used

- Operating software to be supported

- Communications networks

- Database administration

- Process by which applications software is created (or obtained),
  maintained, and managed

IRM in Healthcare

IRM departments in large hospitals typically are hierarchically structured
organizations having several levels of managers with narrow spans of control.
The department generally reports to the chief financial officer where most of
the applications development emphasis has been placed upon financial and
administrative systems with the exception of the implementation of order entry
from nursing units for ancillary services. This has served to provide some
support to nursing services; however, the support to the ancillary services
departments for internal management of work flow and data management has
been limited.

The IRM department organizational model is the same model used for
hospital departmental structures predominantly found in the healthcare
industry. The centralized, hierarchical structure tends to be inflexible in its
ability to respond to the needs of hospital departments. The emergence of
new technology in the form of microcomputers, minicomputers, and vendor
developed applications software has provided the opportunity for hospital
department managers to search for solutions to departmental needs by

deployment of this technology within their departments. The result of this movement away from the centralized IRM department support has been to decentralize computing in the organization without the benefit of an organizational strategic plan.

In a time of rapidly emerging technology, it is important to have an organizational structure that can adapt quickly in response to new opportunities. The CEO and other leaders in hospital administration need to recognize the strategic value of information systems technology to the future success of the hospital. The position of the IRM department within the organizational structure will determine the department's effectiveness in ensuring the appropriate use of information technology to achieve the operational and strategic goals of the hospital.

Large hospitals will continue to use large mainframe computers to support hospital wide software applications, hospital databases and data administration, networking of distributed systems, and telecommunications. It is appropriate and necessary for the chief executives in hospital administration to redefine the IRM department's organizational structure in support of a three-tiered computing and communications strategy that incorporates the integration and networking of microcomputer professionalwork stations, minicomputer departmental systems, and mainframe corporate systems. The individual responsible for the use of these strategic resources should be a senior level executive regardless of the title of the position, and should participate in setting the strategic objectives of the organization.

Questions

1. Should the senior level information systems manager be a part of the hospital's strategic planning process?

2. Why should the CIO be a member of the hospital's executive staff?

3. Why is it important to have a flexible organizational structure in a time of rapid technological change?

4. What has been the driving force behind the trend from centralization to decentralization in computing?

5. What are the principal functions of the information management resources department in a decentralized computing environment?

6. What are the principal functions of the information management resources department in a centralized computing environment?

References

Barone C. (1987). Converging technologies require flexible organizations. *Cause/Effect* 10 (November):20-5.

Davenport, T. H., M. Jammer, and T. J. Metsisto. 1989. How executives can shape their company's information systems. *Harvard Business Review* 67(2):130-1.

Donovan, J. J. 1988. Beyond chief information officer to network manager. *Harvard Business Review* 66(5):134-40.

Hughes S. 1989. Departmental computing as a competitive business tool. *Direction* (a quarterly publication of Applied Learning) (January):7-9.

McLaughlin, G., D. J. Teeter, R. D. Howard, and J. S. Shott. 1987. The influence of policies on data use. *Cause/Effect* 9:6-11.

Penrod, J. I., and M. G. Dolence. 1987. IRM a short lived concept? In *Cause 87—Leveraging Information Technology—Proceedings of the 1987 CAUSE National Conference*, 173-83. Denver: CAUSE.

Robinson, R. 1988. The changing agenda for information services, a leadership challenge, *Cause/Effect* 11(May):12-7.

Select Bibliography

Holland, R. 1989. The IRMing of America, *CIO* (Insights) 2(March):61-2.

Murray, R. 1989. The challenges of the next decade, *Connect (Corporate Perspective)* 2(Spring):26.

Sherron G. T. 1987. Organizing to manage information resources. In *Cause 87—Leveraging Information Technology—Proceedings of the 1987 CAUSE National Conference,* 185-95. Denver: CAUSE.

Weiss, M. 1987. Transformers, *CIO* 1(September/October):37-41.

3
The Corporate Business Plan and Information Systems

Sam Wilson

Long Range System Plan

A hospital's long range information systems plan should be a product of its corporate strategic business plan. In developing the system plan, the fundamental question to be addressed is, "What information does management need in order to implement its business plan?" These information needs then are translated into the applications contained in the long range system plan. In evaluating a long range system plan, the fundamental question is, "What is the business need (information need) that each system addresses?"

If the corporate business plan is inaccessible, incomplete, or nonexistent, the information systems long range planning process becomes more complex and time consuming. Successful results are compromised because the organization has not decided or has minimally documented what its functional business requirements will be in the future. This uncertainty about needs can make planning future computerization goals difficult. Even worse, the final information system development effort may not be in concert with corporate expectations.

Whatever the case, data processing management must estimate current and future requirements. This can be done by interviewing key operational personnel and senior management regarding strategic and operational management information requirements. Time must also be spent studying the requirements of the day to day operations.

The analyst must connect strategic needs with operational needs, balancing the "blue sky" and the "down to earth" perspectives. It may not be possible to develop strategic systems without first putting operational components in place to serve as foundation or platform systems. Despite the difficulties involved, strategic and operational needs must be blended in order to develop a plan and to design a product which will be acceptable when implemented.

In Table 1, goals and objectives are listed in the lefthand column and a check is placed under the systems which could generate information necessary

DESCRIPTION OF GOAL: Description of Objective	General Ledger	Materials Mgt.	Accounts Payable	Pharmacy	A.D.T.	Order Comm. & Results	Payroll Human Res.	Patient Accounting	Cost Accounting	Strategic Database	Decision Support	Financial Forecasting	Patient Classification	Patient Scheduling	Productivity Reporting
Meet identified patient need															
Document program and service need	□								□	□	□	□			
Decentralized O/P service increase access					□	□			□	□	□		□	□	□
Facilitate admission/ registration of patients					□	□								□	
Purchase state of the art equipment	□								□		□	□			□
Develop product line market plan	□					□		□	□	□	□	□	□		
Enhance and retain nursing personnel									□		□	□	□	□	□
Develop employees in general															
Provide adequate levels of supervision, direction, and compensation							□	□			□	□			□
Develop medical staff relations															
Provide facilities, equipment, and personnel to attract (retain) physicians	□	□	□					□	□	□	□	□		□	□
Continue to be financially sound															
Rates should reflect cost and be competitive for comparable services	□					□			□	□	□	□	□		□
Implement productivity reporting standards	□					□	□		□	□	□	□	□		□
Implement a quality assurance program				□			□				□		□		□
Implement severity of illness program															
Assure consistency of budget with strategic plan	□		□				□	□	□	□	□	□	□		□

Table I. Information Systems Required to Support Strategic Goals and Objectives

to meet the the objective. The systems with the most checks are not necessarily the most urgent; urgency must be defined by senior management based upon the information they believe to be most critical to the organization (Figure 1.)

User Involvement

The success of any application is dependent upon how well it meets the needs of the user. Smaller projects enjoy a higher probability of success than larger system efforts. On small projects, data processing personnel work more closely with users, and there are fewer layers of detail. Large projects tend to involve more detail. They also involve more people; hence, there are more organizational layers between the user, senior management, and the application development team, making the translation of user's needs to application development and/or selection more difficult.

When properly applied, the team approach ensures that all persons impacted by a potential system have a voice in its design, development or selection, and installation. However, it may have the disadvantage of diffusing accountability for decision making. For instance, the team may decide to expand the scope and extend the timeframes for a project without considering additional costs. When this decision is made by a group, the project manager cannot be held accountable. Moreover, the team concept may allow team members to authorize increased cost to the project when an increase of the same magnitude for departmental operations might be rejected when going through the budget approval process.

There are two major questions relating to user involvement in the design of a new system. First, have the users signed off as being satisfied with the design of the screens, reports, forms, etc., that they will potentially use? If the users are not satisfied, the project will not be a success. Second, who is accountable for making decisions that extend timeframes or increase the cost of the project? If no one is accountable, there is no incentive to control costs or complete a project successfully within the estimated timeframe. Someone must be ultimately held accountable. If user demands threaten to make increased costs unavoidable, senior management on the steering committee must make the decision whether to approve or disapprove those additional costs.

Project Team Organization

It is impossible to control a project without an organizational structure which defines direct accountability. Figure 2 depicts a structure for project team organization which holds the project leader responsible to the administrative steering committee. Under this structure, the steering committee monitors the entire process, including the data processing technical support as well as the design and review teams. The steering committee is responsible for critical issues relating to the project.

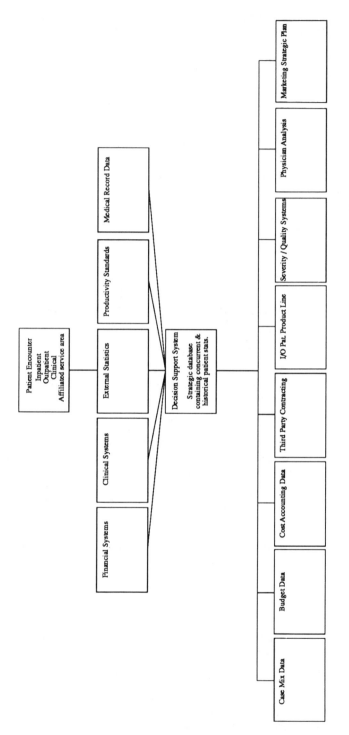

Figure 1. Operational Foundation for Comprehensive Decision Support System

System Project Design Team

The project design team includes staff from all key areas. Medical records, finance, nursing, and data processing departments are involved throughout the entire design process. At the appropriate times, ancillary departments are drawn in to assist in design specifications.

The data processing application programming manager chairs the design team. It is the chair's responsibility to coordinate the plan, monitor and report on its progress, and maintain projected timeframes. This team and the director of information systems are responsible to the administrative steering committee.

The project design team has the primary role in designing and developing requirements for all aspects of the system. Users on the design team are responsible for defining and communicating user needs during the detailed design specification phase. Data processing members are responsible for keeping the team within reasonable information systems standards. In addition, nursing and clinical departments are responsible for developing documentation and conducting education sessions for their departmental colleagues.

Project Review Team

Under the structure in Figure 2, the project review team membership includes the manager for data processing programming and the coordinators for nursing, medical records, and finance. Other departmental coordinators serve on an ad hoc basis. The director of information systems chairs the team. The review team functions as a governing body for the project and defines its priorities and scope. It also resolves any conflicts which do not require the involvement of the steering committee.

Project Leader

The project leader periodically reports the status of the project to the steering committee. A bar chart, comparing completed work with the original estimates, highlights the status of each major task. If a task is behind schedule, the project leader is prepared to explain why. If the problem is outside the review team's control, the steering committee must address the problem, extend the completion date of the project, or limit the project scope.

Project Team Accountability

Just as the project leader is directly responsible to the steering committee, so should each team member be accountable to the project leader. Performance evaluation should directly affect each team member's promotion/merit evaluation within the organization. At the completion of the project,

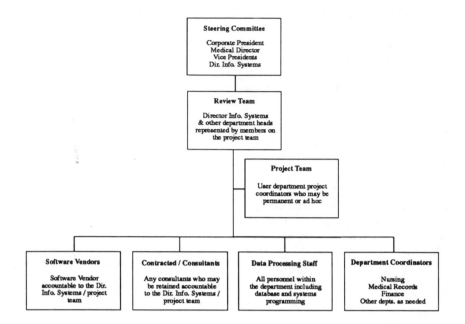

Figure 2. Proposed Steering Committee
Manage and Control Project Scope

all team members would be expected to return to their original jobs within their respective departments.

Individual work programs should be issued to project team members. Without a customized work plan, the team members lose the urgent sense that the project must be completed on a timely basis. Moreover, the project leader cannot hold a team member responsible for time schedules for work which was never formally assigned.

Project control is facilitated when team members report their time back against specific steps in individual work plans. This process highlights problem areas and potential overruns at their source. Identifying problems early allows the project leader to adjust staffing assignments, address problems, and present alternative courses of action to the steering committee before deadlines are missed.

Methodology

The organization should document the methodology for the design, selection, and implementation of new systems. This work plan should list each task to be performed, estimate time required for its completion, and describe it in specific terms. Estimates should be sufficiently detailed to provide the project manager a degree of comfort, if not of reasonable certainty.

The ability to make reasonable estimates is enhanced by using a methodology which provides a step by step chronology for the design and installation of new computer systems. This methodology should identify the physical output at the completion of each step, such as interview notes, a flowchart, a screen design, a program specification, etc. Forecasting the production of tangible outputs tied to specific work steps can make estimates more accurate and monitoring more easily managed. In addition, the physical output can serve as part of the documentation required after the system is installed and turned over for maintenance.

Process

The first step is to document thoroughly everything about the systems (manual or computerized) being considered for installation or revision. All lines of communication involved in each function or procedure are identified, as well as all documents to be used, and any exception to the norm. The review team is consulted to verify accuracy and ensure that all steps in the process are accounted for. Each area is required to designate a contact person to be consulted for specifications and functional details. Consulting confers a sense of system ownership on the departments participating in the design process.

Once the old system is documented, potential automated functions are identified and specifications developed for each function. Specifications compiled by the user team are then examined by the review team. If the review team recommends changes in the design, the design is revised accordingly. This process continues until all functional specifications are approved.

Steering Committee Guidelines

Issues which have the potential to increase the cost and/or extend the timeframe of the project are brought before the steering committee. Every decision involves trade offs; benefits must be weighed against costs. Any decision to drain the organization's cash reserves for unbudgeted expansion of the project should not be made without the involvement of top management.

Prioritizing Applications

Sequencing

Sequencing applications should be based upon the strength of the business need those applications address. The system that meets the most critical business need should be first; the system that meets the least critical business need should be last.

Systems not meeting any business need should not be undertaken. The strength of the business need must be determined by top management, as identified by the business plan, not as interpreted by data processing personnel.

Again, clarity regarding what the organization intends to accomplish with its computerization effort is critical to the success of the project. Developing a clear statement should assist in subsequently determining the approach to accomplishing those organizational goals. It is most important that the organization considers its ultimate goal so that the approach selected does not inhibit the second, third, and fourth steps of its plan. Experience shows that an organization can make a choice in meeting its initial objectives that makes it very difficult to accomplish the remaining steps of its plan.

Return on Investment

Once approved as meeting a business need, a potential computer application should be evaluated in budgetary terms. The method most commonly used is to determine the number of years the system must remain operational in order to recover development, acquisition, and ongoing maintenance costs. This is similar to the number of years payback method used in capital budgeting. If cash flow for benefits, development, and maintenance is discounted at the cost of capital, the methodology becomes identical to the net present value method of capital budgeting.

Although it may be difficult to quantify the benefit of a new system, doing so is analogous to operating a department at a loss. The organization may be willing to absorb an annual loss of one million dollars but balk at three million. At some point, senior management must be willing to quantify the value of the service or new computer application.

The organization needs reasonable assurance regarding project costs and benefits. The key to achieving this is to have a methodology which functions as a checklist, ensuring that all steps are included and steps that require estimates are covered. Assumptions underlying the cost/benefit estimates should be documented. As conditions change, these assumptions and the resulting cost/benefit estimates can be updated.

Again, the assessment of project benefit must satisfy some cost vs. savings relationship, defined by responses to the following questions:

- What are the needs?
- What are the present service levels?
- What is the current cost of the services?
- Are the present services meeting the needs?
- What is the quality of services?
- Are the current services cost effective?
- Is capacity adequate?
- Are there opportunities for improvement?
- Can capacity be better utilized?
- What would it cost to improve capacity?

- What would be the savings to eliminate overhead and improve service function?
- What will the organization's business function be in the next two to five years?

After time and dollar estimates are attached to responses to these questions, some value can generally be placed on the potential return on the investment.

However, this value is meaningful only if the system is designed and implemented to specifications. Users must achieve cost savings by reducing staff or improving productivity consistent with the original justification of the system. If the users are unable to do so, they should be prepared to explain to the steering committee which business functions and/or volumes changed during the implementation period, altering the expected outcome.

Departmental Organization

Organizing a department by functions, as shown in Figure 3, has a number of advantages. The functional organizational structure facilitates

- Assigning new work (new work accrues to the person whose functional area encompasses the new activities)

- Assigning responsibility for both new and ongoing activities

- Developing procedures and standards (individuals can develop standards or procedures for their areas for management review)

- Developing cohesiveness in the organization (staff are more likely to feel they have contributed to the total project scope)

- Assigning one manager to be devoted fulltime to systems programming (if the internal workings of the computer are not fine tuned, even the best written application programs will have poor response times)

- Bringing all analysts and programmers under the same manager, making it easier to rotate staff between maintenance and new systems development online systems and batch program systems

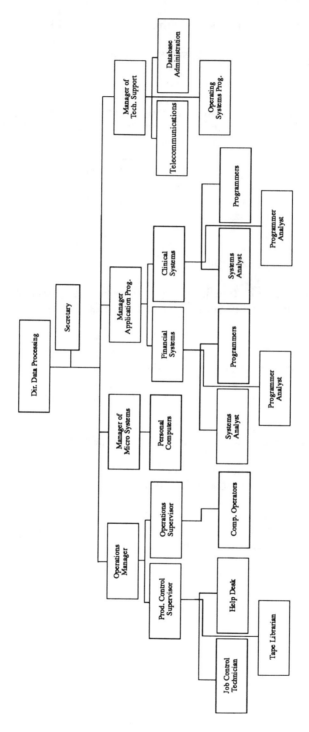

Figure 3. Data Processing Reporting Relationship Functionally Organized

Standards and Procedures

Standards should be developed as guidelines to assist staff in computer systems documentations. Inadequate system documentation increases the time required to perform maintenance or develop new systems which interface with the existing ones. Documentation is the only mechanism that describes what a computer system should do and how it does it.

Characteristically, good systems documentation includes system flows, system narratives, file descriptions, records layouts, program flowcharts, program narratives, definitions of codes and special characters, test plans, test data and test results, and program listings. In addition, documentation should include components which establish

- Standard naming conventions to facilitate both development and maintenance of computer programs

- Standardized programming procedures emphasizing structured logic, common data base calls, paragraph naming conventions, etc.

- Strict enforcement of procedures for protecting production programs

- Procedures for submitting and running jobs and for distributing reports

- Standards requiring recovery/restart or back up procedures be operational before new applications are implemented

- Procedures and training in disaster drills

- Standards for operating documentation which must be met before a system becomes operational

- Standards for user documentation, which must be met before a system becomes operational

- Assignment of responsibilities and work tasks to system programmers and data base team

- Procedures for user sign off for each phase of the project, eliminating any opportunity for creeping scope or major misunderstandings at the project conclusion

Key Issues for Hospital Information Systems Success

The structured process enables the project teams and top management to address the organization's information requirements, beginning with the development of a long range computer plan. The project design team then documents scope and selects the method to achieve the goals. Methods range from complete turnkey (all of the development is done by the selected vendor), to total inhouse development (one in which all of the software development is done by the inhouse programming staff). In today's environment, the best solution generally is somewhere between the two extremes.

The preferred method is to use the design team's definition of scope as a guide for developing a request for proposal (RFP). The organization then uses the RFP to elicit and evaluate proposals from software vendors. Because it is highly unlikely that a single vendor and a single system can meet all identified information requirements, the organization must select various system components/vendors for the best possible fit. Preferably, the system selected will require a minimal number of modifications of the core application programs. The closer the fit with project specifications, the less time and cost are required to install the system. Moreover, fewer organizational adaptations are required, minimizing the difficulty of applying maintenance as future software versions or additional enhancements are released by the vendor.

As a rule, purchased software requires a modification factor computed at a minimum of 20 percent (it generally runs higher if replacing existing automated systems) of the time estimate to develop the software in house. However, if the estimated time requirement for modifying the purchased software exceeds the 20 percent modification factor by a large margin, the search committee probably should continue to look for a more appropriate fit. If software cannot be found which meets the expectations, the organization must elect either to narrow the scope or to develop its own software solution.

When more than one vendor is selected to provide various components (for example, one vendor is selected for billing and accounts receivable and another for general ledger), the expectation should be that the systems should share common data. This sharing process should be some form of automated interface. Generally, the user should not be adversely affected by the integration of the various systems. This integration, beyond interfacing, is most important for eliminating redundant data entry and maintaining the accuracy, consistency, and integrity of data throughout the total system.

The hospital and its board of directors must be provided a clear understanding of the potential implications of the computer implementation plan. This is particularly important when the proposed system has a scope significant enough to possibly have a measurable impact on profitability, cash flow, and resource commitment across the total organization.

A major information systems project is like any major building project. Both may involve construction time spanning several years and require resources totaling hundreds of thousands of dollars before the project is completed and any direct benefits can be realized by the hospital. However, without this investment of time and money in automation, healthcare organizations cannot hope to thrive in an environment that is increasingly competitive and even threatens economic disaster.

Questions

1. Describe the essential elements necessary to develop a long range system plan.

2. Describe how a long range system plan would be used by the organization to manage and control its computer resources.

3. How can the computer plan be developed in the absence of a corporate plan? How might the project be successful without clear corporate direction?

4. Why does the author suggest a team approach to project definition?

5. Describe the composition of the various management teams and their responsibilities to the project.

6. How is the RFP developed?

7. How should project priorities be established, and by whom?

8. How should the information systems department be organized to perform most efficiently?

9. What essential elements are required for information systems managers to ensure consistency and accurate management of the data processing function?

4

Centralized and Distributed Information Systems: Two Architecture Approaches for the 90s

Lawrence A. Sharrott

Centralized versus Distributed Computing

Today there are two major ways of providing data processing services within most businesses, including hospitals. The first approach is centralized computing and involves the acquisition of a large computer typically known as a mainframe. To this computer are attached a number of dumb terminals that do not have any processing power of their own. All of the computing is done on the large machine. The results of the processing are presented either on the terminal or in reports. All of the data necessary for the work being performed are housed on one of the many disk drives that are attached to the mainframe.

The other approach is known as the distributed processing approach. This technique uses a high speed network to connect a number of computers, including machines usually referred to as personal computers or somewhat larger machines typically designated as minicomputers. Each of these machines is intelligent, that is, each has the ability to run programs and manipulate data.

The computers that a person will use to perform work are called workstations. Data may be stored on the user's workstation or on a file server, that is, a computer with large amounts of disk storage which serves as a repository for significant amounts of data.

In centralized computing, all programs and all data are on one machine and all processing shares the same centralized resources. In the distributed approach, data and programs may be located on any of the machines that are connected to the network. In fact, the programs on one workstation may act upon data that are located on another workstation. Each of these approaches has its advantages and disadvantages. Each fills a need in the provision of data processing services.

Advantages of Distributed Computing

There are many reasons for selecting a distributed system to deliver data processing services. The two leading reasons are politics and cost. There are a number of other reasons that also enter into the decision making process, including the best possible reason, functionality of the system.

In many medical centers, there are strong political entities which wield considerable influence and have significant needs for data processing resources. There are powerful reasons for acquiring and managing a data processing center within a department. Control of the budget dollars for data processing improves departmental stature. Departments may argue that locating data processing within their units will free floor space elsewhere in the institution. Most important, controlling the data processing function means controlling the information necessary for a strong negotiating position relative to the rest of the institution. Cost is also a strong motivator for acquiring departmental and distributed processing systems. Several scenarios are possible within a distributed environment, delivering different cost/benefit ratios to the institution.

Three Scenarios for Distributed Computing

Scenario 1: The Controlled Environment. In this scenario, which actually reduces costs, the processing environment is tightly managed and controlled. Departments may select the needed processing software and hardware which fit the functional needs of their departments, but the variety of vendors will probably be restricted.

The management information services (MIS) department may have established a standard hardware platform within which systems may be selected. Today, it is still much easier and less costly to connect multiple machines from the same vendor than to connect a number of disparate machines. In this controlled environment, the networking probably comes from the same vendor as the computing hardware, and departmental processors tend to be on the small side.

This scenario yields most of the benefits of a fully distributed environment. Departmental users may select, within bounds, the computing system that they want for their department. They manage and control their own destiny and have the status, power, and control that they are seeking. In the near future, standards now evolving in the industry will facilitate interconnects will result in a truly seamless interconnect capability. This will permit any machine on the network to easily access data stored on another computer.

Scenario 2: The Uncontrolled Environment. The second scenario for distributed processing does not yield the same level of benefits and may incur a higher level of costs, though costs remain difficult to measure. In this scenario, there is basically no management of the selection and procurement process. No architecture, guidelines, or recommended approaches are outlined for system selection. Departments may choose whatever system they please without regard for factors other than their own requirements. The result can be a costly miasma of many types of computers from a wide variety of vendors.

Such an environment has a critical need for a widely available and standard networking scheme and a standard communication protocol for the interconnection of machines. However, the network hardware is likely to come from a third party and require the use of network software from an additional vendor. With computers from a wide variety of vendors, and hence few vendor discounts for multiple machines at one site, maintenance costs are high.

Support personnel becomes an issue, since a small staff cannot hope to be skilled on a large number of machines from varying vendors. Interfacing the machines and their applications can become more difficult, especially when the machines use different communications techniques. Moreover, if these machines are all located in their respective departments and in dedicated and environmentally controlled space, the institution incurs additional physical plant costs. Many of these costs are hidden and indirect, but they are real costs that drive to the bottom line of the healthcare institution.

Scenario 3: The Partially Controlled Environment. The most realistic scenario is somewhere in between the two described above. Departments are permitted to select the systems they want, but have some constraints in the selection process. The number of vendors is restricted but not absolutely controlled. With equipment from no more than two to three vendors, support can be handled by a small staff.

Minicomputers typically do not require an extensive support staff, and many of the commercially available turnkey systems can be handled by a well trained and interested end user. Operations may still require trained operators, but many of the system setup and technical operations are provided by the vendor under their maintenance contract. However, the issues of providing a proper environment, appropriate backup, maintenance, and service level all still exist in this environment.

As is true of the uncontrolled environment, costs may be hidden in the areas of staffing and of maintaining and operating the equipment. Because the costs of operations and systems administration are pushed into the user departments, the approach may be considered a form of financial accounting chargeback. It also causes departments to have some of their staff increase the breadth of their jobs, as they may be responsible for their normal tasks as well as the care and feeding of the computing system. This may be desirable and improve certain jobs within the institution. It potentially provides a new technically based career path for the department member who wishes to extend the practical use of computers within that particular department.

Selecting an Approach

Comparing the cost effectiveness of a distributed environment versus a centralized environment can be difficult. For an accurate comparison, all of the costs must be captured for both options. Costs will be highly dependent on the variety of computers, the number allowed, and the support requirements for each. The level of indirect costs will increase the difficulty of an accurate comparison between the two competing approaches.

In a distributed environment, costs are incurred across a number of departments and are associated with each computer. Large networks with multiple minicomputers and many workstations can be expensive. Although costs may approach those for a mainframe system, the distributed environment may allow for increased functionality. Costs for a centralized mainframe environment, with simple terminals connected to the mainframe, are easier to track or project. Once all of the costs are captured, the comparison is straight-forward and proceeds strictly from a cost point of view.

Size is an important factor in selecting an approach. With increasing demands on computing resources, the requirements for processing power and storage are growing dramatically. It is becoming increasingly difficult for even large mainframe computers to handle all of the terminals and data storage required by an entire business enterprise. When this occurs, networks of mainframe computers may be called for. This is not a typical case in hospitals today, but it certainly could be so in the not too distant future. As the regulations for reporting on the cost and care of patients increase and as the amount of data collected on each patient increases, the computing resources required will demand increased numbers of mainframes or networked technology.

The difficult issues to face are the perceptions of power, control, and service. In large healthcare institutions, an individual ancillary department such as radiology or laboratory can be a very large operation. The heads of these departments generate significant revenues for the institution and will want to provide their services on a high quality, low cost basis. To satisfy these needs, these departments will demand that the computing solution for them fulfill

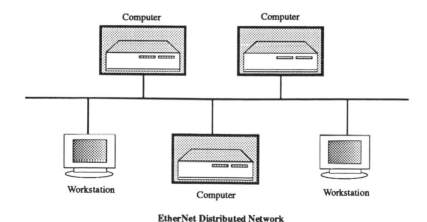

Figure 1. EtherNet Distributed Network

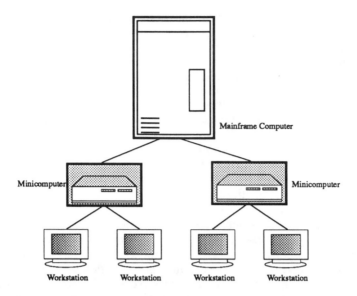

Figure 2. Hierarchical Distributed System

their functional and business needs. Given the systems available, even the most centralized organization in a large institution will probably be faced with distributed processing in these two departments. The requirements in these areas are so unique and the interfaces so specific that the possibility of obtaining a high quality solution from one vendor for the hospital as a whole, including these departments, is not very likely.

Thus, the location and control of the computing resource for these departments will become major issues, to be resolved mainly through the political process. The level of influence wielded by the head of the department will have as dramatic an impact on these issues as the leadership power and influence of the institution's highest management. Cost will be of some concern, but will not become the burning issue over which these questions will be resolved. The managerial and political culture of an institution will likely determine the approach to be taken.

Distributed Processing

Developments

Distributed processing has been a part of the data processing field for some time. The means for accomplishing it have changed during the past five years. Prior to the advent of the personal computer, most distributed computing environments consisted of several computers linked by wire or telephone lines. These connections were rather slow in speed. The logical connections were point to point, with one machine generally connected to only one other machine. Many of the configurations were in either a star topology as shown in Figure 1 or a hierarchical topology as shown in Figure 2.

Personal computers have gradually rendered the traditional networks inadequate. At first, the users of personal computers were content to be isolated. They then demanded that they be connected to the corporate mainframe computers, so that they could obtain data without rekeying. This connection also allowed them to place data back on the mainframe after they manipulated those data with innovative tools on their personal computers. The next phase was to share data and high quality printers or other resources with other personal computer users. Doing this through the mainframe was awkward and, depending on the type of connection, quite slow. When peer to peer communication and full data sharing became the next demand, the need for high speed local area networks (LANs) became evident.

By providing high speed communication over a limited distance, LANs extend new services and techniques. LANs make it possible for groups of personal computers to share data files or expensive components, such as laser printers. Software that is located on one computer can be retrieved and run on another machine located on the same network. When the local area network is connected to a minicomputer or a mainframe, the personal computer becomes a standalone processor, a terminal to the main machine, or a cooperative processor.

In the cooperative processor role, a program can be moved from the main computer and run on the personal computer. The data may still reside on the main machine but be brought to the desktop only as needed. The result is a very versatile environment which allows unique integration of data, processing power, high quality display of information, and a common user interface. As the costs of personal computers and networking have dropped, the demand for Lotus type spreadsheets and Macintosh style presentation graphics has increased dramatically.

The implementation of these new technologies will still be driven by corporate culture, leadership styles, and politics, but the direction based upon end user demand is clear. Distributed processing will continue to increase in all industries. In healthcare, as departmental needs become more complex and software solutions come closer to fulfilling those needs, the number of distributed systems is likely to grow. Continued pressure for more cost effective management and still greater computing power on the desktop will certainly feed the demand for distributed processing.

Issues

Distributed processing is not without its problems. Especially in large distributed environments, it is difficult to guarantee service levels and resolve problems. Since local area networks contain many active electronic components, a methodical approach to the isolation of the problem is required. In many instances, two technicians must work in concert to determine the source of the problem, which can range from a failing personal computer or network card to a segment of damaged cable. (At the Hospital of the University of

Pennsylvania, the most frequent problem is damage to the cable plant caused by construction and maintenance workers. This damage has resulted in anything from a complete outage to slow data transfer or loss of data in transit from one machine to another.)

In a centralized mainframe environment, processor failure is very clear. When the computer fails, everything is down. In the distributed environment, this is not the case. The failure of one CPU on the network may have very little to do with other processors on the network. This failure may be reported by end users in unclear and subtle ways. In all cases, however, end users will clearly state the one position that they understand: the network is down. Integrated network management tools are sorely needed to manage heterogeneous networks. Many of the computer industry's leading firms are working to develop such tools; once these tools are available, they will greatly enhance the ability to manage network, guarantee availability, and resolve problems.

One of the major advantages of a centralized system is the extent to which it makes possible the integration of information. When a system is designed, the analysts who are the architects of the system can define the data elements to be stored within the system. Through the use of advanced relational database techniques, these analysts can easily define relationships among data elements, such as length of stay and attending physician. These architects have many tools at their disposal, such as data modeling and prototyping, and can design the whole structure. As long as they design carefully, the ability to define relationships will not be narrowly restricted.

With a distributed system, developing and providing the ability to manipulate the data required for these relationships can be a difficult task. Distributed processing in healthcare institutions is in its infancy. Thus far only a few vendors have developed the tools and techniques which allow for easy integration of data. Although integration will remain difficult to achieve until standards for data sharing are more firmly embedded in software applications, it is not impossible. With careful analysis and an understanding of the available data, relationaldata bases can be built on a distributed network system which allows the necessary manipulations. This approach is currently available only to those institutions that have the resources or staff to build these facilities. Some of the financial systems in use today can provide some of these capabilities in a networked environment. A good data storage and reporting facility can be built using the historical databases fed by the patient accounting systems and used to provide length of stay and financial forecasting data.

Like any other complex business, healthcare institutions require the use of computing technologies to help manage their business. The general financial trends in healthcare call for the provision of services through fewer resources. If properly planned and implemented, computing can help to provide the services needed at lower cost. Whether the environment is centralized or distributed, the institution absolutely must prioritize its needs as part of its strategic and tactical plans.

Because of its large financial profile, mainframe computing typically has a higher visibility to the management of an institution. Replacing a mainframe may involve spending several million dollars. This level of expenditure will require the development of plans, much discussion, and approval from multiple levels of management, including the board of trustees.

In a distributed environment, the growth of the computing resource can take place with a much lower profile. The addition of a new system may involve adding a small number of personal computers or perhaps a small minicomputer. Because these expenditures may be made with the approval of only the department manager or the controller, there is greater danger of growing a system which does not meet the needs of the institution. A process must be created for developing, rank ordering, and managing to priorities. The temptation to placate a squeaky wheel department with a partial, low cost solution is very real and can lead to chaos.

Mainframe Use

Distributed processing will not mean the death of large mainframe computers. Complex environments will continue to require large scale, high speed processing. High volume billing is a problem for less than a mainframe, and the same may hold true for the storage and manipulation of cost accounting data. If used to provide the administrative functions of admitting, discharge, and transfer, a mainframe can become a part of a distributed environment where the laboratory and radiology have their own machines. On such a network, the mainframe can broadcast the necessary patient demographic and location information to other machines which in turn can transmit data back to the mainframe for the purpose of billing.

With the installation of a transaction oriented database, the mainframe can also be used as a database management machine. As important patient oriented events are captured, they can be transferred to the mainframe database for storage and later manipulation. This technique requires common definition and timely capture of the data elements, but potentially could become the foundation for automated clinical and financial patient records. If interactively available through a network, it could also be used in providing actual treatment to patients. (Despite its potential, such an approach will most like encounter resistance among traditional mainframe computing staff. Distributed databases, remote cooperative computers, and distributed control are not within their technological cultural background.)

In many cases, the model of choice will have the mainframe connected to departmental machines through a local area network, such as IBM's Token Ring. Departments that have traditionally used computers, such as billing, collections, and admitting, will be directly connected to the mainframe computer through ordinary terminals. Other departments such as nursing and clinical ancillary departments will connect their departmental computers to the mainframe through the local area network. Their own processing will be done on the departmental machine that provides the solutions to their particular needs. Data that must be used for institutional reporting will be housed on the mainframe, while data needed for the management of individual departments will be housed on departmental processors. Thus, the needs of the institution will be met by concentrating the appropriate data on the mainframe, and the needs of the individual department through a dedicated departmental computing system.

Benefits

In a distributed environment, benefits will accrue from the improved computing available to departments throughout the healthcare institution. Specialized systems supported by niche vendors will offer individual departments higher functionality than systems provided by a large generic vendor attempting to meet heterogeneous needs. Although hardware acquisitions and software development remain expensive, buying or licensing systems may provide some cost relief from developing systems inhouse. The only caveat is that purchased systems must in fact provide the services that are needed.

Computing will meet less resistance in the workplace as departments are included in the selection process and given a real choice in the system they are to use. As users participate in the installation process, they will realize their reputations are on the line along with those of the MIS department. The probability of success will increase.

Increased functionality should have positive effects on the provision of treatment to patients. Using a single workstation in their office or at the point of care, clinicians will be able to retrieve all clinical data on their patients. With technological advances, it will soon be possible for clinicians to call the hospital on their car phones, and have a computer read to them the current lab results.

The Future

Distributed processing has come about for a number of reasons. Personal computers and the innovative software that runs on them have had a dramatic effect. The lowering of computing costs has made computing technologies more widely available. Computers are now so much a part of our society that we see them in many homes and think it unusual if businesses operate without them.

The result has been a reduced fear of computers and a more defined expectation of what computing should be like. It is not unusual for professionals to expect that their computing work will have a Pacman look and feel to it. Ease of use and availability of information are the future of computing. The WIMPs (windows, icons, mouse, pointing) approach will be common. This will require more intelligent and powerful workstations for people to use.

As image and voice technology improve, the need for higher speed connections between the data (servers) and the users (workstations) will become more important. The implementation of standard protocols for communicating will increase. Transmission Control Protocol/Internetworking protocol (TCP/IP), Open Systems Interconnection (OSI), Ethernet, Token Ring, Health Level 7 (HL/7), and American Standards for Testing Materials (ASTM) will all become common terms in the implementation of computing systems. Each of these will play an important part in allowing diverse computing systems to talk freely with each other.

Because a well designed and implemented distributed system can make available to all users all of the data within the institution, control of the data and security become important issues. However, the factors that have the greatest effect on the implementation of these new technologies are now and will continue to be funding, management, and institutional politics. Only if these issues and factors are addressed can healthcare realize in full the promise of the new technologies.

Questions

1. Can a network designed to support a distributed LAN architecture support the communications requirements of a mainframe environment?

2. What criteria should be applied to determine the cost effectiveness of a distributed LAN environment?

3. Currently the pharmacy is running on a mainframe based application which has been in operation for some time. They are proposing to replace this application with one based on networked personal computers. What should your strategy be for implementing this new pharmacy system?

Select Bibliography

Champine, G. A., with R. D. Coop. 1980. *Distributed computer systems impact on management, design and analysis.* New York: North-Holland Publishing Co.

Chorafas, D. 1984. *Designing and implementing local area networks.* New York: McGraw-Hill.

Martin, J. 1981. *Design and strategy for distributed data processing.* Englewood Cliffs, N.J.: Prentice-Hall.

Stallings, W. 1985. *Tutorial, local network technology,* 2nd ed. Washington, D.C.: IEEE.

Section 2–Managing the Institution

Unit 4—Buying Expertise

Unit Introduction

By necessity risk aversive, healthcare institutions may seek outside expertise to minimize risk in expensive decision areas, among them information technology. Knowing when and how to maximize the value of both consultants and vendors can help ensure success in acquiring, implementing, and managing information systems. This unit advocates a healthy skepticism and advises how the buyer can best beware.

Childs writes from his knowledge as president of a worldwide healthcare publishing and consulting company, providing a candid insider's view of consultants. A young hands-on information specialist who orchestrates installations for a major consulting firm, Ball offers practical advice on managing consultants. Marley, vice president for information systems at a large medical center, provides a different perspective on the same topic. Hammon, president of his consulting firm, explains the acquisition and implementation process, offering detailed guidance for healthcare institutions.

Paying consultants for good advice can be a successful cost containment measure.

1

Consulting: State of the Art

Bill W. Childs

Hospital Information Systems

A number of months ago, an executive vice president and administrator of a large teaching hospital ran into his former director of data processing at a healthcare convention. They chatted about the last two years since the former data processing director had become an independent consultant to other hospitals in the selection and purchase of information systems. Judging from his former employee's grand appearance, the administrator ventured, "You must be doing very well!"

Without hesitating, the consultant said, "Oh, yes, sir, I now bill out at $2,000 per day," a significant promotion from the $200 per day he had been paid previously by the administrator. Impressed, the administrator said, "John, do you suppose we could purchase just ten minutes of your time? I'd like to know where you filed all that documentation you and your staff were supposed to be working on the last two years you were with us."

This is not how the consultant would have liked the negotiation to go, but his former employer was a fairly smart fellow. He knew what he did and did not know, and he knew what he wanted—not a bad start for someone needing a consultant.

The Market: The Dilema

Reported to be in excess of $250 million in 1987, the healthcare consulting market in the United States is big business. Estimates put this figure as exceeding $300 million or $50,000 per hospital in 1990. Why is this market so large and why has it drawn nearly every Big Eight accounting firm into the business? Why also are there so many independent small and large firms in the business?

The answers to these questions are simple, and yet the reasoning behind most of the answers is quite complex. First, the answers. The buyers have demanded more and more consulting time. Consultants have done an

319

outstanding job of marketing their services. Almost all buyers have purchased systems in the past that did not meet their expectations after purchase. Finally, several hospitals have been absolutely burned by vendors that did not deliver as expected.

Because of this last item alone, it is no wonder that buyers are reluctant to make future purchase decisions without the assistance of outside experts to lessen their chance of making a mistake. After all, the cost of today's systems is high, and the potential for error is great.

The healthcare consulting market is actually divided into several segments and specialties. Some consulting firms offer a complete menu of services while others specialize in specific areas such as the clinical laboratory or perhaps the acquisition process only.

As shown in Table 1, there are many specialty areas for healthcare consultants. New areas not on the list continue to emerge. Consultants seem to materialize to fill any need once it is identified. There are also hospital managers who have already decided to go in a specific direction and are looking for a consultant to rubber stamp their decision and give it the seal of approval. After all, if the high priced expert agrees that this is the path to take, then who can fault the buyer?

Choosing a Consultant

How should administrators choose a consultant? The answer to this question is fairly simple and straightforward. Consultants are and should be hired for the following reasons:

- They bring expertise that the administrator does not currently have inhouse. There may be several reasons why these people should not be permanently on staff. The expertise they have may not be needed over the long haul, and it may not be within the administrator's budget except for short durations.
- Consultants can be an addition to the hospital staff for short periods of time or for specific projects. When the need is over, the cost can be over.

Definition of the Consulting Task

Unless the task is predefined, most hospital staffs waste a lot of time and money on consultants. Of course, there is the case where a consultant is brought in to define the task or figure out the problem. These kinds of consulting engagements, by their nature, can be time consuming and costly.

When consultants look at a potential engagement, they most often think of billable hours. There probably is nothing wrong with this because it falls into basic survival needs. The point here is that the buyer needs to be aware that most consultants will create the largest, most comprehensive deal they can.

Table 1. Specialty Areas for Healthcare Consultants: A Partial Listing

General systems consulting	General acquisitions
Request for information (RFI) process	Request for proposal (RFP) process
Needs assessments	Contracting
Implementation	Capital planning
Staffing	Facilities management
Hardware planning and acquisition	Departmental systems
Laboratory	Ambulatory care
Radiology	Other ancillaries
Development	Communications
Integration	Planning
Marketing	Retrofitting

A consulting friend of the author's used to ask, "Did you select and purchase the system you currently have or were you sold the system by some fast talking salesman?" Clearly, administrators should ask themselves this question and be sure to complete a basic needs assessment before they buy consulting services. Whatever the need, the hospital and its administrator will be better off if they define their needs first.

How Should Hospitals Use Consultants?

The Administrator's View. It should be obvious that there is no single view as to how consultants should be used. Consulting may not be the oldest known profession, but it certainly ranks right up there with other professions that are often lauded as the oldest.

After all, it was Moses some 5,000 years ago that could not get his people moving to the promised land because of management problems. It was his father in law, Jethro, who suggested he needed rulers of hundreds and thousands because his span of control was too great. Even earlier, Job had several unwanted consultants give him advice on how to solve his many problems.

In preparation for this chapter, the author interviewed about 15 administrators for their words of wisdom regarding the use and misuse of consultants. Their varied responses are contained in the various sections of this chapter. They concurred in only a few areas: they paid more than planned; the engagement took longer than intended; and accomplishments fell short of what had been desired. Nonetheless, 11 out of 15 were relatively happy with their consultants' work, and all 15 indicated that they would be engaging another consultant within the year to address current or future problems.

In information systems, the largest use of consultants falls in one of three categories: selection of a system; contract negotiations; and implementation. Consultants are offering services in other areas as well.

Buying into Consultants

A practice that is common among vendors is to bring in consultants to provide expert opinions in a given area. Many vendors select projects that the consulting community can work on and request that consultants provide their expertise.

Some things that should not go unnoticed are the obligations consultants set up when they perform vendor and hospital consulting. Some would say consulting for both is not a conflict of interest. A case in New York involving a system failing to meet standards may be instructive, however. Attorneys for the hospital are basing their case in part on the discovery that the consultant recommending the system to the hospital had also reviewed the system for the vendor.

Companies that cannot afford to have consultants pass judgment on their systems are often omitted from consideration for purchase. Several smaller vendors have told the author that in the last several years they have only won contracts when no consultant was involved in the selection process.

Another major potential problem today is the advent of consulting groups setting themselves up as systems integrators. This consulting service often can eliminate those vendors who exclusively offer their own services. Several vendors have complained that, unless they allow outside consultants to get involved in the implementation process, they cannot get any business from the consultants.

Buying into consultants frustrates everyone in the industry, but vendors are reluctant to confront the issue for fear they will be blackballed.

Educating the Consultant

How does one become a consultant? By what process does one become an expert? As with most things in life, there are multiple ways—hard work, brilliance, or luck (being in the right place at the right time). A few individuals even enter consulting when temporarily unemployed.

Twelve years ago, a young systems analyst in the author's organization was fired for lack of both performance and potential. Later that year, he was making almost twice his salary as a consultant for a Big Eight firm. The same year, one of the firm's outstanding vice presidents resigned and opened up an independent consulting group. A capable man, with much to offer his clients, he is still doing very well today. As is true in any field, some consultants are barely mediocre while others are absolutely outstanding and worth every dollar they are paid.

Over the years, how do consultants stay on top of developments in the marketplace? Some consulting groups do an outstanding job while others get by. Certainly a good question for any administrator to ask a potential consulting firm is, "What is the breadth and depth of your knowledge, and by what standard do you measure?"

A few consulting firms conduct annual educational seminars for their staffs. To these seminars they invite company spokesmen and experts in specific markets. Ernst & Young, for example, offers educational seminars characterized by information intensive formats. On the other hand, a few firms engage in the questionable practice of demanding payment by the vendors to come in to corporate headquarters and learn about new products and services.

Because the educational process is problematic, many vendors are hiring people to deal with the consulting community and provide them with the information they need to stay up with current products and services. This past year, this author's firm received videos from over ten vendors, explaining new directions, products, and services.

When selecting consultants, it is always prudent to ask, "Who will be working on my project?" and "What is that individual's background and expertise?"

Recently, a hospital hired a Big Eight consulting firm to find and implement a financial information system for the hospital. The experience of that consulting firm was limited to implementing one system for a particular vendor. After a $300,000 selection fee, the consultants chose the vendor they were most familiar with and then proceeded to implement. The choice may have been right, but the costly selection fee is open to question.

A growing practice among the major consultants is the exclusion of start up and small vendors. The high costs of starting up and sustaining a product over time have driven many smaller companies out of the market. This phenomenon has made consultants much more conservative. Small companies complain that excluding them deprives customers of new technology. Although the pioneers know that leading edge technologies can become bleeding edge, there will always be visionaries that are willing to gamble on future rewards.

Knowledge Couplers and Specialization

Information overload today brings both the blessings and problems inherent in specialization. In healthcare, specialization has been the norm for many years. Physicians began the separation of practice by specialty; nurses and hospitals followed. Inevitably, systems and consultants have had to specialize in order to remain expert in their fields. The problems with specialization are not on the surface, but appear when a given problem does not easily fit within a defined specialty or crosses over between specialties.

Background and specialization affect processes and decisions. The result may not be the best possible solution available but simply the best a given individual can come up with. Within companies and healthcare delivery systems, this phenomenon is often referred to as corporate culture. For certain companies, distinct cultures often come to mind, as shown in Table 2. It does not matter that these companies may excel elsewhere. Where they have made their mark is where they are remembered. Because of investments and expertise, they often have a difficult time moving away from these niche markets.

Table 2. Cultures and Niches Identified with Certain Companies

SMS	Shared systems
McDonnell Douglas	Shared systems sold to American Express
HBO	Inhouse systems
TDS	Medical information systems
Cycare	Ambulatory systems
Sunquest	Laboratory systems
Spectrum (Previously Baxter)	Inhouse IBM mainframe, minicomputer, and microcomputer systems
HMDS	Microbased systems

There is a theory saying, "If you have a hammer in your hand, everything looks like a nail." In healthcare, for instance, psychiatrists think first of the patient's mind, internists are likely to treat with medicine, and surgeons are predisposed to cut something out.

Specialists in any area tend to solve problems based on their specialties. As knowledge bases in healthcare get larger, this tendency becomes more obvious and the specialties grow narrower. Eventually computers will help to couple all of these knowledge bases together. For the moment, though, it is experts in the field who must do so.

When selecting consultants, administrators should be aware of this phenomenon. The consultant educated on mini systems will find it hard to consider mainframe or micro systems. The consultant from a financial systems background will not be as much in tune with the subtleties of medical systems. Likewise, it is rare that someone who has always placed systems inhouse can evaluate the advantages of a time shared, off site system. In short, the key question to ask in finding a good consultant is what that consultant's track record has been and why.

The Challenge

Consulting today is big business in the healthcare market. The complexities of healthcare and of information technology force potential buyers, managers, and systems to go to the market for help. The process is long and costly, and there are many places that it can go off track. Unfortunately, vendors and staff within hospitals often deliver less than originally promised.

It may be tempting to write this failure off as a problem in managing expectations. However, information systems, properly conceived, designed, developed, implemented, and managed, can go a long way toward saving money and improving the quality of care in healthcare. With an eye on service, a mind full of knowledge, and a heart committed to getting the job done, the consultant can provide invaluable assistance in this critical and demanding task.

Questions

1. What are some significant reasons that a hospital should employ a consultant?

2. How should a hospital prepare itself prior to employing a consultant?

3. What are the advantages of employing a free lance consultant as opposed to employing a large consulting firm? What are the advantages of dealing with a large consulting firm?

4. Should the hospital already have a solution to its problems predetermined and only employ a consultant to verify their solution or should a consultant be employed in order to determine the optimum solution?

5. Should a hospital employ a consultant who has been known to have close ties to a vendor bidding on the hospital system? Under what conditions might this be a good idea, under what conditions would this be a poor idea?

2
Maximizing the Benefits of Using Consultants

Elizabeth E. Ball

Healthcare costs account for 12 percent of the United States' gross national product (GNP). As cost containment measures have been implemented to address the high costs of healthcare, acute care facilities have required speedy revenue recovery mechanisms to survive. To run more efficiently, hospitals are turning to information resources management and automating clinical and financial applications which provide administrators with the management information they need to make cost effective decisions. The increased importance and cost of information resources management have spawned the growth of healthcare information systems (HCIS) consulting practices.

How Consulting Firms Work

Consulting firms make money by selling work. To keep their employees utilized and to command high rates, consulting firms must provide services that are of a high quality and caliber. Individual consultants have specialized skills and proven experience; established in their fields, they often have previously worked for a vendor, a hospital, or both.

The consulting firm's goal is to keep the client satisfied and to offer its clients the best services. It is important to realize that there is a finite number of hospitals in the country.

Although one survey notes that 41 percent of the hospital executives see consultants as necessary supplements, hospitals needing healthcare information system consulting services are only a fraction of this 41 percent.

If the consulting firm does not produce what its client requires, the firm will not sell any additional work. The dissatisfied client may look elsewhere; other hospitals may hear of the dissatisfied client. Future sales and utilization will suffer. To stay in business, the consulting firm must keep its clients. To do so, it must have employees who do high quality work and make the firm stand apart from its competitors.

Services Provided by Consultants

Consulting firms rely on the inability of healthcare institutions to keep up with the latest innovations which affect information systems functionality and with developments in other acute care facilities. Consulting firms sell their ability to provide up to date product information and the benefit of experiences in other hospitals. Often the services of consultants protect the client from making the same mistake another institution has already made.

The services that a typical healthcare information systems consultant practice offers are:

- Selection and evaluation of information systems
- Contract negotiations
- Implementation support
- Long range information systems planning
- System testing
- Policy and procedure documentation
- Project management
- Telecommunications/networking
- Quality assurance
- Cost justification
- Reorganization
- Interface support

In retaining information system consultants, healthcare institutions may request the consultants to do any of the following:

Provide Specific Expertise. Often when healthcare institutions lack the specific expertise needed to get a job done, consultants have performed the required task numerous times at other hospitals and are familiar with the vendor or application. Hiring consultants to provide a service that the hospital is not capable of performing inhouse is a common occurrence at acute care facilities.

Perform a Temporary Job. A hospital may have the need for a certain resource for four or six months but not for a full time employee. In these instances it is more cost effective for the institution to pay for a trained individual for the duration of the temporary job or until the backlog is caught up. For example, when converting computer systems most applications are very labor intensive to install, and the hospital does not have the staff to perform all the necessary tasks. After the implementation, there is no longer a need for the resources. This is a common use of consultants.

Provide an Acting Information Systems Director. Hiring management information services directors may be a time consuming process. Consulting firms often provide acting directors until an acceptable candidate is found. This service protects the hospital from the degradation of information service when the director leaves. It also takes the pressure off the hospital to hire someone immediately rather than taking the time necessary to recruit and hire the best candidate.

Review and Evaluate Organizational Structures or System Definition. Consultants are hired in this capacity for their objectivity and neutrality. When evaluating past work or current organizational structures, inhouse hospital staff may be unable to assume an objective viewpoint. Again, since consultants are not biased by the political history or personalities within the hospital, they can make recommendations which are in the best interest of the hospital.

Ensure Successful Implementations. Stories of disastrous implementations are abundant. Administrators often hire consultants to prevent them from making the same mistakes other hospitals made and to protect the hospital from being taken advantage of by the vendor. Consultants are hired for their experience with implementations and to increase the chances for successful outcomes.

Do the Work No One Else Wants to Do. For example, the Joint Commission on the Accreditation of Health Organizations (JCAHO) requires hospitals to have written policies and procedures in place. Typically no one wants to write the policies and procedures, so consultants are hired to finish the job in compliance with JCAHO.

Meet Time Constraints. Time constraints are often the reason for hospitals to hire consultants. When a task needs to be completed in a tight timeframe consultants provide the bodies to get the job done. For example, when looking for a new hospital information system, an institution may choose to expedite the process by hiring a consultant to assist in identifying the required functionalities and writing the request for proposal.

Assist in Project Management. Administrators may not have enough time to devote to project management or may fear that a project that they approved, or are responsible for, is not running smoothly. They may then hire consultants to assist or to warn of possible complications. On occasion, an administrator may hire a consultant as a security blanket or a scapegoat. If the project is a success, the administrator and the consultant both win. However, if the project fails, the administrator may place the blame on the consultant.

Avoid Making Costly Mistakes. As the financial portfolios of hospitals are becoming bleaker, hospitals cannot afford to make mistakes nor do they have the time to correct mistakes. As automation has become critical to an institution's ability to survive, hospitals are under pressure and must make decisions that are right the first time. Many hospitals hire healthcare information system consultants because they cannot afford to take the risk of making a mistake. More hospitals should.

Getting the Most Value from Consultants

Before hiring a firm, the hospital should arrange to meet the individual consultants from the firm who will be assigned to the project. The client should make sure those consultants are experienced and capable of discussing specific experiences with other hospitals. There should be no learning curve to prevent immediate results from the consultants. For example, if implementation assistance is required, the individual consultant should be familiar with not only the application but also the vendor. Checking references will also ensure that the most value is received from the consultants.

The hospital should stipulate deliverables with due dates and identify a series of continuing checkpoints before the project begins. Granting extensions for deliverables sets a bad precedent and should not be done. As clients, the hospital should clearly define the scope of the project and establish that the estimated hours will not exceed a certain dollar amount. The individual(s) directing the consultant should prepare a list of all items that are to be completed and share it with the consultant.

If the consultants are local, the hospital should request that they work on site at the hospital. There they will get more done for the client than they would at their own offices. The hospital should also ask the consultants for weekly status reports and make sure they know to alert the hospital immediately of any potential delays. To benefit from the engagement, the hospital must let the consultants know what its requirements and expectations are. This means, quite simply, that the hospital must function as a responsible client and present an organized account of what is to be accomplished by the consultants.

The Future for Healthcare Information Systems Consulting

In addition to the established trends toward decreased hardware costs and increased software costs, information resources management shows great increases in installation costs. Trends also suggest that the percentage of the total hospital budget devoted to management information systems will increase in the future.

Information resources management has become a critical factor in the ability of a hospital to survive. In order to survive in this era of cost containment, hospitals must be able to identify profitable services and growing markets. Without information systems, hospitals can neither run efficiently nor produce the information administrators need. Consultants are engaged to address many issues associated with information resources management.

The dependence of healthcare institutions upon their information systems and the increasing complexity of technology combine to make healthcare information systems consulting a growing and profitable market.

Questions

1. What reasons would you give to your administrator to justify using consultants?

2. What would you look for in hiring a consultant?

3. Name four services that healthcare information systems consultants provide.

4. What are the trends in making the best use of consulting firms and their employees?

3
Managing Consulting Services: A Guide for the CIO

Amelia Lee Marley

The chief information officer (CIO) is responsible for the provision of information within the healthcare organization. This responsibility encompasses the accuracy, adequacy, availability, assimilation, and cost effectiveness of information as the needs of the organization evolve and dictate. The resources to meet the organization's information systems requirements include computer hardware, computer software, internal personnel, vendor personnel, and consulting personnel. The personnel costs of implementing and maintaining new technology are a significant component of the total cost equation. Effective management of these personnel costs is key to maximization of information systems resources.

Cost effective utilization of consultants is a skill essential to the success of the CIO. Of hospital executives surveyed, 41 percent saw consultants as necessary supplements to internal resources but only 29 percent believed consultants' fees are cost justified (Packter 1987). Executives are leery of using consultants because they are an expensive resource and inappropriate use of consultants is extremely costly. Therefore, the CIO must be a prudent buyer of consulting services. Effectively used, consultants can greatly enhance the investment made in information systems.

The key to effectively using consultants is understanding how to evaluate, select, and manage consulting services. This chapter provides insights into how consulting firms work and gives practical guidelines for using consultants.

Understanding How Consulting Firms Work

Consulting is a service industry in the purest sense. A consulting firm's primary assets are its personnel. These assets produce revenue by providing services to clients. Services are usually billed at a negotiated hourly rate. Within a practice, individual consultants are monitored in terms of their utilization rate, that is, the percentage of their time which is billed to clients.

331

A practice is monitored in terms of its revenue contributions. The consultant's goal is to stay utilized; the practice's goal is to contribute revenues at a level defined in the firm's business plan.

To meet these goals, consulting firms attempt to convince potential clients of needs which can be met by the personnel of the consulting firm. The marketing of consulting services is largely a process of needs identification. Needs identified are likely to be related to systems planning, systems selection, systems implementation, or systems use evaluation. It is during the consulting marketing cycle that the potential consumer can become quite confused. The CIO must discern the difference between the creation of a perceived need and a legitimate lack of resources to meet a stated goal.

Evaluating the Need for Consulting Services

There are five key questions the CIO should answer when determining whether or not to use consulting services.

How do the services being proposed fit into the overall information systems plan? The CIO should evaluate how the project being proposed by the consulting firm fits into the overall information systems plan. It may be that there is no plan. If so, the first and most critical step is to develop one. An information systems plan is essential. A CIO operating without a plan has no way of knowing what the overall blueprint for change is. Without a plan, it is impossible to determine whether the organization's information systems needs and priorities are being met. The proposed services should be considered only if the services are relevant to the information systems plan or if the plan is changed to reflect a shift in priorities.

Are the services being proposed critical to the implementation of the information systems plan? The CIO should evaluate how critical the proposed project is to the success of the information systems plan. If the project relates to the plan but is not essential to its success, then it probably is not worth pursuing. For example, a consulting firm might propose to conduct an extensive needs analysis prior to the selection of a radiology system. The selection of a radiology system might be part of the plan, but it may also be that the director of radiology understands radiology systems sufficiently that a needs analysis would be neither necessary nor welcome.

How aggressive are the dates incorporated in the information systems plan and how committed in the organization to these dates? It is important to consider how aggressive the organization is relative to the deadlines incorporated in the information systems plan. If the timelines are generous or the dates are flexible, there is less need to staff aggressively. If the organization is on a tight time schedule and the dates are inflexible, then adequate personnel resources must be quickly obtained. A consulting firm, being a provider of short term manpower, is an appropriate resource to utilize in this scenario.

What risks are inherent in the information systems plan? The CIO should consider the degree of risk inherent in the institution's information systems plan. The implementation of new technology includes higher associated risks. It may be appropriate to involve consultants during the implementation of a pilot system to assist in managing the associated risks. For example, it would be appropriate to hire a consultant to perform extensive software testing on software which is newly developed. However, using a consulting firm to test mature software would probably not be critical to the success of the project.

Are there less costly resources available to accomplish the objectives to be met by the consulting firm? The CIO should also determine whether there is staff available, internal or third party, to perform the tasks of the project at a lesser cost. If so, these resources might be used in place of consultants. However, this involves the careful examination of the skill set of internal staff as well as a solid understanding of what contributions systems vendors can make. Consultants are a potential solution if internal personnel and vendor personnel cannot provide the resources needed to successfully meet the goals of the information systems plan (Gigiulio 1984).

Selecting a Consulting Firm

Once it is determined that there is a need for consulting services, the next step is to select a firm. Answering the following questions should address the key areas to be considered:

- What kinds of experience and skills do the specific individuals assigned to the engagement have which are critical to the success of the project team?

- What resources are available to the project team from across the consulting firm which could be utilized as needed on the engagement?

- Has the consulting firm demonstrated a commitment to the potential client by providing services before a formal agreement is made?

- Does the consulting firm lend credibility at the board and departmental level?

- Does the executive consultant or partner who is marketing the engagement demonstrate a sincere interest in the success of the CIO's goals?

- Will the consulting staff assigned to the engagement blend well with internal staff and with any associated vendors?

In essence, the questions posed above relate to the experience, expertise, commitment, and compatibility of the consulting firm being evaluated. To be further considered, the consulting firm must have personnel available for the engagement who have the knowledge and skills to meet the demands of the project. If these criteria are met, it is simply a matter of cost and selecting the organization with which to do business. It is important that there is a positive business relationship between the client and the consultant. This can occur only when there is a fundamental compatibility between the two.

Managing the Consulting Firm

A letter of agreement finalizes the understanding between the client and the consultant. In the letter of agreement, the scope, work plan, personnel, deliverables, and fees should be defined. If any of these items are missing from an engagement letter, the client should request that they be added. Each of these items is described below.

Scope: A general description of the project which sets forth the direction and boundaries for what will be included as part of the engagement. It is important that the scope be stated so that the consultant and client conceptually agree to what is included as part of the engagement. Typically, the scope of the engagement should not change. However, if a change in scope is proposed, the evaluation process is the same as that used for evaluating any prospective consulting services.

Work Plan: The definition of tasks to be performed and the associated dates of completion. The work plan is important to ensure that the engagement has been well thought out and to monitor progress once work begins.

Personnel: The identification and qualifications of specific individuals to be assigned to an engagement. It is important to state in writing that the individuals specified in the letter of understanding will not be substituted with other personnel unless expressly agreed to before the fact by the client.

Deliverables: Any product which will be produced during the course of the engagement. This would include any reports or other performance commitments stated in the letter of agreement. The due dates of deliverables should be outlined in the work plan.

Fees: Usually stated as an hourly rate. The key point here is that consulting firms have standard rates which are typically negotiated downward. The client might wish to establish an upper dollar cap for the project to protect against budget overruns. However, the hourly rate is generally not as negotiable when caps are incorporated in the letter of agreement. The client's negotiating strategy must be assessed on a basis specific to the needs of the organization.

Once the engagement begins, it is important to monitor progress. One of the best techniques for doing this is by regularly polling internal staff as to how they perceive the progress of the project. Also, discussing the engagement progress with consulting personnel and referencing the letter of agreement helps ensure open lines of communication.

In managing consultants, the CIO must constantly evaluate the need for consulting services. The consulting firm should be discharged if the service does not meet expectations or is determined unnecessary to the successful implementation of the information systems plan.

Dealing with Future Trends

Technology is changing the information systems environment at a pace which challenges those in the industry to keep up. It makes sense to use outside resources, consultant or vendor, when lack of internal staff expertise prohibits an organization from using information as a competitive advantage. The rate of technology change will continue to accelerate resulting in the availability of new products. The major challenge will be how to assimilate these new products into the organization's culture in order to capitalize on new technologies. As this occurs and is recognized, healthcare organizations will increasingly turn to consultants to meet this challenge.

An editorial titled "The High Cost of Consulting" warned of the pitfalls in using consultants (Childs 1989), and cost does make executives cautious in using consulting services. Difficult though it may be, knowing when and how to use consultants can greatly enhance the organization's utilization of information and literally mean the difference between success and failure. Guidelines for the CIO include the following:

- Recognize that consulting firms survive by keeping staff on engagements. Therefore, there is an incentive for the firm to identify a client need which can best be met by the consulting firm's resources.

- Evaluate the need for consulting firms in reference to an information systems plan. The services must be relevant and critical to the success of the plan.

- Select a consulting firm by assessing the skills of the consultants and determining the compatibility of the consulting firm with the CIO's organization.

- Manage the use of a consulting firm by establishing mutual expectations with the consultant and by monitoring, as client, the progress of the engagement.

Questions

1. Explain the importance of knowing how to be a prudent buyer of consulting services.

2. Describe why the marketing process used by consulting firms may lead to confusion on the part of a potential client.

3. What is the key reference which should be used in the evaluation of the need for consulting services?

4. Describe several key areas of consideration in the selection of a consulting firm.

References

Packter, C. L. 1987. Executives wary of info systems consultants. *Hospitals* 61:91.

Gigiulio, L. 1984. Who should plan for the implementation of a hospital information system? *Health Care Strategic Management* 2:28-31.

Childs, B. W. 1989. The high cost of consulting, *U.S. Healthcare* 6:8.

4
Understanding the Purchasing and Installation Process

Gary L. Hammon

In the current technological environment, a healthcare organization can and should work with vendors of information technology. Planning is key to producing a climate conducive to the successful integration of products. The management of the information resources department must be aware of the pitfalls to be avoided or overcome. Also, the steps involving the review of product offerings, the selection process, procurement procedures, site visits, demonstrations, contract negotiations, and final award must be handled in a professional manner. Faced with a plethora of vendors and products, the information systems manager has to choose wisely in order to meet the needs of the organization and to achieve the integrated information solution at the least cost and with the greatest benefit.

The selection, acquisition, and purchase of the product or products may be the easiest part of the task. Contract negotiations can be difficult, but the healthcare organization must be firm and reasonable. Once the hardware and/or software is delivered, the real challenge begins. Will the new technology work in a standalone mode? Will the new technology work with existing technology (hardware/software integration)? Will the new technology, in conjunction with the existing technology, meet the needs as expected (data and information integration)? Will the vendor perform (both delivery and installation) as specified in the purchasing documents? There are no ironclad guarantees.

The integration of new software with existing mainframe software poses fewer hardware issues than the installation of a complete standalone hardware/software system utilizing a network for communications with existing system(s). However, the same concerns over inhouse personnel capabilities, vendor personnel, contractual terms, and relationship with the vendor(s) apply and need to be addressed.

337

The information resources department must work with the vendors, both current and new, to ensure success. They must forge a partnership arrangement with the vendors for the good of the healthcare institution.

Preliminary Considerations

In a few cases, a healthcare organization has a staff that is large enough and possesses the requisite training and experience to meet the management and technical requirements for a successful (on time and within budget) selection and integration of technologies. Some information resources managers underestimate the size and complexity of the task. An institution is ill advised to rely on a vendor to safeguard the institution's interest, and unrealistic to have this expectation.

Most healthcare organizations do not have staff with the requisite training and experience for a successful selection, management of the process, and integration of technologies. What do they do to protect the organization's investment and deliver the service to the end user?

The preliminary work sets the stage for a successful or unsuccessful installation. If the details of the various activities are not monitored and verified, the probability of difficulties in the future increases.

Planning Considerations

Once the healthcare organization makes the decision and commitment to move toward an integrated healthcare information system environment, a plan must be developed to chart the necessary steps and budget implications of each step to meet the goal. Evaluation points should be identified within the plan to ensure a timely and on budget completion of the project. The healthcare institution should share this information with potential vendors so they understand the organization's expectations. This step will not remove all the substandard vendors, but can be used in the event of nonperformance or other difficulties.

As part of the planning process, the senior management of the healthcare organization must determine whether the existing data processing (information resources) department has the quantity and quality of staff to meet the technological and managerial requirements of the undertaking. This is an important step, and an unduly optimistic or unwarranted positive evaluation can be harmful to the success of the project and the bottom line of the institution.

For the implementation of an integrated system to succeed, important technical decisions must be made prior to selection and acquisition of hardware and software. If the expertise is not available inhouse, the institution should employ an experienced integration consultant to assist with this phase of the effort. This will save time and money for the institution.

Some of the technology related data gathering and performance decisions to be made early in the process are the following:

- What are the requirements of the currently installed systems regarding an interface (one way and two way) to another system?
  Electrical signal?
  Bit stream?
  Use of start and stop bits?
  Packet switching available?
  Handling of and requirements for received information?
  Procedure(s) and requirements for transmitting information?

- How should the existing and planned systems be physically connected?
  Direct connect?
  Protocol converters?
  Peer to peer?
  Local area network?
  Telephone switch?
  A combination of the above?

- What is the targeted response time for attached terminals or PCs?

- What is considered a reasonable amount of overhead per interface within the network? How much overhead can the network and the user tolerate?

- What is the desirable approach or methodology to balancing throughput within the network without unfairly loading one or more of the component machines?

There are other considerations, but the detail in these areas alone documents the need to have or engage personnel with the expertise to address technology choices and to protect purchasing organizations and their users. Responses to technical questions are invaluable, assisting in the evaluation of vendor offerings during the purchasing process and later in the assessment of vendor performance.

If the inhouse staff does not have the expertise to install the new system and make it operational, a budget should be allocated to employ a third party to handle this responsibility. In the long run, this will be considered an investment and not an expense. Both the timely installation of the new system and the integration of existing systems will benefit the institution and the end users.

Contractual Considerations

It has been said that a contract is like a good fence—it makes better neighbors. A contract cannot guarantee that the vendor will perform as expected, but it can define the institution's expectations, requirements, time schedules, and monetary considerations. A responsible vendor will want a contract that spells out this information in order to prevent misunderstandings. A lawsuit will not ensure the system will be installed on schedule and within budget and should be the last resort, after all other efforts have failed. Delay dollar penalties, on the other hand, can offset some of the monetary losses of the organization and place pressure on the vendor to perform.

Purchase documents should be explicitly cited in the contract and should contain the specifications and performance data used in the selection process. The institution should state

- Expected date of delivery and installation

- Expected date of system turnover to the information resources department for acceptance testing

- Expected system operational (go live) date, following acceptance testing and correction of errors and bugs

For each of these three items, the healthcare institution should require the assessment of dollar penalties in the event the vendor cannot meet or exceed these requirements. Since the vendor will probably require the institution to accept the same penalty in the event the delay is the fault of the purchaser, the institution should carefully evaluate possible exposure. Other contract sections should stipulate

- Performance criteria as outlined in the purchasing documents attached to and cited in the contract

- Procedures for the vendor to clear up performance discrepancies, correct malfunctions, and address other shortcomings, including an escalation procedure (names and telephone numbers for several levels of management above the local office) in the event local staff is not responsive

- Procedures to handle fingerpointing when problems arise, assigning responsibility to the major contractor or vendor for conflict resolution and involving the institution as an interested party, but not in the middle of the problem

- A provision to ensure that the integration scheme follows a current standard and not a one of a kind vendor oriented standard, protecting future upgrades

A checklist for contract negotiations is reproduced in Table 1.

Table 1. A Checklist for Users

According to Touche Ross & Co. analyst Lee Gruenfeld, once you've done a comprehensive requirements analysis for a systems integration project, and you're ready to sign an agreement that parcels out the responsibilities, liabilities and risks, make sure you:

- Include as many important system performance specifications as possible in the contract. The integrator may not like it, but usually he'll agree to it.

- Insist on seeing the contracts between the primary integrator and any secondary equipment suppliers he may be using. Prices should be specified. And make sure the primary integrator has access to source code and a license that allows him to modify and upgrade software as required. Consider signing a separate agreement with each vendor on the job.

- Review the contract's liability limitations. Who's going to pay if something goes wrong or if the project turns out to require more, or more expensive, hardware?

- Consider ways to expedite dispute resolution. Approaches such as out-of-court arbitration can reduce legal expenses and allow work to continue while disputes are settled.

- Plan for what will happen if your integrator is gobbled up in a merger or acquisition or if he goes out of business. Who becomes responsible for finishing the job? Can you get the source code?

- Make sure the integrator and his employees are specifically prohibited from disclosing any confidential, competitive information they may pick up on the job.

- Prohibit the integrator from raiding your shop for IS talent. Experienced analysts are the life blood of consultants and integrators. And they usually get them from you-know-who.

Source: Excerpted with permission from *DATAMATION,* May 15, 1989, Cahners Publishing Company.

Another Consideration

The local representative and the immediate manager of the vendor with the preferred system should have made a favorable impression prior to the start of the final selection process. In the event that the vendor personnel are not professional, responsive, and likeable, the institution should reconsider the vendor's product. As far as the institution is concerned, the local personnel are the vendor. If the information resources manager and/or the departmental personnel do not respect and/or like the vendor's personnel, the chances of success are diminished. When misunderstandings and difficulties occur, as they will, relationships will not have the foundation of trust to allow a reasonable, timely solution. The healthcare organization cannot and will not benefit from an adversary relationship. A carefully drawn purchasing document and contract are important, but the gray areas and misunderstandings can be handled in a professional manner for rapid closure. People and not companies make things happen!

If the desired system is the only system which meets the expressed needs of the institution, there is an alternative. Depending upon vendor organization and the level of personnel who are cause for concern, the healthcare institution can empower an executive level officer and the information resources manager to meet with the vendor's local or regional manager. The next step depends upon the results of the meeting. If the vendor agrees to replace the personnel in question, the institution should take some time to become acquainted with the replacement. Only then should the institution decide on the selection issue. However, if the vendor will not make a replacement, the institution should reconsider the vendor's system and look at other alternatives.

After the above process, if the institution decides to acquire the vendor's system in spite of the personnel assigned to the account, then the purchasing document and contract become even more important. The institution must meticulously delineate each and every specification, since the working relationship with the vendor personnel will most likely not be of a nature which allows the institution to recover from items omitted in error.

Ongoing Considerations

During installation, acceptance testing, error correction, and time periods for going live, the manager of information resources should meet with the senior onsite vendor representative at least daily. This should be a formal session, formally recorded by a designated notetaker. Proceedings should be published for all participants and used to check the status of project activities to review open items from previous meetings, and to discuss new items and other project related questions or concerns. Two way communication is vital; effectively handled, it can establish rapport and prevent misunderstandings or the build up of hostile feelings. The daily sessions should focus on both information exchange and problem solving.

After the operational system has been accepted, the manager of information resources should meet with the vendor's local manager and/or senior maintenance technician and software specialist on a monthly basis. It might be useful to invite the sales representative also. Again, this should be a formal session, formally recorded. The published record should be used in reviewing maintenance history for hardware and software over the previous 30 days and open item maintenance lists from previous meetings. The record should also assist in the discussion of new hardware and software upgrades and of any questions or concerns. Again, effective two way communication with vendor personnel is vital for the healthcare organization.

If the open item list continues to grow without apparent resolution, the institution should contact the manager of the person with whom the ongoing meetings have been held and request a meeting to review the situation and resolve it. If resolution is not forthcoming in a reasonable time, the next step is to escalate the problems to the next level of management, and all the way to the president of the company if necessary. Such escalation is unfortunate, but probably will not have to occur a second time with the same local management staff. A word of caution, however: to preserve a working relationship with local vendor staff, the institution should not call the president until all the other levels of management have had a chance to act, or unless the situation is so desperate that immediate resolution is needed.

By building rapport with the assigned vendor personnel, the information resources manager can benefit from shared brainstorming and planning sessions. Of course, these sessions will reflect the vendor's bias, but can provide useful information for comparing products and developing alternative strategies. This is one more resource for the manager to use in meeting continuing planning responsibilities.

Conclusion

The manager of the information resources department begins to set the stage for dealing with vendor personnel at the initial contact with a sales representative. Then the review of products activity, selection process, contract negotiations, installation, and acceptance testing build upon this base. Good vendor relationships are not accidental. They are carefully constructed and are vital to a successful project and to ongoing installation.

Questions

1. If an institution can find the right system, the vendor will be happy to take responsibility for the successful installation. [ ] Yes [ ] No

2. The institution will not have to be involved with the implementation process once the contract is signed. [ ] Yes [ ] No

3. The information resources department will not have to be concerned with the preparation of a contract since the vendor usually has a standard contract. [ ] Yes [ ] No

4. If the information resources department does not like the vendor's contract, then the healthcare organization's legal staff or firm can handle the development of a suitable contract without assistance from Information Resources. [ ] Yes [ ] No

5. If the assigned vendor personnel are not cooperative and supportive, then just run them off and do all the work inhouse. [ ] Yes [ ] No

6. In the event the inhouse staff is not experienced with the proposed technology, it is better to make some mistakes while learning and save money by not hiring a consultant. [ ] Yes [ ] No

7. The selection and installation of a network is a good time to train the staff in the new technology. [ ] Yes [ ] No

8. The institution can turn over all the planning, selection, acquisition, and installation of a new system to the consultant and forget the problems. [ ] Yes [ ] No

9. The vendor of the selected new system will be concerned over the possible impact of interface overhead on the existing systems. [ ] Yes [ ] No

Suggested Periodicals for Further Readings

Serial publications are the best source today for continuing to learn more about the area of integration. There may be textbooks published in the future, as the methodology for integration is undergoing definition. Some current serials to read are:

Monthly Journals

Datamation
PC Resources
PC Computing

Weekly News Publications

Computerworld
InfoWorld

Index

Contributors

JAMES W. ALBRIGHT, M.H.A.
President and Chief Executive Officer, Bayfront Medical Center,
St. Petersburg, Florida

WILLIAM ANLYAN, M.D.
Chancellor, Duke University, Durham, North Carolina

ELIZABETH E. BALL, M.A.
Manager, Healthcare Information Systems, Ernst & Young,
New York, New York

MARION J. BALL, Ed.D.
Associate Vice President for Information Resources, University of
Maryland at Baltimore, Baltimore, Maryland

CAROLE A. BARONE, Ph.D.
Vice President for Information Systems and Computing, Syracuse
University, Syracuse, New York

GRACE H. CHICKADONZ, R.N., Ph.D.
Dean and Professor of Nursing, Syracuse University, Syracuse, New York

BILL W. CHILDS, M.S.
President and Chief Executive Officer, Health Data Analysis Corporation,
Lakewood, Colorado

MORRIS F. COLLEN, M.D.
Consultant and Director Emeritus, Division of Research, Kaiser
Permanente Medical Group, Oakland, California

RICHARD A. CORRELL, M.B.A.
President, Center for Healthcare Information Management, Chicago,
Illinois

JUDITH V. DOUGLAS, M.H.S.
Associate Director, Information Resources Management, University of
Maryland at Baltimore, Baltimore, Maryland

JANE G. ELCHLEPP, M.D., Ph.D.
Associate Professor of Pathology and Assistant to the Chancellor for
Health Affairs, Duke University Medical Center, Durham, North Carolina

BENJAMIN FLOSSIE, B.S., B.B.
Supervisor, Transfusion Department, Department of Pathology and
Laboratory Medicine, Akron General Medical Center, Akron, Ohio

JAMES M. GABLER, M.S.
Chief Information Officer, Santa Rosa Healthcare Corporation,
San Antonio, Texas

ANDREW C. GARLING, M.D.
Vice President of Medical Affairs, TDS Healthcare Systems Corporation,
Atlanta, Georgia

CHARLES F. GENRE, M.D.
Chairman, Pathology Department, and Clinic Laboratory Director, Ochsner
Foundation Hospital, New Orleans, Louisiana

MARILYN GORE, R.N., B.N.
Nursing Systems Development Analyst, Calgary General Hospital, Calgary,
Alberta, Canada

GARY L. HAMMON, B.S.B.A.
Manager, Superior Consultant Company, Inc., San Antonio, Texas

KATHRYN J. HANNAH, R.N., Ph.D.
Professor, Faculty of Nursing, University of Calgary, Calgary, Alberta,
Canada

KEVIN J. HARLEN, M.S.P.H.
Vice President, Patient Care Management, Bayfront Medical Center,
St. Petersburg, Florida

BETSY S. HERSHER, B.S.
President, Health Care Consulting, Hersher Associates, Ltd., Northbrook,
Illinois

THOMAS M. JENKINS, Ph.D.
President, Human Assets Incorporated, Newark, Delaware

G. FREDERICK KESSLER, JR., M.D.
Chief, Clinical Laboratory Services, Department of Pathology and
Laboratory Medicine, Akron General Medical Center, Akron, Ohio

LINDA KOCK, B.S.N., M.S.
Director of Special Projects, Patient Care, Parkview Memorial Hospital,
Fort Wayne, Indiana

THOMAS W. MAGRAW, M.S.
Vice President of Support Services, Bayfront Medical Center,
St. Petersburg, Florida

BRIAN T. MALEC, Ph.D.
Chairman, Division of Health Administration, Governors State University,
University Park, Illinois

AMELIA LEE MARLEY, B.S., M.H.A.
Vice President, Information Systems, Bayfront Medical Center,
St. Petersburg, Florida

PATSY B. MARR, R.N., M.S.N.
Director, Hospital Information Systems, New York University Medical
Center, New York, New York

MICHAEL MCLOONE
Chief Executive Officer, Beaumont Hospital, Dublin, Ireland

JOHN A. MELVIN, M.S., M.B.A.
Manager, Information Technology Services, Price Waterhouse, Toronto,
Ontario, Canada

MICHAEL J. MESTROVICH, Ph.D.
Deputy Assistant Secretary of Defense, Health Management Systems, Falls
Church, Virginia

MARY ETTA MILLS, R.N., Sc.D., C.N.A.A.
Associate Professor, School of Nursing, University of Maryland at
Baltimore, Baltimore, Maryland

BYRON B. OBERST, M.D., F.A.A.P.
Medical Advisor and Independent Contractor, Medical Computer
Management, Inc., Omaha, Nebraska

ROBERT I. O'DESKY, Ph.D.
President, RIO Consultants, Columbia, Missouri

SHARON O'KEEFE, M.S.
Vice President of Nursing, University of Maryland Medical System,
Baltimore Maryland

JAMES I. PENROD, Ed.D.
Vice President for Information Resources Management, California State
University, Los Angeles, California

PETER PETERSON, M.D.
Private Practice of Pulmonary Diseases, Denver, Colorado

ROBERT J. PICKTON, MBA
Vice President, Management Systems, Moses H. Cone Memorial Hospital,
Greensboro, North Carolina

PATRICK F. PLEMMONS, M.H.A.
Partner, Lamalie Associates, Inc., Atlanta, Georgia

WES RADULSKI, R.N., B.N.
Nursing Systems Development Analyst, Calgary General Hospital, Calgary,
Alberta, Canada

ARTHUR E. RAPPOPORT, M.D.
Consultant to the Clinical Laboratory, Vero Beach, Florida

SHERI ROSS, R.N.
Masterfiles Analyst, Calgary General Hospital, Calgary, Alberta, Canada

DOUGLAS A. RYCKMAN, M.H.A.
Partner and Regional Industry Director, Andersen Consulting, Arthur
Andersen & Co., Tampa, Florida

HOMER H. SCHMITZ, Ph.D.
Chief Financial Officer, The James Clinic, St. Louis, Missouri

ROGER H. SHANNON, M.D.
Director, Radiology Service, Veterans Health Service and Research
Administration, Department of Veterans Affairs, Durham, North Carolina

LAWRENCE H. SHARROTT, M.S.
Director, Healthcare Information Services Planning, Bell Atlantic
Enterprises Corporation, Philadelphia, Pennsylvania

EDWARD H. SHORTLIFFE, M.D., Ph.D.
Professor of Medicine and Computer Science, Stanford University,
Stanford, California

MARY NELL SPRABERRY, Dr.P.H.
Healthcare Specialist, Computer Task Group, Inc., Leeds, Alabama

WILLIAM W. STEAD, M.D.
Associate Professor of Medicine, Director, Medical Center Information
Systems, Duke University Medical Center, Durham, North Carolina

DAVID E. SUTHERLAND II, Ph.D.
Assistant Professor, Department of Information Systems, University of
Maryland Baltimore County, Baltimore, Maryland

TERESE M. TIMM, B.A.
Manager and Instructor, Office of Medical Informatics, St. Joseph Hospital, Denver, Colorado

RUSSELL E. TRANBARGER, R.N., C.N.A.A.
Professor, School of Nursing, University of North Carolina at Greensboro, Greensboro, North Carolina

MICHAEL S. VICTOROFF, M.D.
Family Practice Physician, Denver, Colorado

ANN WARNOCK-MATHERON, R.N., M.N.
Coordinator of Nursing Systems, Calgary General Hospital, Calgary, Alberta, Canada

SAM WILSON, B.S.
Director of Management Information Systems, Lutheran Medical Center, Wheat Ridge, Colorado

ROBERT G. WINFREE, M.A.
Associate Vice President for Health Affairs, Duke University Medical Center, Durham, North Carolina

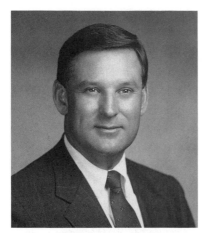

James W. Albright

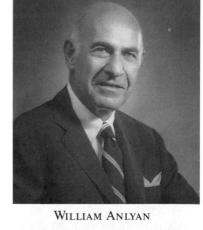

William Anlyan

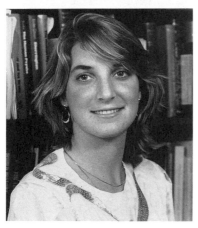

Elizabeth E. Ball

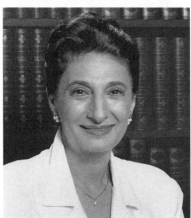

Marion J. Ball

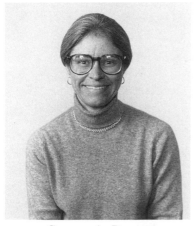

Carole A. Barone

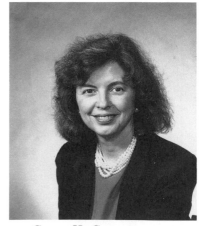

Grace H. Chickadonz

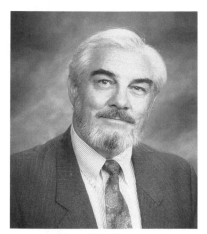

BILL W. CHILDS

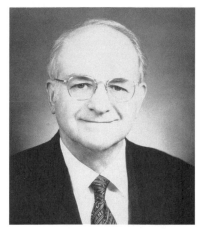

MORRIS F. COLLEN

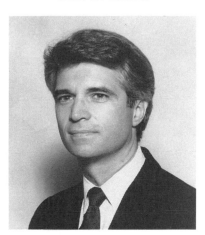

RICHARD A. CORRELL

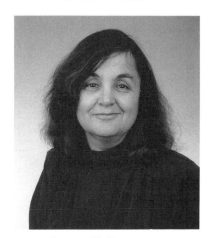

JUDITH V. DOUGLAS

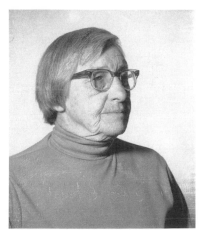

JANE G. ELCHLEPP

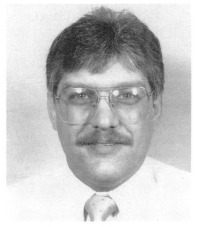

BENJAMIN FLOSSIE

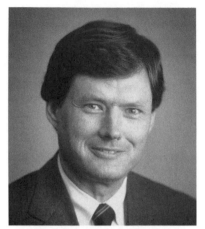

JAMES M. GABLER

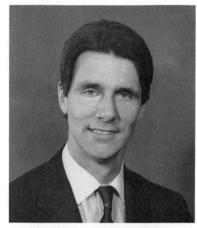

ANDREW C. GARLING

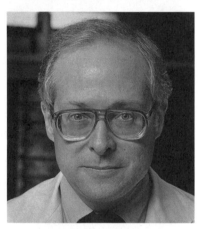

CHARLES F. GENRE

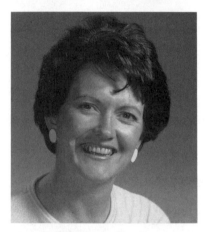

MARILYN GORE

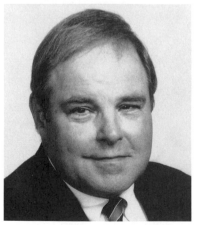

GARY L. HAMMON

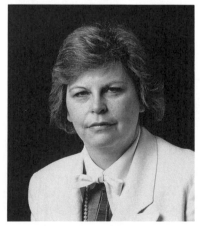

KATHRYN J. HANNAH

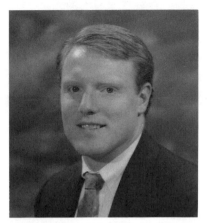

KEVIN J. HARLEN

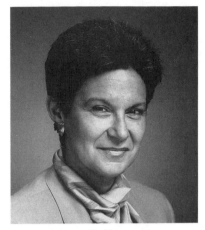

BETSY S. HERSHER

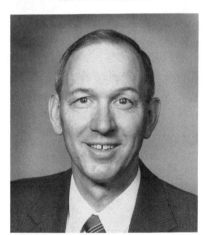

THOMAS M. JENKINS

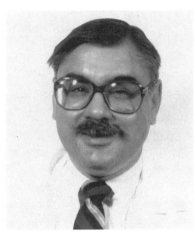

G. FREDERICK KESSLER, JR.

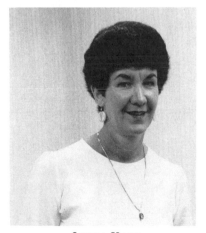

LINDA KOCK

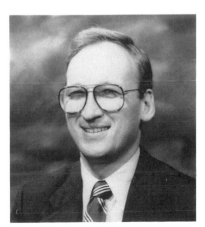

THOMAS W. MAGRAW

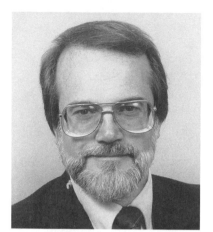

Brian T. Malec

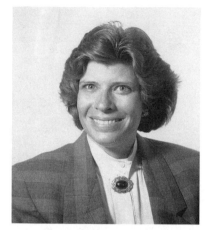

Amelia Lee Marley

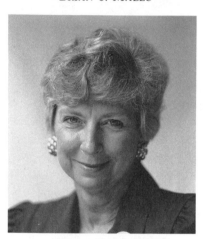

Patsy B. Marr

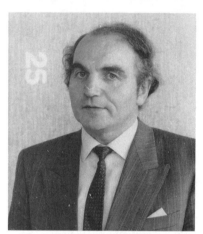

Michael McLoone

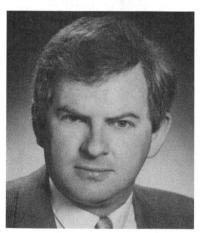

John A. Melvin

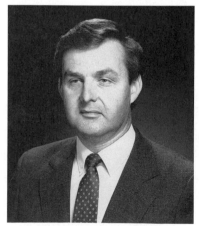

Michael J. Mestrovich

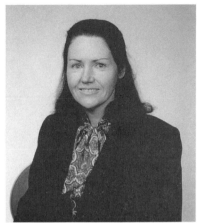

Mary Etta Mills

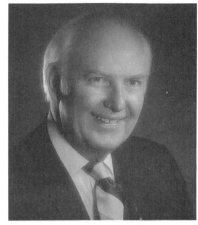

Byron B. Oberst

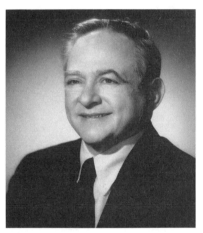

Robert I. O'Desky

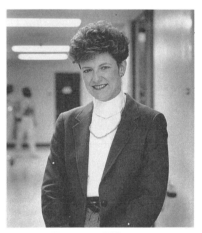

Sharon O'Keefe

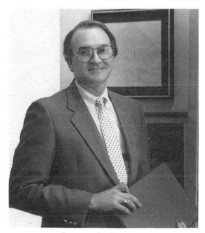

James I. Penrod

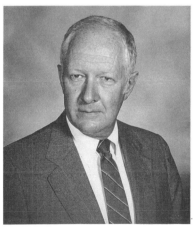

Peter Peterson

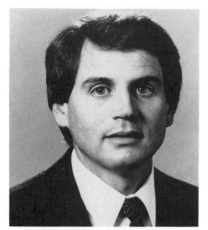

Robert J. Pickton

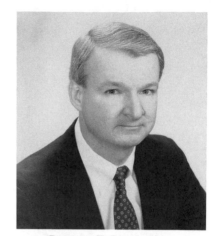

Patrick F. Plemmons

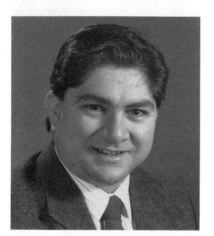

Wes Radulski

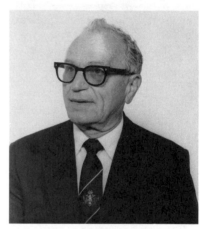

Arthur E. Rappoport

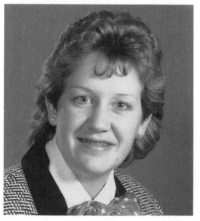

Sheri Ross

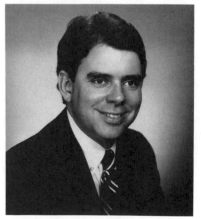

Douglas A. Ryckman

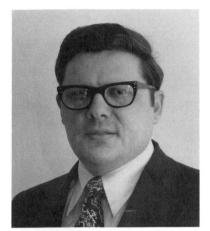

HOMER H. SCHMITZ

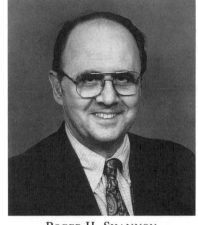

ROGER H. SHANNON

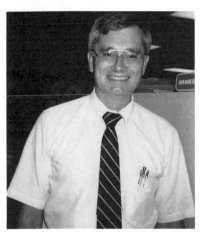

LAWRENCE H. SHARROTT

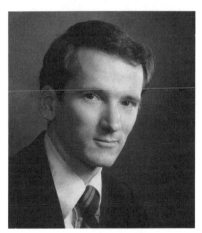

EDWARD H. SHORTLIFFE

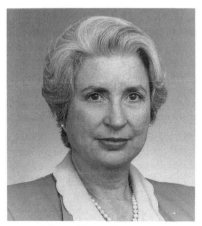

MARY NELL SPRABERRY

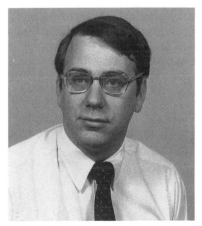

WILLIAM W. STEAD

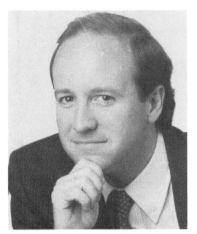

David E. Sutherland II

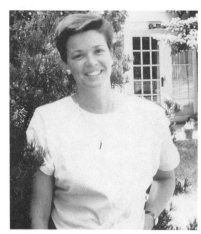

Terese M. Timm

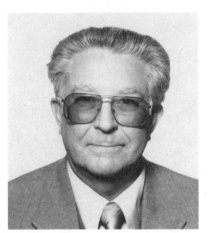

Russell E. Tranbarger

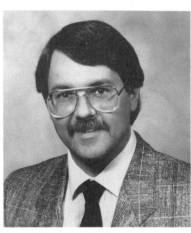

Michael S. Victoroff

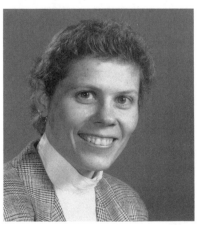

Ann Warnock-Matheron

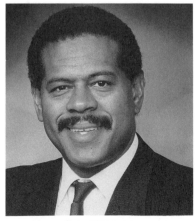

Sam Wilson

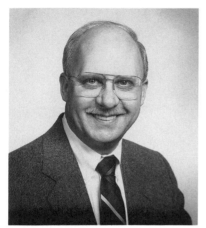

Robert G. Winfree